Рис. 4

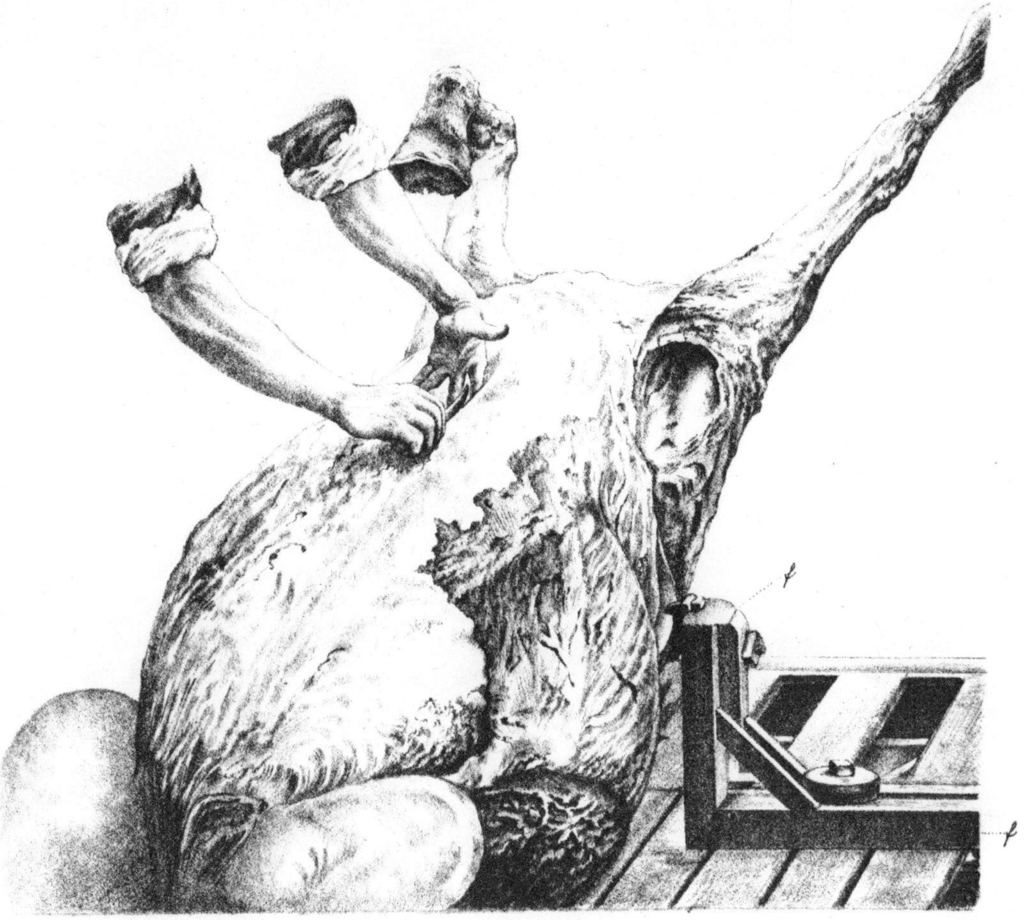

f

f

Рис. Э. Споріусъ

Казань. Лит. В. Ключникова

Veterinary Pathology in Russia, 1860–1930

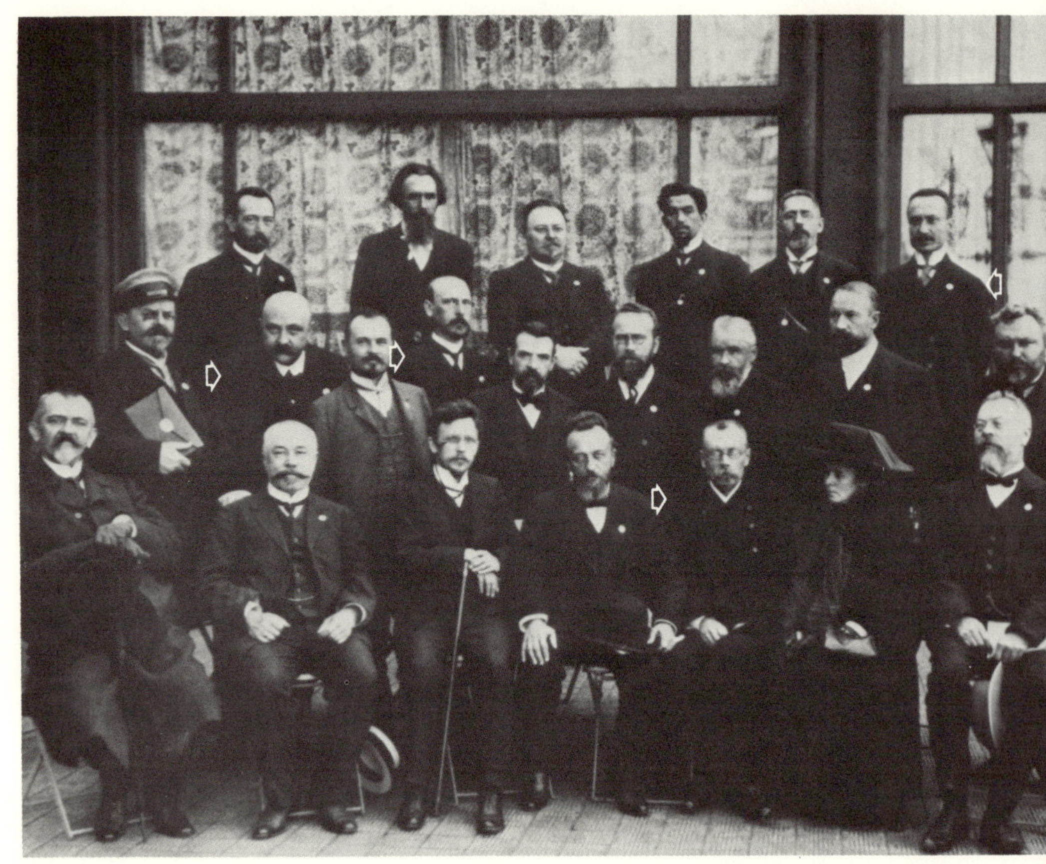

The Russian delegation to the Ninth International Veterinary Congress, The Hague, 1909, included four pathologists. Identified in the picture by arrows, they are, from left to right: I. I. Shukevich, K. H. Bohl, N. N. Mari, and N. D. Ball. To the right of Bohl is A. A. Vladimirov, who is also mentioned in this book.

VETERINARY PATHOLOGY IN RUSSIA, 1860–1930

LEON Z. SAUNDERS

CORNELL UNIVERSITY PRESS

ITHACA AND LONDON

THIS BOOK HAS BEEN PUBLISHED WITH THE AID OF A GRANT FROM
THE HULL MEMORIAL PUBLICATION FUND OF CORNELL UNIVERSITY.

First published 1980 by Cornell University Press.
Published in the United Kingdom by Cornell University Press Ltd.,
2-4 Brook Street, London W1Y 1AA.

International Standard Book Number 0-8014-1191-2
Library of Congress Catalog Card Number 79-52502
Printed in the United States of America
Librarians: Library of Congress cataloging information appears on the last page of the book.

Endpapers: Illustrations from Constantin Blumberg's book *Sektsionnaya Tekhnika,* Kazan, 1895.

Contents

Contents

Preface

Why does a veterinarian venture into history? History should be written "to prevent virtuous actions from being forgotten, and that evil words and deeds should fear an infamous reputation with posterity," said Tacitus. "A noble employment to rescue from oblivion those who deserve to be remembered," Pliny the Younger described the work of the historian. Not everyone, of course, has shared these lofty views. Konrad Adenauer derided history as merely "the sum total of things that could have been avoided." Tolstoy called it "a collection of fables and useless trifles," and, as history has been written in the Soviet Union for the past several decades, his description is both apt and prescient. Lest anyone doubt that virtuous actions are indeed forgotten, the chronicle that follows should convince the skeptic. The task of rescuing deserving people from oblivion is a necessary one in veterinary pathology as in other walks of life.

Perhaps I should explain specifically why I have dwelt on the particular aspect of history treated in this book. A number of years ago, I began to gather materials for a biographical history of veterinary pathology and, whether by chance or not, to file them by countries rather than alphabetically. I thus became aware early in my research that I had no folder for Russia.

Once aware of this lacuna, I made some desultory effort to fill it, but found that the requisite information was hard to come by and that its acquisition would yield only to a determined effort. I considered the possibility that any Russian contributions to veterinary pathology I might unearth would be too meager to warrant the effort. In that event I could work on the biographical history, ignoring Russians without any detriment to the project. Pursuing this course involved the risk of omitting contributions of value, however—a potential injustice to the individuals concerned and a disservice to readers of the book.

I therefore made the decision—not without initial skepticism—to invest some time and effort against the risk that the results would not be commensurate with the investment. As the work progressed, I developed an interest in the personalities concerned; also the sheer difficulty of obtaining information of any kind became a challenge that spurred me on. Besides, as Mary Renault has said, "The past is no dream; like Everest it is there,"[441] and, like a climber, I could not resist its challenge. The subproject thus developed a momentum of its own, in the face of which the major enterprise—while not forgotton—was temporarily sidetracked.

In setting out the facts on the veterinary pathologists, I have found it necessary to provide some minimal background of historical information on Russian veterinary medicine, veterinary education, Russian history in general, and the history of pathology. Events chronicled under each of these categories were, of course, crucial in shaping developments in Russian veterinary pathology. While I have deemed it necessary to deviate slightly from my main theme in this way, I should emphasize that the outline provided by these few bits of background information is deliberately sketchy. To have attempted more would have been to exceed my ability and lose the thread of the story. Some of the major events in Russian history and in the history of pathology that occurred during the period covered are alluded to in the text, and others are listed in the section "Some Historical Events."

To spare others some of the difficulties I have encountered, I have appended some bibliographic material at the end of the book. I hope that these references will prove helpful to those who have occasion to refer to Russian veterinary literature. Material elaborating on certain footnotes, which would have made the latter too voluminous and broken the thread of the story, appears in the appendixes. Those readers who do not require supporting documentation or background information can ignore the reference list and the appendixes without detriment to their understanding of the text.

Finally, a word about the illustrations. In reading about nineteenth-century Russia, I found that pictures were evocative of impressions to an extent that descriptions never were. Often, after reading an article or a book and pondering on what a place was really like, I would find the mental image I had formed incongruent with that depicted in drawings or photographs. I therefore opted for the inclusion of enough pictures to provide some background imagery and to spare the reader the labor of seeking these pictures in scattered and inaccessible sources. I hope that these illustrations will form a useful and interesting supplement to the text.

Many people have helped me in compiling this book. Mr. Vladimir Rimsky-Korsakoff of the Brookhaven National Laboratory was kind enough to translate some Russian literature for me many years ago. A distant relative of the composer and a worthy representative of the best in Russian culture, he was never too busy to drop his work to aid a colleague. I look back on our association with pleasure.

I am greatly indebted to Dr. George W. Lucyszyn of the Smith Kline and French Laboratories. His knowledge of the Polish, Ukrainian, and Russian languages was always cheerfully put at my disposal during the several years that this book was being written. His wide acquaintance with émigré Ukrainian scholars and his indefatigable efforts to obtain information from them have aided me immeasurably. Of these scholars, Professor Ivan Chinchenko of Winnipeg and the late Professor Vasyl Plushch of Munich were particularly helpful.

Dr. Svend W. Nielsen of the University of Connecticut kindly translated two Danish historical papers for me. Dr. Stuart Young of Colorado State University helped me pick up the trail of a Russian veterinarian who worked in Colorado before World War I. Miss Ruzica Popovitch, of the Slavic Reference Department, and Dr. R. V. Allen, Soviet Specialist, at the Library of Congress in Washington, D.C., provided advice and help with bibliographic searches. I am grateful for their interest and assistance. Dr. K. Baresel, Director of the Library at the Veterinary College of Hanover, Germany, kindly provided a copy of a calligraphed address from the archives of the College. I am most grateful for the opportunity to publish this valuable historical document.

The Commonwealth Bureau of Animal Health in Weybridge, England, has the largest collection of Russian veterinary publications in the English-speaking world. Mr. Roy Mack, F.R.C.V.S., Director of the Bureau and author of the very useful *Russian-English Veterinary Dictionary,* graciously put his extensive collection at my disposal. I am most grateful for the hospitality and help he extended to me during my visits.

Dr. W. Girolla, Director of the Library at the Vienna Veterinary University, Miss Margarita Åkesson, formerly Librarian at the Royal Veterinary College in Stockholm, and Dr. I. Katić, Research Librarian at the Royal Veterinary and Agricultural College in Copenhagen, hospitably extended the use of these collections to me on several occasions. My best thanks to these colleagues for their friendly and knowledgeable help. Miss Judy Bitting and Mrs. Alice Dempsey of the Smith Kline and French Research Library in Philadelphia patiently obtained many interlibrary loans and successfully negotiated with sometimes reluctant librarians in a few institutions. My grateful thanks for their efforts.

The staff of the National Library of Medicine in Bethesda, Maryland, has been particularly helpful, from the Director, Dr. M. M. Cummings, to the people in the several divisions. I would like to thank him, Mr. A. M. Berkowitz, Chief of the Reference Division, Mrs. Edith Blair of this division, and Mr. P. Dore, Mrs. Dorothy Hankes, and Mrs. Lucinda Keister of the History of Medicine Division.

Obtaining photographs has been a special problem. I regret that so few of the ones in this book are of the quality that I would like. Good originals were almost never obtainable. Messrs. Thomas Covatta and Michael Henry of the Smith Kline and French Laboratories helped me in the darkroom. Mr. Robert Epp converted some poor photographs into drawings. My sincere thanks to all of them.

Mrs. Murdoth Biddle typed the first dozen drafts and kept the numerous loose ends together at the inception of the project. Miss Patricia Fogarty typed the several "final" drafts of the manuscript and helped see it through the press. My grateful thanks to both of them for their unfailing patience and help.

Professor B. Hörning of the University of Bern has helped with copies of articles, tips, information, encouragement, advice, and proofreading. He also provided me with a copy of an unpublished report by Professor Dr. Nöller of a study trip to the Soviet Union made in 1929, just before the close of the period I am covering here. For all of this kindness my best thanks are given.

L. Z. S.

Philadelphia

Some Historical Events

1858–1930

Year	Russian History	Pathology, Veterinary Medicine
1858		Carmine staining introduced by Josef Gerlach.
1861	Freeing of the serfs. Student riots at Kazan University.	
1863	Polish uprising suppressed with bloodshed and exile.	First International Veterinary Congress, held in Hamburg.
1865	Introduction of *zemstvo* (elected local council) government.	Alum hematoxylin introduced for tissue staining by Friedrich Böhmer of Würzburg. Second Int. Vet. Congr., Vienna. Epithelial origin of epithelial tumors proved by Carl Thiersch of Erlangen.
1867	Alaska sold to the United States for $7,200,000.	Diapadesis of leukocytes in inflammation described by Julius Conheim. Third Int. Vet. Congr., Zurich.
1869	Russians living in Zurich begin plotting revolutionary activity. Tolstoy publishes *War and Peace*. Mendeleev publishes periodic table of elements.	Paraffin embedding introduced by Edwin Klebs. Pancreatic islets described by Paul Langerhans.
1870		Pathology of bovine pleuropneumonia described by Joseph Woodward.

1871

Bacteria first stained in tissue sections by Carl Weigert, Leipzig.

Abbe condenser devised by Ernst Abbe, Jena.

1872

Moscow University and Military-Medical Academy in St. Petersburg begin admission of women.

Occurrence of metastasis of tumors by embolism via blood or lymphatic vessels shown by Wilhelm Waldeyer of Strassburg.

1873

Russia, Germany, and Austria conclude three emperors' pact in Berlin.

Freezing microtome introduced by William Rutherford.

1876

Kazan University admits women.

Eosin introduced as histological stain.

1878

Russians win the Russo-Turkish War.

Death of Carl Rokitansky in Vienna.

Fecal examination for the diagnosis of hookworms introduced by Giovanni Bassi.

1879

Verminous bronchitis of dogs described by William Osler.

1881

Alexander II assassinated.

Sliding microtome devised by pathologist Richard Thoma, constructed by Robert Jung of Heidelberg.

1882

Igor Stravinsky born.

Student riots in St. Petersburg and Kazan Universities.

Censorship of newspapers tightened.

Myelin sheath stain devised by Carl Weigert.

Tubercle bacillus discovered by Robert Koch.

Glanders bacillus discovered by Friedrich Loeffler.

1883

Ivan Turgenev dies.

Karl Marx dies.

Intensification of russification in Polish schools and University of Warsaw begins.

Cholera bacillus discovered by Robert Koch.

Diphtheria bacillus discovered by Edwin Klebs.

Veterinary division of Military-Medical Academy in St. Petersburg closed.

Fourth Int. Vet. Congr., Brussels.

1884

Russification of Baltic provinces intensifies.

Stain for fibrin devised by Carl Weigert.

Theory of phagocytosis introduced by Ilya Mechnikov.

Stain for bacteria devised by Hans Christian Gram.

1886

Elastic stain devised by Carl Weigert.

1887

Secret defense treaty with Germany.

Marc Chagall born.

Student riots at Odessa and Kharkov universities.

Bacillus of Malta fever discovered by David Bruce.

1888

Rimsky-Korsakoff writes "Scheherazade."

1889

Fifth Int. Vet. Congr., Paris.

1891

Sergei Prokofiev born.

Famine in Russia.

Use of rubber gloves introduced in surgery by W. S. Halsted, Baltimore.

1892

Trans-Siberian Railway begun.

Bacillus of gas gangrene discovered by William Welch, Baltimore.

1893

Peter Tchaikovsky composes his *Symphonie Pathétique.* He dies of cholera contracted from contaminated drinking water.

Formaldehyde solution advocated for fixation by F. and J. Blum of Frankfurt a.M.

Atrioventricular bundle described by Wilhelm His.

Protozoal nature of Texas fever discovered by Theobald Smith.

First filterable virus (foot and mouth disease) demonstrated by Loeffler and Frosch.

Some Historical Events

1894

Tsar Alexander III dies. Accession of Nicholas II.

Zenker's fluid introduced by Konrad Zenker of Erlangen.

1895

Lenin arrested for revolutionary activities and (in 1897) exiled to Siberia.

Tsetse fly transmission of sleeping sickness discovered by David Bruce.

Theodor Kitt publishes his *Lehrbuch der Pathologischen Anatomie der Haustiere.*

Sixth Int. Vet. Congr., Bern.

1896

First strike in St. Petersburg; 30,000 workers participate.

1899

Student disorders in universities begin.

First book on veterinary neuropathology, *Die Nervenkrankheiten des Pferdes,* written by Hermann Dexler.

1900

Lenin returns from exile.

Blood groups discovered by Karl Landsteiner.

1902

Minister for Public Instruction assassinated.

1903

First all-Russian meeting of veterinarians, Petrograd.

Protozoa in kala-azar discovered by William Leishman.

Rabies inclusion bodies discovered by Adelchi Negri.

1904

Nobel prize to Ivan Pavlov.

Anton Chekhov dies.

Death of Rudolf Virchow.

1904–1905

Russo-Japanese War.

1905

Bloody Sunday massacre in St. Petersburg. General strikes and uprising.

Canine distemper virus discovered by Henri Carré.

Eighth Int. Vet. Congr., Budapest.

1906

First Duma (parliament) convened —and dismissed.

Role of megakaryocytes in forming platelets discovered by James Wright, Boston.

1907

Second Duma convened and dissolved.

Lenin flees abroad.

1909

Second all-Russian meeting of veterinarians, Moscow.

Ninth Int. Vet. Congr., The Hague.

1910

Tsar Nicholas signs pact in Potsdam with Kaiser Wilhelm.

Death of Robert Koch.

1911

Borna encephalitis described by Ernst Joest.

1914

World War I begins.

Third all-Russian meeting of veterinarians, Kharkov.

1915

Vitamin A demonstrated by Elmer McCollum and Marguerite Davis, Baltimore.

1917

March—abdication of Tsar; democratic government set up. October—seizure of government by Bolsheviks. Beginning of Red Terror of Cheka.

Study of large number of glanders cases on the eastern front by Erich Eberbeck, pathologist of Veterinary Laboratory "East" of the German Army Veterinary Corps.

1918

Beginning of Civil War and of foreign intervention; end of World War I; May to July—capture of Penza, Chelyabinsk, Irkutsk, and Omsk by Czechoslovak Legion.

Publication by Erich Eberbeck of extensive research work on the pathology of glanders.

Damage to buildings and equipment of Kazan Veterinary Institute by Red Army troops.

1920

36,000 wooden houses destroyed in Petrograd to provide fuel. Roads in city destroyed because people removed the wooden paving blocks to heat their houses.[395]

Publication by Ernst Joest of *Handbuch der pathologischen Anatomie der Haustiere,* the first encyclopedic, multiauthor treatise on veterinary pathology.

1921

Water transport at a standstill because barges and rowboats have been demolished for fuel.[395] End of Civil War; beginning of famine.

Bacterial cultures *freeze* in the incubators in Military Veterinary Bacteriological Laboratory in Moscow.

1922

Famine—relief by Herbert Hoover's American Relief Administration.

Interference with clotting discovered as cause of sweet clover poisoning of calves by Frank Schofield, Guelph.

1926

Stalin undisputed head of U.S.S.R.

Death of Ernst Joest.

1928

Rationing of bread introduced in cities.

1929

Beginning of forced collectivization of peasants.

B.C.G. tuberculosis vaccine introduced by Albert Calmette.

1930

Peasants fight back and destroy much of their livestock.

Death of Professor N. D. Ball.

Introduction

Very few things happen at the right time, and the rest do not happen at all; the conscientious historian will correct these defects.

—Herodotus

The second half of the nineteenth century was the formative period for veterinary pathology in Europe. As a consequence of the epochal work of Virchow, pathology was emerging as an independent discipline in many Continental medical schools, and this trend was also discernible among veterinary schools. During these five decades, chairs of pathology, with this discipline as the incumbent's major or sole responsibility, were established in one veterinary school after another: Vienna, 1849 (Röll); Turin, 1858 (Perroncito); Utrecht, 1869 (Reynders); Berlin, 1870 (Schütz); Bern, 1871 (Anacker); Pisa, 1871 (Rivolta); Munich, 1874 (Bollinger); Hanover, 1875 (Rabe); Copenhagen, 1879 (Bang); Dresden, 1879 (Johne).

The historical facts about the Western veterinary pathologists are either well known or available in readily obtainable journals or books. Parallel developments were taking place in the Russian Empire—then as now a conglomerate of non-Russian states held by Russia[35]—but these developments have either not been documented at all or else are described only in scattered fragments in Russian publications. Most of the libraries of North America and Western Europe do not have these publications.

Veterinary pathology appears to be a thriving discipline in the Soviet Union today, as evidenced by the proceedings of the second meeting of veterinary pathologists, attended by 126 people, the third, at which 182 papers were given (*Path. Vet. 4:* 289–298, 1967), and the fourth with 236! Veterinary pathologists also participate in scientific meetings of human pathologists; I have identified a dozen of them in a list of participants at a meeting in 1954.[163] It would appear that veterinary pathology is looked upon as an important discipline and enjoys considerable official support in the U.S.S.R. today.[4,251,417]

Such was not always the case, however. I have attempted to trace the modest beginning of the specialty in the last century, identify the people who played a role in it, and follow it to 1930. This is a historically logical breaking point, because one of the two founders of contemporary veterinary pathology (Nikolai D. Ball) died then. It is also a useful point since I am unable to view more recent events in adequate perspective. Because the other founder (Karl H. Bohl) enjoyed an exceptionally long life, I have carried my account of it until his death in 1959 and have likewise traced P. N. Krakht-Paleev's career to its end in 1949. Otherwise the cutoff point is as noted.

Insofar as I can determine, Russian veterinary pathology during the last half of the nineteenth century and the first 20 years of the twentieth was essentially a non-Russian—chiefly a German—science, despite the fact that most of the educated class spoke French rather than German. The revolution in March of 1917 and the seizure of power by the Bolsheviks in October did little to change this situation, since the handful of veterinary pathologists who served in tsarist Russia continued to hold the same or better posts under the Soviet regime.* Thus, before beginning to relate the story of

*Carmichael[131] (p. 232) states that after the Civil War the Bolsheviks found themselves at the helm of a ruined state, their problem of organizing it exacerbated by the emigration of two million Russians of the educated classes. [Westwood[623] (p. 263) puts the figure at only half that.]

veterinary pathology in Russia, I must first discuss the reasons for the pervasive German influence on it.

These émigrés included some of the cream of Russian creative talent: painters (Chagall, Kandinsky), authors (Nabokov), composers (Rachmaninov, Stravinsky), conductors (Koussevitsky), choreographers (Fokine, Balanchine), and engineers (Seversky, Sikorsky). They also included may scientists who left Russia and contributed their knowledge to the countries of their adoption,[223] but no veterinary pathologists were among them. All of the latter cast their lots with the new regime, whether from conviction, expediency, or necessity, I do not know. The reasons may have differed in individual cases, or the motivation may have been a patriotism for the motherland which transcended allegiance to the regime that happened to have seized power. Only in the case of K. H. Bohl have I encountered an indication; Gizatullin et al.[181] state, "He took the side of Soviet power from the first days of the revolution," but this does not tell us what motivated him to do so. Many of the intelligentsia were people of liberal ideas, who welcomed the throwing off of the autocratic restrictions. But by the time some scientists who did not flee at the outset realized that tsarist tyranny had been replaced by an even more barbarous Bolshevik one, it was too late to leave; facile emigration was possible only for a short while after 1918. For example, Gutmann[204] relates that the Tartu Veterinary Faculty tried to get Professor Holzmann to come from Kazan to teach anatomy in the early 1920s; but despite repeated requests from Estonia, the Soviet government denied him an exit permit. Finally (in 1922), like many others at that time, he died of typhus.

1 The German Influence on Veterinary Pathology

Russians Educated in Germany

Veterinary pathology—like veterinary medicine in general and like human pathology—was during the earlier half of the era 1860 to 1930 predominantly a German science. The reason was German leadership in the medical sciences—men like Virchow and his pupils or Koch attracted an unending stream of physicians from all over the world; the custom arose that a medical scholar had not completed his education until he had made the pilgrimage to Germany. For example, N. Ivanovskii, speaking at the unveiling of the bust of M. M. Rudnev in St. Petersburg, said: "At this time, [the 1860s], the attention of the whole scientific world was directed at Berlin, where R. Virchow took pathology along the new path of cellular pathology."[216] The tremendous influence of Virchow on Russian pathology is vividly described by Sacharoff.[453] Although the influence of his ideas was worldwide, Virchow himself was particularly cordial to Russian medicine and to Russians who came to work with him.[162]

The German influence in human pathology continued unabated in the twentieth century, despite the fact that Russia and Germany had fought as enemies during World War I. Professor Otto Lubarsch of Berlin wrote that the Russian Society of Pathologists was founded in 1909 after the model of the German one.[307] Many of its members not only read German, but spoke it fluently. In 1923 both Lubarsch and Professor Ludwig Aschoff of Freiburg were invited to the first postwar meeting of the Russian Society in Petrograd.[645] Lubarsch[307] mentioned that he was acquainted with some of the Russian pathologists attending this meeting because they had repeatedly visited Berlin and that he soon made the acquaintance of others. He states further, "One noted that all of them [the German-speaking Russians, since Lubarsch spoke no Russian], had an inner need to again join forces with German science, its spirit and its forms." He and Aschoff were elected honorary members of the Russian Society of Pathologists. Lubarsch was also invited to the subsequent meetings of this society (Moscow, 1925; Kiev, 1927), but was unable to attend until 1930, when he and Dr. Hamperl represented German pathology at the meeting in Baku. The meeting in Kiev had been designated as the Virchow Memorial Meeting (see Appendix I).[348]

The Russian veterinary pathologists were attracted by such men as Johne, Schütz, Kitt, and Joest, although several (Blumberg, Bohl, Ravich, Rudnev, and Kolesnikov, the latter two medical pathologists with comparative interests) studied under Virchow himself, whose interest in both veterinary medicine and comparative pathology was considerable.*

Those veterinary pathologists who wanted to further their scientific education, including McFadyean† (Edinburgh) and Frothingham (Harvard) in the 1890s and Innes (Cambridge)

*See, for example, his polemics with Semmer about tuberculosis.[622] See also Ravich.[436] Völker-Caprin[623] relates some of Virchow's veterinary activities, but no one has compiled a list of veterinarians who studied under him, and the fact that the above named Russians did is perhaps only the "tip of the iceberg." Schütz and Ostertag, two people who reached world fame in German veterinary pathology, worked or studied under Virchow.

†McFadyean relates visiting Bang in Copenhagen as well as the three Germans—Schütz, Johne, and Kitt—in a single summer.[310]

and Olafson (Cornell) in the 1930s, went to Germany to do so, whether they were Americans, Britons, or Russians.

Thus J. I. Ravich, Professor of Pathology in the veterinary division of the Imperial Medico-Surgical Academy at St. Petersburg, studied in Germany under Virchow in 1860–1862. The Kazan Veterinary Institute similarly began a system of professorial stipends for study abroad as early as the nineteenth century,[21] but the practice was not restricted to Kazan. As we shall see later, the Warsaw Veterinary Institute sent Ball to Berlin to work with Schütz, and the Kharkov Veterinary Institute sent Krakht-Paleev there a few years later as well as to Dresden and Munich to study under Joest and Kitt.

By the time of the 1917 Revolution, the Veterinary Laboratory of the Ministry of Internal Affairs, forerunner of the All-Union Institute of Experimental Veterinary Medicine (VIEV), had sent 15 scientific workers abroad for advanced study for periods of up to two years.[39] The countries were not mentioned, but from other sources (such as Nosik,[372] p. 9, the *Bolshaya Meditsinskaya Entsiklopediya, Veterinarnaya Entsiklopediya*) one knows that the parasitologists often went to France and the bacteriologists and pathologists to France, Germany, Austria, Switzerland, and Denmark. This was still going on near the end of the period covered here. Thus, in 1929, B. G. Ivanov, for 30 years head of the pathology department of VIEV, studied in Germany, in the laboratories of Karl Nieberle (Leipzig) and J. Dobberstein (Berlin).[531]

The presence of Russians in German universities was not always a one-way street. Some gave more than they got. Olga Mechnikov[35] (p. 46) relates that working in Rudolf Leuckart's (1822–1898) laboratory during the latter's absence on vacation, her husband Ilya discovered the phenomenon of alternation of generations in nematodes. When the famous zoologist returned, he was at first incredulous but later proposed to Mechnikov that they continue the work and publish it jointly. When Mechnikov exhausted himself in this pursuit, Leuckart advised him to take a rest, which he did in Switzerland. While he rested, Leuckart published Mechnikov's work under his own name—a dismal example of the greed for fame and lack of scruple in attaining it which marred his character.

Preeminence of German Books and Journals

In the nineteenth century and early twentieth, pathology in both North America and Russia was taught—like most veterinary subjects—either from German textbooks or from translations of German textbooks.* Thus, Kitt's *General Pathology* in the English translation (by Cadbury of Philadelphia) was widely used in the United States at the turn of the century, and Friedberger and Fröhner's *Pathology* in the English translation (by Captain Hayes of London) just before that. Mohler, Eichorn, and Herzog translated Hutyra and Marek's *Spezielle Pathologie und Therapie der Haustiere* into English and Willenz did so into Russian (published by *Veterinarnaya Zhizn,* Moscow, 1913). When the Danish veterinarian Engelsen visited Dorpat in 1885, pathology was being taught from Bruckmüller's textbook.[235]

The authors of such books, Kitt, Joest, Nieberle, Dobberstein, and Hutyra and Marek,† attracted postgraduate students from the countries which had no international figures. Additional prominence was gained by German veterinary

*As late as 1929, an advertisement of the publishing house Novaya Derevnya, Moscow, at the back of N. N. Marï's book on meat inspection, listed 12 books for sale in the series "Veterinarnaya Biblioteka." Half of these were foreign, 5 translated from German, and 1 from French.

†After the first (Hungarian) edition in 1894 their book appeared in numerous editions only in German, never again in Hungarian.

pathologists who served as editors of journals, for example, *Ergebnisse der allgemeinen Pathologie,* which always had at least one veterinarian (Dexler, Casper, Cohrs) on its editorial board, *Zeitschrift für Infektionskrankheiten, parasitäre Krankheiten und Hygiene der Haustiere,* edited by Joest, *Monatshefte für praktische Tierheilkunde,* edited by Kitt, and *Archiv für wissenschaftliche und praktische Tierheilkunde,* edited by Schütz. These journals, like the books, were read all over the world. After the turn of the century, when German veterinary educators had fought and won an equal status with others in the academic world, the teaching of German veterinary medicine chiefly in universities rather than in separate schools kept the German veterinary pathologists in contact with their medical confreres and other biological scientists and added to their professional knowledge and status.

In Russia, many German medical and even more veterinary books eventually were translated and became available in the Russian language. A book often underwent several editions in its original German before a translation could be brought out, however, and those who wished to get the information fairly fresh were obliged to read German. In order to ensure that its students would be able to read German books and journals, at least one Russian medical school, the Imperial Medico-Chirurgical Academy in St. Petersburg, taught German as an obligatory course during the third and fourth semesters (Ivanovskii[217], p. 309).

The internationally known German veterinarians to whom the Russians came for postgraduate study also had outstanding, well-equipped laboratories and clinics. Thus we can readily understand why it was Germany, rather than other European countries or the United States, at which envious eyes were cast from the Soviet Union. In the report of the Kharkov Veterinary Institute of 1929, the dean, Professor Ponirovskii, points out that in 1926, in economically troubled times and while Germany was burdened with 700,000,000 marks of reparation payments, the Berlin Veterinary College had been allotted 1,3000,000 gold marks for a new surgical clinic and 800,000 gold marks for a new pathological institute. He also deplored that the German schools, in Leipzig and Berlin, received more generous operating budgets than were available to the Ukrainian schools.[427] His candor may have cost him his job, or even his head; whether by coincidence or not, I find no mention of this man's name in any subsequent publication from the Kharkov Veterinary Institute.

In 1929, the Hanover Veterinary College celebrated its 150th anniversary. Figure 1 illustrates the German half of a calligraphic parchment scroll presented to the College by the veterinary faculty of the Zootechnical Institute in Moscow. If my translation of its text (below) seems a bit stilted, it is because the original is even more so! Nevertheless, there is no doubt about the sincerity of the sentiments expressed.

> The Veterinary Faculty of the Moscow Zootechnical Institute considers it its pleasant duty to greet, with profound respect, the significant jubilee of one of the first nurseries of veterinary knowledge—the Veterinary College of Hanover.
>
> By its highly fruitful activity in the course of one and one-half centuries, the Veterinary College of Hanover advanced the development of veterinary knowledge, and brought veterinary medicine to the heights it deserved, not only in its homeland, but also in numerous countries far removed from Hanover.
>
> A whole series of Russian veterinarians of the earlier and the present generations obtained their knowledge in the course of many long years to a great extent from the textbooks, manuals, and scientific works which thrived under the creativity of the scientific workers at the Hanover Veterinary College.
>
> With this constantly in mind, the Moscow Veterinary College expresses its deepest thanks to all former and presently active colleagues, in the name of the Russian veterinary fraternity, for the immeasurable benefits which the Veterinary College of Hanover has already brought and will bring in

Das Veterinär-Fakultät des Zootechnischen Instituts zu Moskau hält es für seine verbindliche und angenehme Pflicht mit tiefer Ehrfurcht das bedeutungsvolle Jubiläum einer der ersten Pflanzstätten der veterinärischen Kenntnisse - die Tierärztliche Hochschule zu Hannover zu begrüssen.

Mit ihrer höchst fruchtbringenden Tätigkeit im Laufe von anderthalb Jahrhunderten förderte die Tierärztliche Hochschule zu Hannover die Entwicklung der tierärztlichen Kenntnisse und brachte das Veterinärwesen auf die ihr gebührende Höhe nicht nur in ihrer Heimat, sondern auch in zahlreichen von Hannover veitlegenen Ländern.

Eine ganze Reihe russischer Veterinär-Arzte der früheren und heutigen Generationen schöpften ihre Kenntnisse im Laufe langer Jahren in grossem Masse aus den Lehrbüchern, Leitfaden und wissenschaftlichen Werken, die unter der Feder der wissenschaftlichen Mitwirker an der Tierärztlichen Hochschule zu Hannover gediehen.

Dies ständig im Auge habend, drückt die Moskauer Tierärztliche Hochschule allen gewesenen und heute tätigen Kollegen ihren innigsten Dank aus im Namen der russischen Veterinär-Korporation für den unermesslichen Nutzen die sie schon gebracht und ferner noch bringen werden auf dem Gebiete der wissenschaftlichen und praktischen Veterinär-Medizin der ganzen Welt und wünscht auch ein künftiges Weiterblühen dieser ältesten Stätte der wissenschaftlichen tierärztlichen Kenntnisse.

Dekan professor [illegible]

Figure 1. Calligraphic scroll presented to the Hanover Veterinary College.

the future in scientific and practical veterinary medicine to the whole world. The Moscow Veterinary College also extends its wishes for the continued flourishing in the future of this oldest facility of scientific veterinary knowledge.

Professor A. Klimov, Dean

Publication in German Journals

In addition to the purely German journals, such as the *Berliner tierärztliche Wochenschrift* and *Deutsche tierärzliche Wochenschrift,* which always published a few papers by veterinarians from Slavic countries, other German veterinary journals (such as *Deutsche Zeitschrift für Thiermedizin, Archiv für wissenschaftliche und praktische Tierheilkunde*) carried an international (European) editorial board, usually including at least one Russian professor. These Russians were German-oriented and steered their own and their colleagues' papers to the German journals. Thus, from their inception in the nineteenth century, the major German veterinary journals published contributions by Russian authors. Eugen Semmer (Dorpat) served on the editorial board of the *Deut. Z. Thiermed.* from 1882 and N. D. Ball (Leningrad) on the *Arch. Tierheilk.* from 1928 to 1930. Both of them wrote German abstracts of Russian articles for the *Jahresbericht Veterinärmedizin,* and Ball had his assistants Belkin and Valentin Z. Chernyak do so as well. M. G. Tartakovskii served on the editorial board of this journal as well as writing abstracts.

A few Russians also republished their monographic length articles in German as small books. For example, Ravich introduced his booklet on anthrax in 1872 by saying that he had already published it in Russian in 1870, but had been hindered by illness from translating it into German and thus communicating it to his esteemed colleagues outside of Russia. In two other of his books translated from Russian into

German he stressed his desire to reach his German colleagues thereby.[440]

This custom continued unchanged from Tsarist into Soviet times, until the German invasion of Russia. In the 1920s and 1930s many Russians published in the *Tierärztliche Rundschau,* the *Berliner tierärztliche Wochenschrift,* the *Deutsche tierärztliche Wochenschrift,* the *Zeitschrift für Infektionskrankheiten der Haustiere,* and the *Archiv für Tierheilkunde.* During the first three years (1939–1941) of World War II, before this invasion, there were still numerous papers by Russians to be found in the German veterinary journals. And a few years before that, in 1928, one finds in a Russian veterinary publication (*Uchenye Zapiski Kazanskogo Gosudarstvennogo Veterinarnogo Instituta* vol. 38) that frontispiece portraits of German veterinarians—Professor W. Ellenberger and Professor E. Fröhner—appeared on the occasion of their birthdays, clear evidence of continuing Russian respect for and cordiality toward German veterinary science. A congratulatory article with the portraits in a somewhat less prominent position also appeared on this occasion in the White Russian journal *Belaruskaya Veterynariya.*[600] The scientific proceedings of both the Kazan and the Leningrad Veterinary Colleges were subtitled in German: *Wissenschaftliche Berichte des Vet. Institutes zu Kazan* and *Annalen der Staatlichen Tierärztlichen Hochschule zu Leningrad* through the 1920s and 1930s. The summaries of articles, when in a foreign language, were almost invariably in German (rarely in French).

Additional evidence of the respect for German veterinary medicine is the inclusion of 200 hours of German language in the Soviet veterinary curriculum in 1930. This compared with 124 hours for pathologic anatomy and histology and only 60 hours for Leninism![49] That year a German-Russian dictionary for medical and veterinary doctors also was published by Bogdanov and Pavlov,[75] and the *Vestnik Sovremennoi Veterinarii,* the U.S.S.R.'s leading veterinary journal, carried a four-page article on the Leipzig veterinary school.[550] As an indication of reciprocal interest, the *Deutsche tierärztliche Wochenschrift* in 1930 carried a brief "historical" note on the first half-decade of the Byelorussian Veterinary Institute in Vitebsk.[592]

The Baltic-German Influence

There is another reason for the dominance of German in Russian veterinary pathology. Of the four veterinary schools that remained in the Russian Empire after the one in St. Petersburg closed in 1883, only one, at Kazan, was in Russia proper.* The others were in Warsaw, Kharkov, and Dorpat (*Yurev* [Russian], *Tartu* [Estonian]). Instruction in Warsaw was in Polish until 1865, when the school was russified as a reprisal for the Polish uprising, and in Dorpat it was in German.

At the University of Dorpat, a chair of veterinary medicine existed from 1804 to 1820, occupied by Dr. C. F. Deutsch (1768–1843), a German physician. It is not clear either from mention of this chair[606] or from Levitsky's[296] biography of Deutsch† that much time was actually devoted by him to

*There had also been departments of veterinary medicine during the nineteenth century in two other institutions of medical instruction of the empire, the Military-Medical Academies of Moscow and Vilna, but these had closed (see pp. 17–18), leaving the largest cities without veterinary schools.

†Christian Frederick Deutsch was born in Frankfurt an der Oder, Germany, September 27, 1768. He graduated in medicine from the University of Halle on November 10, 1792, with an M.D. dissertation on abdominal pregnancy. In 1796, he was appointed extraordinary professor in the medical faculty of the University of Erlangen; his specialty in that appointment is not stated. He was appointed ordinary professor of obstetrics (human) and veterinary science in the medical faculty of the University of Dorpat and apparently spent most of his time practicing and teaching obstetrics (until 1835) rather than in veterinary activities. What his qualifications

veterinary medicine. At that time it was still considered in Russia that physicians could teach medical students veterinary medicine by lecturing to them for a few hours. The chair of veterinary medicine was abolished in 1820, but 28 years later an independent veterinary school was created in this city.

From the time of its founding in 1848 until 1890, the language of instruction of the Dorpat Veterinary School (later Institute) was German, as it was also during this time at the University of Dorpat, which had the medical faculty. German was the native language of the landed gentry who formed the ruling class of the Baltic provinces, and therefore was the language of instruction in the middle and high schools in all of these provinces, not just Estonia. Instruction at the University of Dorpat and at the Veterinary Institute (which was not a part of the University) obviously had to follow in the same language. Russian was used at the Dorpat Veterinary Institute only to the extent that it was studied as a foreign language. Russification of the educational institutions in Estonia was begun in 1864, but a request for a progress report by the imperial government in 1873 showed that not much had occurred.

It is amusing to read Tehver's account[589] of the imperial government's demands that the veterinary instruction be given in Russian and the faculty's demurring, with the contention that the students could not understand it and that there were no textbooks in Russian. In fact, several of the faculty could not lecture in Russian, because they were Estonians or Latvians who had been educated in German and not bothered (or found it necessary) to learn Russian. Russification of the Dorpat Veterinary Institute, again demanded by

were for teaching veterinary subjects I do not know. Deutsch returned to Germany after 1835, celebrated the fiftieth anniversary of his M.D. degree in 1842, and died in Dresden on April 5, 1843.

the government in 1873, was almost complete by 1890; however, German was used until the retirement of the last non-Russian speaking professor in 1893*. The Veterinary Institute was thus treated more leniently than the University of Dorpat, which was closed as an institution giving instruction in German in 1893, to be replaced by the Russian Yuryev University.[526]

From the standpoint of veterinary pathology, the Dorpat school was the most important of the four, since directly or indirectly it supplied most of the pathologists for the other veterinary schools. After 1883, it was also the only veterinary school in the Russian Empire which enjoyed an international reputation, because of the scientific eminence of its teaching faculty. In this respect, it completely eclipsed the other three schools in the empire from its founding until 1917 and left an imprint on Russian (and European) veterinary science still discernible a century later. Its faculty had close ties with that of the Berlin Veterinary College, which appreciated the bastion of German culture within the Slavic empire.[467] The Dorpat faculty also maintained professional relations with that of the Vienna Veterinary College, publishing in Austrian journals and honoring Viennese professors with associate membership of their faculty.

The first pathologist at the Dorpat Veterinary Institute was Friedrich Brauell, a German. The second, Eugen Semmer, a Latvian, who at first specialized in microscopic anatomy under Brauell's tutelage, published his dissertation[474] in 1865 and most of his earlier works in German,

*This was Professor A. Rosenberg, a graduate of the medical faculty of Dorpat University, who taught veterinary anatomy. Tehver merely states that the German language disappeared as a medium of instruction with Rosenberg's retirement in 1893. However, Schmaltz[471] goes a step further and tells us that Rosenberg had refused to lecture in the Russian language. He had thus successfully resisted almost a quarter of a century of pressure to do so.

turning to Russian only later,[610] a fact which is glossed over in silence by his Soviet biographers.[229] Thus, for most of the second half of the nineteenth century, most of the veterinary pathologists (there were only eight* in Russia at the outbreak of the 1917 Revolution[151,251] were either graduates of the German-speaking Dorpat school or had been trained by men who were. The 94-year-old parasitologist, K. I. Skryabin, who was active as a scientist until his death in 1972, graduated from Dorpat in 1905 and published several of his early scientific contributions in the field of pathology before turning to parasitology.[417] The recollection of his early days at Dorpat, in his autobiography written in 1969, is a lively account of those times.[553]

The esteem in which the Dorpat Veterinary Institute was held in Germany is shown by the greetings it received on the occasion of its fiftieth anniversary in 1898. Professor H. Möller, who taught surgery at the Berlin Veterinary College, dedicated the third (1898) edition of his ophthalmology book to the Dorpat Institute. Professor R. Schmaltz, the anatomist, attended the anniversary celebration in Dorpat as the representative of the Berlin Veterinary College.† Upon his return, Schmaltz described the colorful ceremonies in fascinating detail in the *Berliner tierärztliche Wochenschrift.*[467] The address he himself delivered did not appear in print until 20 years later, when he was editor of the journal and another author (Zalewsky[647]) included it in an article on Dorpat. Schmaltz's interest in the Dorpat Veterinary Institute continued unabated at least until 1924, when he expressed concern because its existence was threatened by economic difficulties in

*Ball in Warsaw, Bohl in Kazan, Mari, Shukevich, and Tartakovskii in St. Petersburg, Waldmann in Dorpat, Ostapenko and Krakht-Paleev in Kharkov.

†He thus reciprocated the visit eight years previously of Professor Semmer, who had attended the centenary celebration of the Berlin Veterinary Institute as the representative of the Dorpat faculty.

the new and struggling republic of Estonia.[468,470] Perusal of these papers reveals several interesting points.

Although I have not enough information to judge with assurance, there is evidence that the enforced switch to the Russian language in teaching and publication merely represented a façade of token compliance, behind which most of the Dorpat faculty members, although politically loyal to the Tsar, culturally continued to "think German." For example, in 1907, when the faculty commenced publication of the *Zhurnal Nauchnoi i Prakticheskoi Veterinarnoi Meditsiny,* it was subtitled in German *Zeitschrift für wissenschaftliche und praktische Veterinärmedicin.* Of the 16 articles in the first volume that carried a summary in a foreign language, 13 were in German and 3 in French. Further evidence that russification had not completely effaced German culture in Dorpat is in the article by the German military veterinarian, Zalewsky,[647] written while Estonia was under German occupation in 1918. He is urging the occupation authorities to provide for the reopening of the Dorpat Veterinary Institute, and part of his plea was:

> Eine Kulturstätte ihres Ranges kann man nicht einfach mit einem Federstrich für alle Zeiten vernichten. Es ist vielmehr unsere Pflicht, eine ehemalige kerndeutsche Hochschule, die, trotz aller Russifizierungsversuche und Anfechtungen, in ihrem Wesen deutsch geblieben ist, wieder zur Blüte zu erwecken.
>
> Wir deutschen Tierärzte wünschen unserer baltischen hohen Schule, die stets als wohlberufene Vertreterin der tierärztlichen Wissenschaft im Osten deutsches Wesen, Kultur und Wissen hochgeschätzt und in Ehren gehalten hat, Glück und Segen auf ihrem neuen Lebensweg. Sie möge in ihrem 4. Geschichtsabschnitt weiter blühen und gedeihen als festes Glied in der Reihe deutscher tierärztlicher Bildungsstätten und als starkes Bollwerk deutscher Kultur gen Osten.

A cultural center of this rank cannot simply be destroyed forever with a stroke of the pen. It is rather our duty to bring this once thoroughly German university to flourish again, which despite all attacks and attempts at russification has in essence remained German.

We German veterinarians wish our Baltic college (which has always, in the high calling as representative of veterinary science in the East, maintained the German spirit, culture, and knowledge in high esteem and honor) luck and blessing on its new road of life. May it continue to bloom and thrive in the 4th period of its history as a solid member in the series of German veterinary educational institutions and as a strong bulwark of German culture against the East.

The Dorpat Veterinary Institute reopened but a few short weeks under German occupation and then the war was over. When Estonia gained her independence from Russia in 1919, veterinary medicine was taught in the veterinary faculty of Tartu University, some subjects in German and the rest in Estonian. A brave and noble nation had prevailed

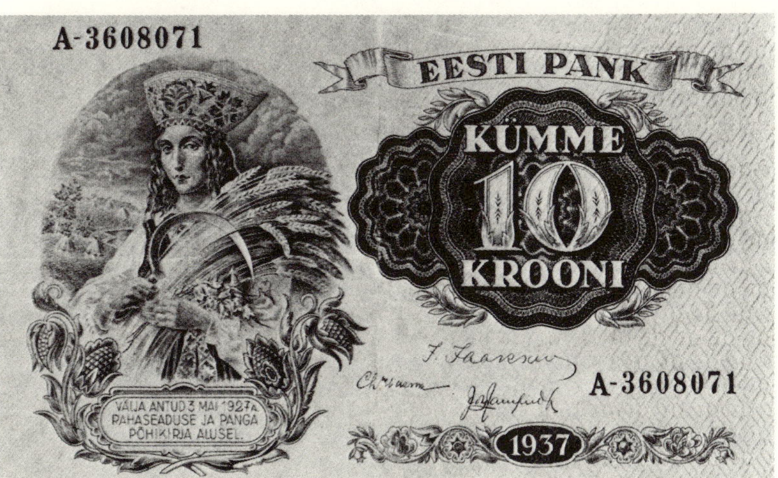

Figure 2. Ten-crown banknote of the Estonian Bank.

against seemingly overwhelming odds to assert its right to exist unshackled (Fig. 2).

Summary

In the nineteenth and 20th centuries, almost all of the Russian teachers of veterinary pathology were educated in Germany. In addition, German textbooks and journals exercised a continuing influence on them. Three of these teachers also served on the editorial boards and all of them published articles in these journals. The effect of all of this was that the ideas of German veterinary medicine permeated Russian veterinary pathology and exerted a tremendous influence on it. When one adds that in the scientifically most important veterinary school, instruction for many years during the nineteenth century was not in Russian but German, the reasons for the prevalence of German ideas in Russian veterinary pathology (and in Russian veterinary medicine in general) emerge clearly.

This situation prevailed during most of the period covered by this book, although it began to wane in the last decade. Nevertheless, in 1930, at the end of this period, German was still being taught as part of the veterinary curriculum, a German-Russian veterinary dictionary had just been published, and the German journals carried numerous articles by Russian veterinary pathologists.

2 Some Early Veterinary Schools

Veterinary Education in Moscow

Veterinary education in Russia itself—as distinct from the Russian Empire—began with a chair of "cattle medicine" at Moscow University in 1805. The following year, a chair of veterinary science was established at the Moscow Medico-Chirurgical Academy.[180] The former chair, renamed veterinary medicine, was occupied between 1810 and 1812 by Theobald Renner (1779–1850), a German veterinarian.[116] It was apparently abolished in 1812, after he left Russia. The latter chair grew into a veterinary department with several teachers. There was no separate discipline of veterinary pathology at the Moscow Medico-Chirurgical Academy during the years that veterinarians were educated there (1806 to 1842, according to Pinus[417]). Pathology itself had not yet emerged as a separate discipline in medical schools, either in Russia or elsewhere, but what might be considered the precursor discipline, pathological zootomy, was taught by Professor B. Milhausen.[264] The veterinary department of the Moscow Medico-Chirurgical Academy was closed in 1842, whereupon that city entered an era of 80 years without a veterinary educational institution, although almost all cities of comparable importance in Europe had one.

*Veterinary Education in Vilna**

Millak[356] (p. 376) relates that veterinary science was first taught in the territory of the Kingdom of Poland in 1823. The teacher was Professor L. H. Bojanus, the first holder of the chair in this discipline at the University of Vilna. Millak states that "this school was closed down in 1832, together with the University of Vilna in consequence of the miscarriage of the Polish national uprising of 1831."

Veterinary education was available in Vilna also in its Medico-Chirurgical Academy, which had a veterinary department. The latter existed only between 1818 and 1843 (according to Koropov[264]; to 1842 according to Millak[356]), and, as in Moscow, pathology did not yet exist as a separate discipline. When the veterinary department was closed, its anatomical and embryological collections and its equipment were sent to the University of Dorpat; they were put to use upon the founding of the Dorpat Veterinary Institute five years later.[589] Someone in a ministry in St. Petersburg was obviously anticipating this founding and planning ahead for it. It would be interesting to know who, in a government not noted for its foresight (or for that matter even its hindsight, see Appendix V) was envisioning the broad picture of veterinary educational needs for the empire as a whole and providing for them, but I have not been able to determine this.

Between November 3, 1838, and May 30, 1841, Friedrich Brauell, a German veterinarian who made important contributions to veterinary pathology, worked in Vilna as a teacher in the veterinary department of the Medico-Chirurgical Academy. His career is discussed in Chapter 3 on the Dorpat Veterinary Institute, where he spent most of his professional life.

*The city of Vilna, subsequently in Lithuania, was then within the piece of partitioned Poland which had been allotted to the Russian Empire.

3 The Dorpat Veterinary Institute

Between the large regions inhabited by compact German, Italian, and Russian-speaking populations live a number of peoples whose lands have been alternately enriched and laid waste by the ebb and flow of empires.

—Hugh Seton-Watson

At the Dorpat Veterinary Institute (Fig. 3), pathology was first taught—in German—by Friedrich August Brauell (1807–1882) from its founding in 1848. Born in Weimar on December 11, 1807, Brauell (Fig. 4) studied medicine and veterinary medicine in Jena, Berlin, and Copenhagen. He worked for a time as veterinarian for a Weimar horse-breeding establishment, then took a Ph.D. degree at Erlangen in 1834. This was during the era when the Russian government was looking for more German scientists to staff its slowly growing educational institutions, and in 1837 Brauell was appointed to the teaching staff of the veterinary department of the Medico-Chirurgical Academy of Vilna. While teaching there he took the examination and obtained the M.D. degree.*

Brauell next was appointed to the chair of veterinary science at Kazan University in 1841, where he remained until 1848. From there he was sent to join the original faculty of

*These degrees are mentioned by both Müller[363] and Tehver;[589] however, I have been unable to confirm either of them in the published compilations of German or Russian university dissertations.

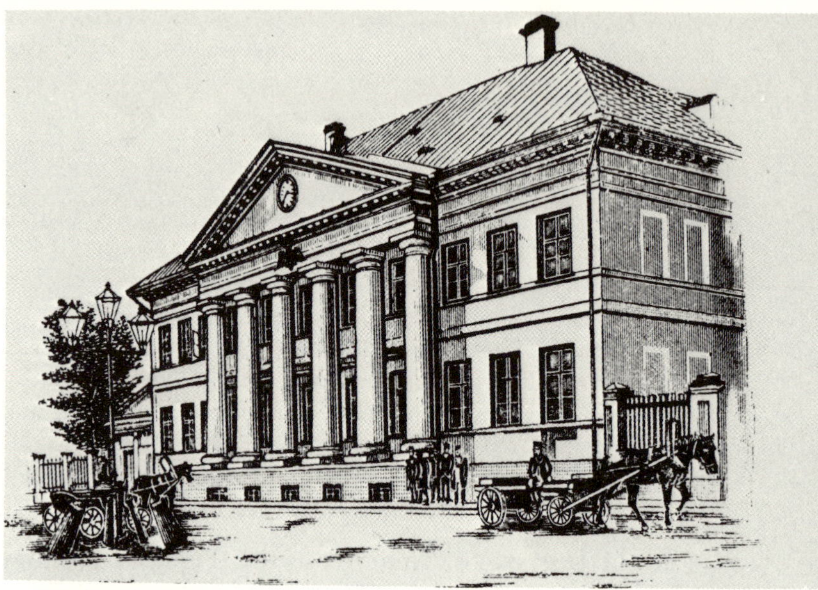

Figure 3. The Dorpat Veterinary Institute as it appeared in 1898.

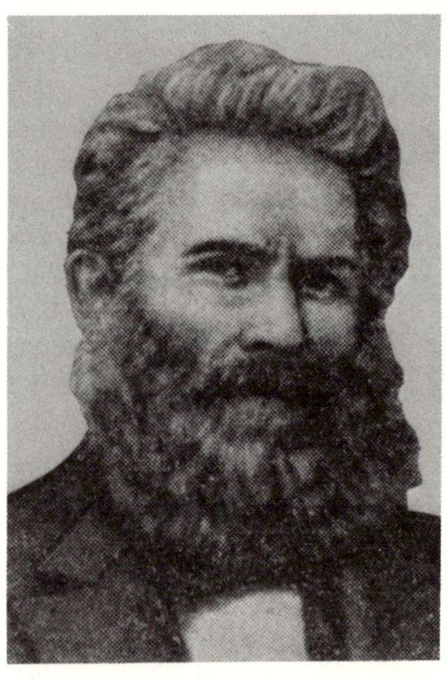

Figure 4. Friedrich Brauell.

the new Dorpat Veterinary Institute for what was to be a twenty-year sojourn. According to Müller, Brauell had difficulties in getting along with his colleagues at Dorpat because of his boisterous manner. I have no other source from which I might check this statement, but judging by one example of his writing,[120] whoever crossed swords with him in print was unlikely to emerge from the fray unscarred or lacking respect for his adversary's mettle! This article pertained to the intemperate criticism of one of Brauell's histological papers by someone using only gross observations. Brauell demolished his adversary with a blast of withering scorn. Even more revealing of his literary talents were the words he used in another more serious instance, when he contended that Professor Albert Krause (1813–1880), a German physician who taught therapeutics at the University of Dorpat from 1850 to 1856, had obtained Brauell's data on experimental anthrax under false pretenses and published them without permission. Here we see Brauell at his most vitriolic. Even in an age when acrimonious polemics had evolved to a high art, Brauell's letter to the editor of the *Deutsche Klinik*[118] must surely rank as an exceptionally lacerating example of the genre.*

The text of Brauell's protest letter follows here in its original German. I have also given it in English, although its flavor of outrage loses much in translation—at least it eluded capture in my version. Its English title can be rendered as: "An observation concerning a peculiar hypertrophic degeneration of the impudence-organ." Brauell was a fine

*Whether this unscrupulous act was responsible for Krause's leaving the University of Dorpat I do not know. The two events occurred during the same year (1856), and the biographical lexicon of the university faculty[296] is strangely silent on the reason for Krause's departure. The biographical lexicon of German physicians mentions that Krause was dismissed from a subsequent post in Saxony in 1879, but does not give the reason.[202]

anatomist, whose talents also enabled him to invent a figurative organ when he needed one as a target for his rhetoric.

EINE BEOBACHTUNG, BETREFFEND EINE EIGENTHÜMLICHE HYPERTROPHISCHE ENTARTUNG DES DREISTIGKEITS-ORGANS.

Da diese Zeitung für Beobachtungen aus deutschen Kliniken und Krankenhäusern bestimmt ist, so wird die geehrte Redaction derselben wohl so freundlich sein, nachstehende, in dieser Zeitung, in der "Deutschen Klinik" selbst, gemachte Beobachtung in ihre Spalten aufzunehmen.

Nachdem ich mich vorigen Winter längere Zeit mit Versuchen, betreffend die Inoculation des Milzbrandes, sowie mit mikroskopischen Untersuchungen des durch Milzbrand veränderten Blutes beschäftigt hatte, erschien eines Morgens Hr. Krause, damals noch Professor in Dorpat, bei mir, und bat mich um nähere Mittheilungen über die von mir angestellten Versuche und Untersuchungen. Ich erklärte dem Hrn. Prof. Krause, dass ich selbst meine Untersuchungen, sobald sie abgeschlossen seien, zu veröffentlichen beabsichtige, in der Voraussetzung, dass Hr. Prof. Krause diesen leicht verständlichen Wink beachten and von seinem Wunsche abstehen werde. Hr. Prof. Krause liess sich aber durch diese Erklärung nicht stören, versicherte mir, dass er meinem Vorhaben durchaus nicht vorgreifen, sondern nur seine Wissbegierde befriedigen wolle, drang mit verschiedenen wiederholten Fragen in mich, und veranlasste mich so, ihm einige wenige unzusammenhängende Bruchstücke mitzutheilen, ohne mich, weder damals noch zu anderer Zeit, um die Erlaubniss zu bitten, von denselben öffentlich Gebrauch machen zu dürfen.—Vor Kurzem nun von einer grösseren Reise zurückgekehrt, finde ich in No. 24 dieser Zeitschrift einen Aufsatz von Hrn. Professor Krause unter der Aufschrift "Die Uebertragung des Milzbrandes von Thieren auf Menschen und vom "Menschen auf Thiere", und in diesem, zu meinem nicht geringen Erstaunen, auch Mittheilungen über meine Versuche und Untersuchungen, zum Theil wenigstens dieselben, welche Hr. Krause mir abgelockt hatte.

Hr. Prof. Krause macht also öffentlichen Gebrauch von meinen Mittheilungen, trotz der ihm von mir gegebenen

Erklärung, dass ich meine Untersuchungen selbst veröffentlichen werde!—Er macht von denselben öffentlichen Gebrauch, trotz seiner Versicherung, dass er meinem Vorhaben nicht vorgreifen, sondern sich nur selbst unterrichten wolle!—Er macht von denselben öffentlichen Gebrauch, ohne von mir dazu autorisirt worden zu sein, ohne mich um die Erlaubniss dazu gebeten, und ohne dieselbe, wie sich von selbst versteht, von mir erhalten zu haben!—

Ich überlasse dem, nicht die gleichen Principien mit Hrn. Professor Krause theilenden, Leser die Epikrise dieser Beobachtung; ich überlasse ihm die Beurtheilung des Hrn. Krause und der von ihm verübten Schmuggelei mit fremdem Eigenthum; desavouire aber:

1) den Hrn. Prof. Krause als meinen Plenipotenten oder Stellvertreter, als welchen er sich unbefugter Weise gerirt hat, mit der Versicherung: dass meine Wahl nie auf Hrn. Krause gefallen wäre, wenn ich eines Stellvertreters bedurft hätte;—und desavouire:
2) auch die von ihm unter meinem (falsch angegebenen) Namen gemachten Mittheilungen als von unbefugter Hand ausgegangene, sehr unvollständige, durch mehrfache Unrichtigkeiten entstellte, und mit grosser Leichtfertigkeit hingeworfene Fragmente.

Schliesslich sei mir noch die Bemerkung erlaubt, dass der an der blauen Blatter gestorbene Mann, um den es sich in dem citirten Aufsatz des Hrn. Prof. Krause handelt, nich "Subb", wie ihn Herr Krause nennt, sondern "Schuppe" hiess, und dass derselbe nicht Veterinärgehülfe war, wie Hr. Krause angiebt, sondern nur Calefactor im zootomischen Theater.

Dorpat, den 20. Oct. 1856. Dr. Brauell.

An Observation Concerning a Peculiar Hypertrophic Degeneration of the Impudence-Organ

Since this newspaper is for observations from German clinics and hospitals, would its honored editorial office be kind enough to accept the following observation in its columns, i.e. in the "German Clinic" itself.

Last winter I occupied considerable time in investigations

on the inoculation of anthrax and on microscopic examination of the blood as altered by anthrax. One morning Mr. Krause, who at that time was still professor in Dorpat, appeared in my laboratory and asked me for detailed information on my ongoing experiments and investigations. I explained to Professor Krause that I intended to publish the results of my research as soon as it was completed, in the hope that he would take cognizance of this easily understandable hint and would desist from questioning me. Professor Krause, however, was not deterred by this explanation; he assured me that he would not encroach on my intentions but merely wished to satisfy his curiosity. He persisted with repeated questions and caused me to give him a few partial and unrelated details; he did not ask my permission either then or at any other time to make public use of this information.

Having recently returned from a long trip I found in number 24 of this journal an article by Professor Krause entitled "The Transmission of Anthrax from Animals to Man and from Man to Animals." In this article I found, with no little astonishment, information about my experiments and investigations, at least part of which Mr. Krause had forced out of me.

Professor Krause thus is making public use of my information despite the explanation I gave him that I would publish my investigations myself! He is making public use of my data despite his assurance that he does not want to forestall me but merely to inform himself! He is making public use of it without having been authorized to do so by me, without having asked my permission, and without, as is self-evident, having received it from me!

I leave it to those readers who do not share the same principles as Professor Krause to determine the final outcome of this observation. I also leave it to the reader to judge Mr. Krause and the smuggling which he has carried out with somebody else's property. However, I disavow:

1) that Professor Krause is my plenipotentiary or representative, in which unauthorized capacity he has been acting, with the assurance that my choice would never have fallen on Mr. Krause had I needed a representative.
2) I further disavow the communication which he falsely made under my name as having come from an unauthorized

> source, and to consist of very incomplete portions, containing numerous errors and tossed out in an ill-considered manner.
>
> Finally, please permit me to remark that the man who died of anthrax and who is mentioned in the cited article by Professor Krause, was not called "Subb" as Mr. Krause named him, but "Schuppe," and that this person was not a veterinary assistant as Mr. Krause states but only the caretaker in the post-mortem room.
>
> Dorpat, 20 Oct. 1856 Dr. Brauell

When Brauell began teaching at Dorpat, he was responsible for the subjects of anatomy, physiology, and pathologic anatomy. As the latter developed into an independent discipline, he devoted proportionately more of his efforts to it. Brauell's scientific career is marked by two periods—at the beginning and at the end—in which anatomical contributions predominated. In the time between these periods he worked and published on pathologic anatomy and pathogenic bacteriology. He also wrote one paper on the history of veterinary medicine in Russia[116].

Like many teachers of veterinary pathology at midcentury, Brauell worked not only in pathology but also in bacteriology and epizootiology, none of which had yet evolved as the more strictly delineated specialities they would later become. Brauell's work in 1862 on the pathology of rinderpest* (Fig. 5), cited by both Ravich and Semmer as the pioneer contribution, and his later work *Pathologisch-anatomische Notizen,* published in 1871,[123] however, leave no doubt that even by today's more specialized standards he was a highly competent practicing pathologist. His original turn of mind resulted in advances in our understanding of the pathology of several diseases. Although not a Russian, he was (in my opinion) the

*This monograph[122] received recognition abroad; Sanderson, of the British Royal Commission on Cattle Plague, called it a "comprehensive and exact treatise on pathological anatomy."[8]

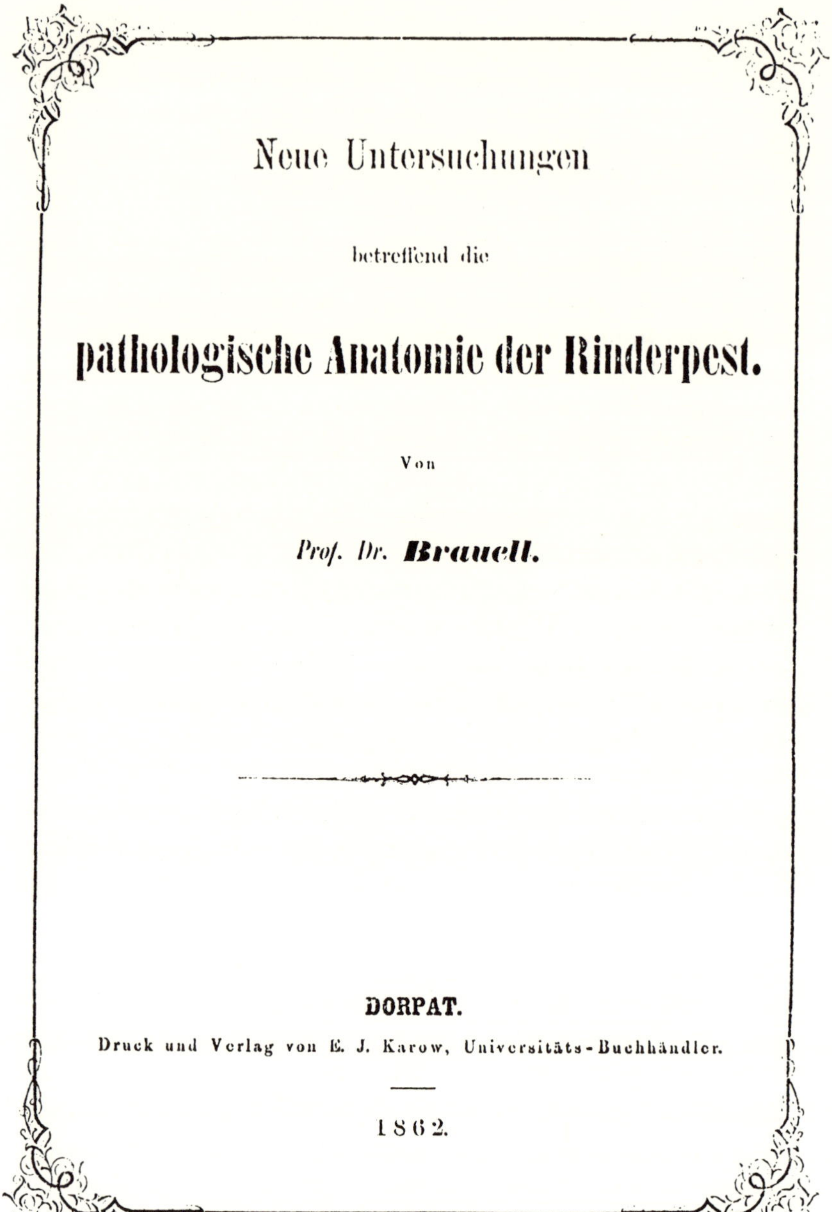

Neue Untersuchungen

betreffend die

pathologische Anatomie der Rinderpest.

Von

Prof. Dr. ***Brauell.***

DORPAT.

Druck und Verlag von E. J. Karow, Universitäts-Buchhändler.

1862.

Figure 5. Title page of "New Investigations Concerning the Pathologic Anatomy of Rinderpest," by F. Brauell. This is the first monograph to report histopathologic changes in an important epizootic disease.

first identifiable veterinary pathologist in the Russian Empire, and his German nationality is not remarkable at a time when the Imperial Academy of Sciences in St. Petersburg was still composed of more foreigners (chiefly Germans) than Russians.[187,236]

Brauell's work in bacteriology did not get adequate recognition in the nineteenth century,[396] which may explain why I have been unable to find a contemporary obituary. Today, however, Brauell is (justly) famous, chiefly for his original contributions to determining the etiology of anthrax. This complicated historical matter has been confused by many writers—indulging in chauvinism (French, German, and Russian), sloppy scholarship, or both—and clarified by only one, Müller, whose work I have paraphrased below.[363]

Brauell's lasting claim to fame is without any doubt his earlier work on anthrax, and, as Müller points out, this claim is nonetheless secure because some of his later work on this disease was of lesser quality. Brauell found anthrax bacilli by microscopic examination of the blood of Carl Shuppe, an anatomy "Diener" at the Veterinary Institute, who had died 33 hours previously of anthrax. This man had assisted at the autopsy of three animals dead of anthrax. Professor Albert Krause, who conducted the autopsy of the unfortunate worker, removed some venous blood from the body and sent it to Professor Brauell for the inoculation of animals. (It was already known at that time that anthrax could be transmitted by animal inoculation, even though its cause was not known.)

Brauell reported finding nonmotile rods both in the blood taken postmortem from Carl Shuppe and in the blood drawn from the sheep which died following inoculation with the former. He described the rods as similar to those which had been reported by Pollender, but emphasized that his finding was an independent one and that he had only read Pollender's work after making it. Pollender's paper appeared about nine months prior to Brauell's discovery, but he stated that "unter den hiesigen Verhältnissen, welche einen raschen Empfang deutscher Zeitschriften nicht gestatten" (Under the local conditions, which do not permit a swift receipt of German journals),* he had received the one with Pollender's paper only after completing his own work.[119]

According to Müller, Brauell is entitled to credit for four major accomplishments, made at a time when bacteriology had not yet become established as a scientific discipline: (1) He was the first to see pathogenic bacteria in the blood of a human being, even though the blood was not taken during life. (2) His chief discovery is that he found anthrax bacilli in the blood of living animals, in one case eight to ten hours before its death, and therefore knew that these could not be bacilli which arose in the course of decomposition of the

*Whether he was speaking of delays in the transportation of printed matter, or the screening of it for suitability before delivery by the Russian censors, or both, is not clear to me. According to Vucinich,[624] the Russian government in 1848 (the year of Brauell's appointment to Dorpat), noting that "minds were being contaminated by imported books being circulated surreptitiously," tightened the censorship regulations pertaining to what could be brought into the country. These remained in force until 1859.[626] Wilson,[635] however, mentions that as late as 1890, copies of the American *Century Magazine,* containing George Kennan's articles critical of the Siberian exile system, "were severely censored" when they reached Russia, "whole pages being blacked out." I imagine that this must have been a time-consuming process. We should not forget also that Brauell's work in 1857 was done before the convening of the postal convention in Bern in 1874 to alleviate the chaotic conditions that had prevailed for years in the international mails. The combination of slow delivery of mail and slow screening of it by lethargic censors probably accounts for Brauell's delay in getting the journal with Pollender's paper, as well as for his cryptic way of alluding to it.

How little things have changed in Russia from Tsarist to Communist times, say, from 1908 to 1978, can be seen from Karl Baedeker's travel guide to Russia, published (in English translation) in 1914. In advising his readers on clearing through the customs examination, he writes: "Unprinted paper only should be used for packing, to avoid any cause of suspicion." Printed matter is still listed under prohibited items in 1978 travel books on the Soviet Union.

animal postmortem. (3) During the decade following his observations of the bacilli in the blood, he repeatedly pointed out that their occurrence was constant, thus encouraging others to look for them. But he also emphasized that such bacilli did not occur in the blood of animals dying from diseases other than anthrax, either ante- or immediately postmortem. He was thus the first person to postulate the thesis (in 1857) *that the presence of bacteria could be used in establishing the diagnosis of a disease.* (4) He determined that the placenta was able to protect the fetus from invasion of bacilli from the blood of the dam.*

Müller says that these four accomplishments, which furthered the beginning of bacteriology as a science, must not obscure the fact that Brauell also made some serious mistakes which retarded rather than advanced bacteriological knowledge. These mistakes are attributable to the fact that the proper techniques necessary for careful bacteriological work had not yet been developed. To examine the mistakes would take us too far afield here; suffice it to say that Brauell's accomplishments with respect to anthrax considerably outweigh them. When one adds to these his contributions to anatomy and to pathological anatomy and histology, he appears clearly as an outstanding figure at the Dorpat Veterinary Institute, one of the ones responsible for the fine reputation it deservedly enjoyed both in Russia and abroad.

An important contribution of Brauell's was the education he imparted to his pupil Eugen Semmer (1843–1906), as well as the example he set for him. The extent of Brauell's influ-

*To the above Peebsen[396] has added that Brauell was the first to describe the bacterial spore, in the reports of his anthrax experiments. I have found this description, but I do not know enough about the history of either bacteriology or microscopy to know whether it is indeed the first. The very thorough and meticulously detailed paper of Müller[363] does not mention it—he might have overlooked it or not considered it important enough to mention.

ence, however, is something I have only been able to surmise rather than determine. Semmer studied under Brauell as an undergraduate and the latter must have had some influence in getting him to stay on to do an M.V.Sc. dissertation* and to enter academic work. In his dissertation on the pharyngeal muscles of animals, dated October 1865, Semmer thanks his "highly honored teacher, Prof. Dr. Brauell," for advice and for help in conducting the work. While the work was Semmer's, it bore the marks of Brauell's influence in its careful and meticulous attention to the details of the dissected organs and its equally careful citation of the work of others. A decade later, in 1875, Semmer paid his respects again when he wrote in his book "On the Pathologic Anatomy of Rinderpest:"[482] "Die ersten eingehenden microscopischen Forschungen auf dem Gebiete der Rinderpest wurden von Brauell 1861 angestellt." (The first thorough microscopic research on rinderpest was conducted by Brauell in 1861.) As already pointed out, Brauell received considerable recognition for first investigating the histopathology of rinderpest, both in Russia and in Germany and England.

Semmer followed in the footsteps of his teacher in investigating the same disease—a very important one in Russia—

*The *Magister Veterinarnykh Nauk* (Master of Veterinary Science) degree was a mandatory requirement for veterinarians who wished to follow an academic career in nineteenth-century Russia and until the 1920s. The doctorate was not open to veterinarians, a situation against which both Semmer[521] and Gryuner[194] railed, but only in articles published abroad! I have compared a dozen Russian M.D. dissertations of that period with as many M.V.Sc. dissertations, and I consider them indistinguishable in scientific content. In fact, several physicians obtained the M.D. with dissertations on *veterinary* subjects, ones as diverse as the anatomy of the horse (Vsevolodov[150]) or rabies in the dog.[259] Uspensky's M.D. dissertation on the histopathology of pulmonary glanders in horses, for example, is a considerably more flimsy contribution to knowledge than most of the M.V.Sc. theses contemporary to it.[608]

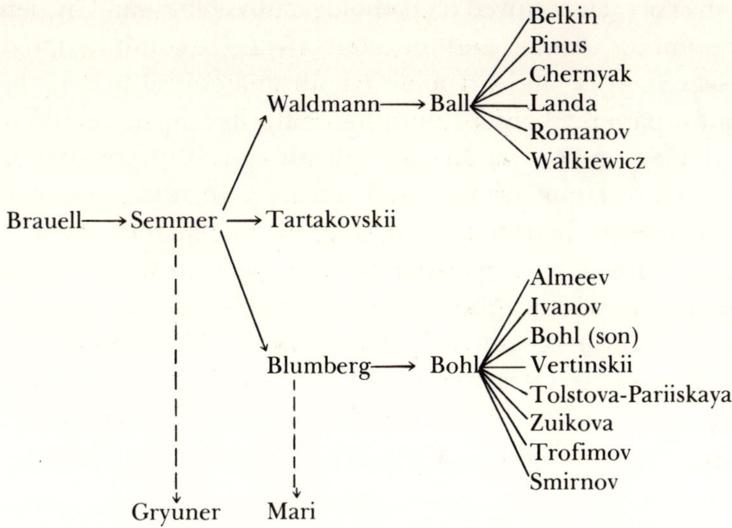

Chart 1. Scientific lineage of veterinary pathologists in Russia.

as well as in taking over his chair. I believe, therefore, that one can trace a direct line of scientific descent as in Chart 1. The tracing of this lineage leads us to the founders of the Leningrad school of veterinary pathologists, N. D. Ball, and the Kazan school, K. H. Bohl, respectively, and indicates that Brauell deserves credit over and above what is his due for his work on anthrax. He is, in fact, the father of veterinary pathology in Russia, in the sense that he left scientific descendants, which Ravich—who had been designated by Pinus as deserving of this title—did not do.

Brauell left Dorpat in 1868, at what Müller terms "the then customary academic retirement age," with a pension of 1,700 rubles. Perhaps this age (60) was the customary one for retirement of foreigners; other professors remained at Dorpat (and elsewhere in Russian institutions) until they were 65 or 70 years old. He returned to Germany and in 1869 was appointed honorary professor in the medical faculty of Leipzig

University. He lectured on pathology, physiology, and hygiene of domestic animals and retired in 1871. He continued to do research work and to publish both anatomical and pathological papers[123] almost until his death in Leipzig in 1882.

Sixteen years after Brauell's death and 30 years after his retirement from the Dorpat Veterinary Institute, a leading German veterinary educator compiled a "balance sheet" of the Institute's accomplishments in its first 50 years. Its text follows this paragraph.* This is not the place to discuss which of the founding faculty members had done the most to bring the DVI its well-deserved scientific reputation, but the Russian government obviously had done well for itself when it had "imported" the 30-year-old Friedrich Brauell back in 1837.

> Und nun gestatten Eure Exzellenz, daß ich dem noch einige Worte Hinzufüge.
>
> Was dieses Institut der Wissenschaft bedeutet, das werden Sie heute von neuem klar erkennen an den Ovationen, die Ihnen hier dargebracht werden, an den Kundgebungen, die aus allen großen Staaten Europas Ihnen Zugehen.
>
> Ewig denkwürdig wird die Stätte bleiben, wo zum erstenmal ein pathogener Mikroorganismus im Versteck seiner verderblichen Tätigkeit von einem durchdringenden Forscherblick—dem Brauells—erspäht wurde.
>
> Zu den Kampfmitteln, mit denen die modernste Medizin gegen die Tierseuchen uns ausgerüstet hat, haben russische Veterinäre das Mallein gefügt und unvergessen wird es bleiben, daß für diese Entdeckung hier ein Gelehrter in den Tod gegangen ist.
>
> Was heute von Afrika aus als etwas angeblich Neues das große Weltpublikum in Staunen setzt—die Rinderpestimpfung, das ist schon vor langer Zeit hier gelehrt und geübt worden.

*Portion of text of speech held by Professor R. Schmaltz, of the Berlin Veterinary College, at the 50-year celebration of the Dorpat Veterinary Institute, in Dorpat in 1898. (From the paper by Zalewsky,[647] published in 1918.)

Die Tätigkeit dieses Instituts hat unzweifelhaft wesentlich mit die russische Veterinärpolizei befähigt, ihre schwierigen Aufgaben so vorzüglich zu erfüllen, daß heute von diesem weiten Reich ein Teil, so groß and größer als mein Heimatland, von der gefährlichsten aller Tierseuchen gänzlich befreit ist, und daß andere Seuchen erfolgreich bekämpft werden.

Die Professoren des hiesigen Veterinärs-Instituts haben mit uns stets wissenschaftliche Verbindung gehalten, erst kürzlich in einem großen, mit Beifall begrüßten Werke, seit lange in Zahlreichen journalistischen Arbeiten.

Die Dorpater Dissertationen erfreuen sich eines begründeten Rufs. Sie zeigen zugleich, daß die Lehrer es sich angelegen sein lassen und verstehen, ihren Geist auf die jüngeren Generationen zu übertragen und Schule zu machen, und daß durch die Tüchtigkeit der Schüler die Zukunft des Instituts gesichert ist.

Aber nicht, um alles das Ihnen zu sagen, kam ich her. Die Dorpater Professoren haben mehr getan, als uns sich wissenschaftlich verbunden. Die Mehrzahl von Ihnen—Sie, Exzellenz, allen voran—haben mit uns auch persönliche Beziehungen angeknüpft.

Sie sind häufige und stets willkommene Gäste in Berlin gewesen. Zu eifrigen Studien kamen sie hin; berzliche Freundschaften sind dabei entstanden.

Und so hat mich heute nicht bloß ein kühles nobile officium hierher getrieben, sondern dem Zuge des Herzens bin ich gefolgt, um diese Freundschaft zu betätigen. Und aus vollem Herzen quellen die Wünsche, die ich ihnen zurufe: Möge das Veterinär-Institut zu Jurjew Blühen und sich stetig fortentwickeln. Möge es ihm vergönnt sein, unter friedlichem Szepter rüstig weiter zu schaffen zum Nutzen seines großen Vaterlandes und zur Förderung der Wissenschaft. Und möge es für die Veterinärmedizin bleiben, was es war und ist: Ein Stern im Osten, der leuchtende Morgenstern am Firmament unserer Wissenschaft.

And now, please permit me, your excellency, to add a few words.

What this institute means to science you will have clearly recognized from the ovations which you have received here and from the testimonials which have been sent to you by all of the great states of Europe.

We will always remain grateful to the institution where the damaging activity of a pathogenic microorganism was detected for the first time by the penetrating view of a research worker—Brauell.

Russian veterinarians have contributed to the protective measures with which our most modern medicine has armed us in the fight against animal plagues. They have discovered mallein, and we will never forget that a scientist paid with his life in the course of this discovery.

Something that comes from Africa and is amazing the world public as supposedly new—rinderpest vaccination—has been taught and practiced here for a long time.

The activity of this institute has without a doubt enabled the Russian veterinary officials to fulfill their obligations so well that today a large part of this empire, larger than my homeland, is completely free of the most dangerous animal plague, and other animal plagues in it are being successfully controlled.

The professors of the local veterinary institute have always maintained scientific relationships with us, recently in a large work which had been greeted with accolades, and for many years in numerous journal articles.

The dissertations from Dorpat enjoy a well-earned reputation. They show simultaneously that the teachers here understand how to convey their spirit to the younger generation, and also that the future of this institute is secure through the quality of the students.

I have not come here, however, in order to say all of this to you. The professors in Dorpat have done more than to ally themselves with us scientifically. The majority of them, and you, your excellency, ahead of all the others, have also taken up personal relationships with us. You have been frequent and always welcome guests in Berlin. You came there for the purpose of undertaking studies; warm friendships have evolved therefrom.

And so what has brought me here today is not merely the cool exercise of an official act, but rather I have followed my

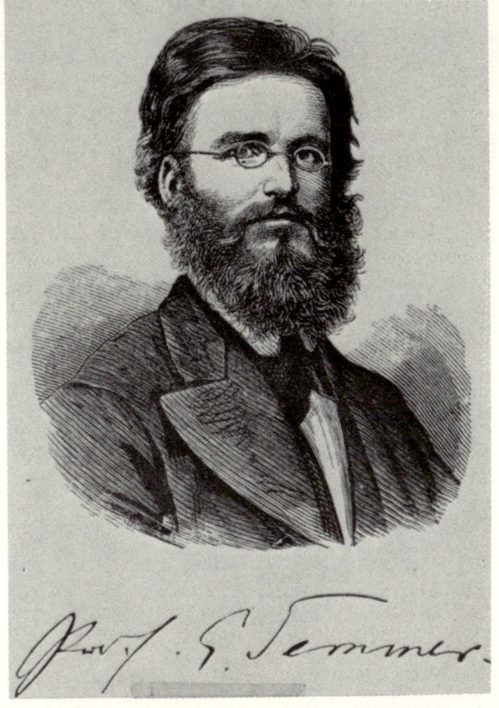

Figure 6. Eugen Semmer.

heart in order to further activate this friendship. And the wishes which I extend to you from the bottom of my heart are these: May the Veterinary Institute in Yuryev flower and continue to develop further, may it be granted to the institute under a peaceful scepter to actively work further for the benefit of its great fatherland and the advance of science, and may it remain for veterinary medicine what it has been and is: a star in the east, the illuminating morning star in the firmament of our science.

We turn now from Brauell to consider the life of Eugen Semmer* in more detail.[3] Semmer (Fig. 6) was a Latvian, born on the Adfer estate in the town of Volmar (now known

*His name appears as Zemmer in Russian publications; however, since he was not a Russian, I have amalgamated all citation of his work in the reference list under Semmer, the way it is spelled in Latvian.

as Valmiera) in Latvia on October 27, 1843. He received his early education in the Volmar Elementary School between 1852 and 1858. From there he transferred to the fifth grade of the classical high school in Dorpat. After completion of the seventh grade there, he enrolled in the Dorpat Veterinary School (as it was then known) as the recipient of a public scholarship. He graduated in 1865 with the degree Master of Veterinary Science, after defending his dissertation (Fig. 7).

Assigned to the military district of Turkestan for duty with the army, he received new orders during his trip there, rescinding this assignment and appointing him prosector in the anatomy department of the Dorpat Veterinary Institute. In addition to these duties, he taught the courses in general pathology, pathologic anatomy, autopsy technique, and microscopy, beginning with January 1869, right after Professor Brauell's departure from Dorpat. In this year, Semmer also began research work in pathogenic bacteriology, which, of course, was still a dozen years removed from becoming established as a formal scientific discipline. Semmer thus carried an extraordinarily heavy teaching load of several subjects while conducting research and writing. In the latter field he was the most fruitful and prolific of the veterinary pathologists in Russia during the late nineteenth century.

In 1890, Semmer published a brief report on the fifth International Veterinary Congress in Paris in the *Arkhiv Veterinarnykh Nauk,* for the benefit of the veterinary profession in Russia.[514] It dealt chiefly with control of infectious diseases, particularly tuberculosis. To my disappointment, this is a dry-as-dust factual summation devoid of value judgments and lacking his usual lively style. From having found Semmer's picture in a group of delegates to this congress (Fig. 60), I know that he met at least one of the men he had previously (1880) attacked in print, Professor Perroncito of Turin. Very likely he met Toussaint and Pasteur, too, but there was no hint in the article about his impressions of individuals or of what he thought of the Congress as a whole.

Die

Schlundmuskeln

der

Hausthiere.

Inaugural-Abhandlung,

welche

mit Genehmigung des Hochverordneten Conseils

der Dorpatschen Veterinairanstalt

zur Erlangung der Würde eines

Magisters

der Veterinairwissenschaften

öffentlich vertheidigen wird

Eugen Nicolai Semmer

aus Livland.

Mit einer lithographirten Tafel.

Dorpat.

Druck von C. Mattiesen.

1865.

Figure 7. Title page of Semmer's dissertation.

Semmer taught at the Dorpat Veterinary Institute from 1870 until he left in 1892 to head the epizootic department of the Institute for Experimental Medicine in St. Petersburg. His work in the latter Institute is described in Chapters 4 and 11. While he was in Dorpat, he published a considerable number of case reports of his postmortem observations, and it is apparent from reading these that even back in the 1870s his autopsy technique was meticulous and thorough. One is particularly impressed that he was going to the trouble of examining the central nervous system at a time when even doing a partial autopsy had not yet caught on[472].*

While in St. Petersburg, Semmer was able to develop an effective vaccine against rinderpest. Semmer is regarded by Chernyak[151] as the father of Russian veterinary pathology, since, unlike Ravich, he did leave scientific descendants. With all due respect to Chernyak, who, writing as a native of the country, is perhaps better qualified to award titles, my choice is Brauell.

Waldmann's obituary of Semmer lists a goodly number of papers—over 100. Examination of this list shows that they are unequally divided between publications in German (about 60 percent), Russian (about 38 percent), and Estonian or Latvian (about 2 percent). Of the Russian articles, several are in newspapers or popular agricultural journals, the scientific contributions in Russian being only about 20 percent of the total. Perhaps in his favoring of the German language over the Russian lies the root of some of the troubles that dogged Semmer's footsteps, discussed later in this chapter.

Following the lead of his teacher, Brauell, Semmer published a small book on the pathologic anatomy of rinderpest in 1875 (Fig. 8).[482] In 1881, he followed this with a large

*Schütz[472] relates that in Berlin in 1870 the custom was for the clinician to decide which organ to examine postmortem. The autopsy would proceed only until that organ had been reached and then stop!

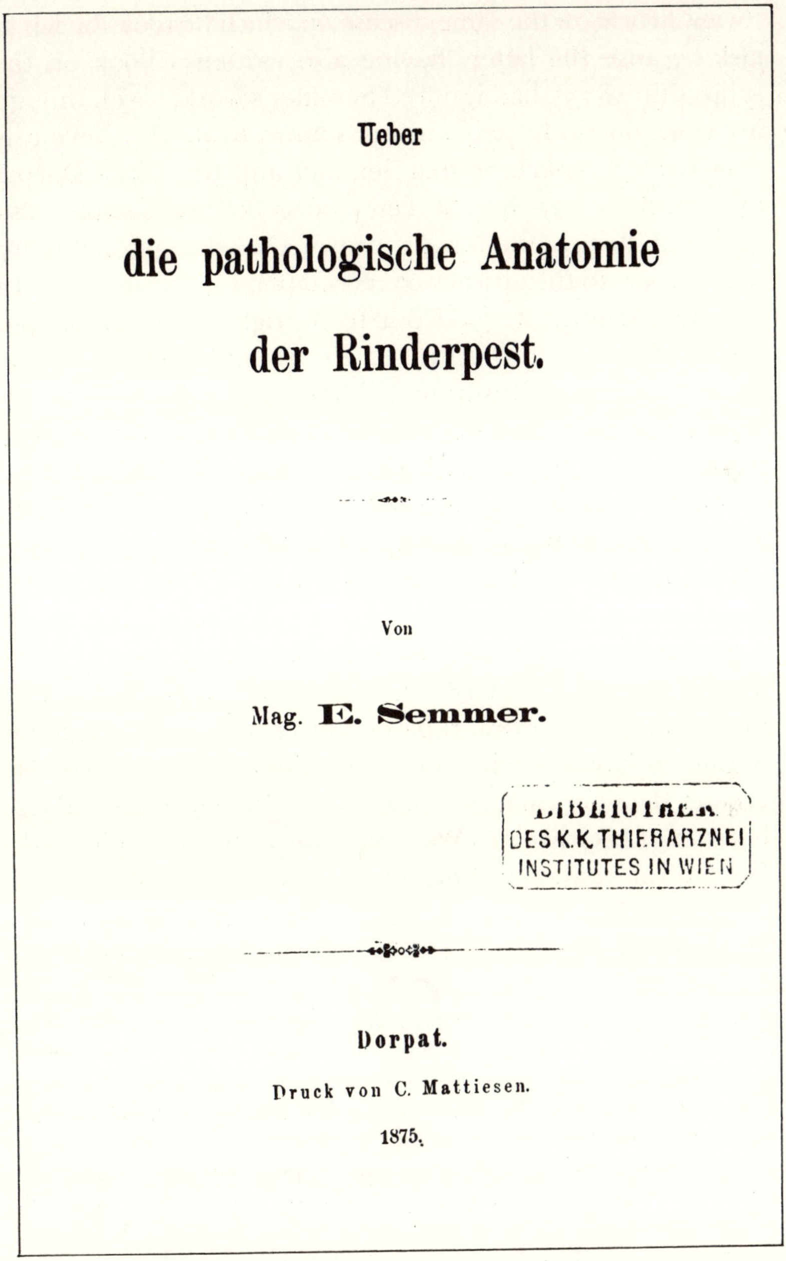

Ueber

die pathologische Anatomie

der Rinderpest.

Von

Mag. **E. Semmer.**

Dorpat.

Druck von C. Mattiesen.

1875.

Figure 8. Title page of Semmer's book on the pathology of rinderpest.

review article on the same disease, in which he took Ravich to task because the latter, having also written a book on the subject (in 1875), had ignored Semmer's work, "even though my work on rinderpest was not known to R." I believe it is reasonable to conclude that Semmer and Brauell in Dorpat were rivals of Ravich in St. Petersburg, because Semmer also criticized Ravich for having drawn the wrong conclusions with respect to the efficacy of vaccination for this disease.* In the end, Semmer turned out to be right—vaccination *was* useful. Semmer also criticized the second director of the Dorpat Veterinary Institute, F. Unterberger, for having contributed to a decision to close the rinderpest vaccine experiment stations in Russia.† On his part, Ravich criticized Brauell with respect to his work on the histology of the hoof, a criticism so sharp as to suggest the above-mentioned intercity rivalry to me. I have developed this theme further on page 191.

Semmer, the most famous of the Dorpat veterinary faculty during the 1880s and 1890s, earned his renown because of his original discoveries in pathology and bacteriology. Some of this work on fowl cholera and on rinderpest is discussed in greater detail in Chapter 10. He was well known abroad also because of his travels to Western Europe, for example, to the fourth International Veterinary Congress in Brussels in 1883, the Fifth in Paris in 1889,[610] the Sixth in Bern in 1895, and because he contributed to German journals and refer-

*P. Jessen, director of the Dorpat Veterinary Institute, who had served on the Rinderpest Commission with Ravich, also castigated him (and the people sitting in offices in St. Petersburg) for being obdurate about vaccination. He did so carefully, however, in a German journal, which he probably hoped would not be read in St. Petersburg.[220]

†Semmer was not afraid to tilt his lance in print, but mostly in German rather than Russian publications. He hit Raevski,[517] the antiveterinary bias of the medical establishment with regard to M.V.Sc. theses,[521] the ignorance of the "so-called" veterinary committee in St. Petersburg, as well as Perroncito, Toussaint, and Pasteur.[500]

ence books and served on their editorial boards.* His obituary in two Austrian journals and one French one shows the esteem in which he was held abroad.[249,562,627]

Semmer was one of the founders (1884) and editors of *Novosti Veterinarnoi Literatury Otechestvennoi i Inostrannoi* (News of Domestic and Foreign Veterinary Literature), which brought the advances as reflected (chiefly) in the Western veterinary books and journals to the profession in Russia. This abstracting journal was short-lived and ended publication the following year.[300] Since it is now almost unknown, even in Russia, I am reproducing the title page from one issue as a historical curiosity (Fig. 9).

The year 1895 was just a couple of years after the first filterable virus had been shown to be the cause of a disease. The precise nature of the agent that causes rinderpest had not yet been discovered. In this year, Semmer retired from the Institute for Experimental Medicine and was able to get a few things off his chest, although even then he felt safe in doing so only through the medium of a foreign journal, the German *Zeitschrift für Thiermedizin*.[518] This paper is very revealing, not only of the state of Russian veterinary science, fumbling its way, with that of other countries, into the era of virology, but also of Semmer's personal attributes and of some of the indignities he had been obliged to endure in the course of his scientific career.

Semmer reviewed the literature of the various attempts by domestic and foreign scientists to incriminate bacteria as the

*For example, *Jahresbericht über die Leistungen der Veterinärmedizin*. Semmer was on the editorial board from the inception of this abstracting journal until 1896, and whatever Russian literature appeared in its columns did so through the medium of his selection and translation. He was also on the editorial board of the *Deutsche Zeitschrift für Thiermedizin* and abstracted the Russian literature for the *Zeitschrift für vergleichende Augenheilkunde* from 1882 to 1885. He also published news of Russian veterinary meetings in Austrian journals.[524]

НОВОСТИ

ВЕТЕРИНАРНОЙ ЛИТЕРАТУРЫ

ОТЕЧЕСТВЕННОЙ и ИНОСТРАННОЙ.

ВЫХОДЯТЪ ЕЖЕМѢСЯЧНО,

подъ редакціей **А. И. Алексѣева.**

Августъ **№ 8.** **1884 г.**

Подписка принимается въ конторѣ редакціи: Кабинетская, № 5.
Цѣна въ годъ **ТРИ** рубля, для подписчиковъ на «Ветеринарное Дѣло» **ДВА** рубля.

Рефераты по иностранной литературѣ составляются Орд. Проф. Дерптскаго Ветеринарнаго Института **Е. М. Земмеромъ**, а по русской литературѣ Адъюнктъ-Проф. Н. Ф. **Колесниковымъ**.

Въ теченіи лѣтнихъ мѣсяцевъ рефераты по русской литературѣ будутъ составляться **Г. Печковскимъ**, за отсутствіемъ Проф. Н. Ф. **Колесникова**.

СОДЕРЖАНІЕ № 8: I. Рефераты по иностранной ветеринарной журналистикѣ: **Röckl**. Pneumonomycosis. — **Schlampp**. Смерть лошади отъ разрыва воздушнаго мѣшка.—**Hiller**. Бромъ противъ дифтерита.—**Lechner**. Кровавая моча у рогатаго скота на горахъ. — **Siedamgrotzky**. Употребленіе нафталина противъ коросты.—**Fonssagrives**. Леченіе бородавокъ.—**Ziehl**. О микрококахъ въ мокротѣ при воспаленіи легкихъ.—**Anacker**. О дискразической кровавой мочѣ лошадей.—**Ponfick**. О гемоглобинеміи и ея послѣдствіяхъ.—**Cantiget**. О размягченіи костей у рогатаго скота. — **Vernant**. Острыя колики съ головокруженіемъ у 6-мѣсячнаго жеребенка съ смертельнымъ исходомъ. — **Masse**. Пузырчатыя глисты у рогатаго скота въ Сиріи.—**Chicoli**. Желтая горячка у рогатаго скота въ Сициліи. — **Larcher**. О ломотѣ у птицъ.—**Trasbot**. Прививаніе сапа морскимъ свинкамъ.—**Mollière**. Pustula maligna отъ укушенія мухою.—**Fehleisen**. Микрококи рожи, ихъ культивированіе и прививаніе человѣку. — **Gibier**. О дѣйствіи чеснока и пилокарпина противъ бѣшенства.—**Liard**. Къ вопросу о переходѣ бѣшенства отъ матери на зародышъ.—**Abadie**. Случаи слишкомъ ранней зрѣлости у лошадей и рогатаго скота. — **Munk**. Движеніе и отдѣленіе молока. — **Cagny**. О замедленіи родовъ.—**Meisse** и **Strohmer**. Образованіе жировъ изъ углеводовъ въ животномъ организмѣ.—**Pröger**. Заболѣваніе овецъ на ржаномъ полѣ.—**Bre**. Энзоотическіе выкидыши у коровъ. — **Parrot** и **Martin**. Опыты превращенія зараз. туберкулъ въ безвредныя инородныя тѣла. — **Trasbot**. Прививаніе сапа морскимъ свинкамъ.—**Hertwig**. Грибокъ Actinomyces въ свиньѣ.

II. Отвѣтъ на критику г-на Печковскаго, Магистра **Краевскаго**.

III. Объявленія.

Рефераты по иностранной ветеринарной журналистикѣ.

Röckl. *Pneumonomycosis*.

Röckl нашелъ при изслѣдованіи легкихъ коровы ткань, пронизанную узелками величиною въ конопляное зерно. Узелки были ярко ограничены и содержали въ рединѣ сплетенія грибковыхъ нитей. Легочная ткань между узелками была гепатизирована, плевра воспалена и покрыта фибринознымъ выпотѣніемъ и сосуды тромбозированы,

Figure 9. Title page of the journal *Novosti Veterinarnoi Literatury*.

cause of rinderpest. Among the authors he mentioned were Kolesnikov and Mechnikov, both of whom had reported that *bacteria* had caused the disease. Nevertheless, Semmer did not spare himself. He pointed out that the findings reported by himself and Archangelskii[5,10] that certain bacteria caused rinderpest had been demonstrated to be erroneous. He added that another report by himself, stating that streptococci caused rinderpest, was also erroneous—such streptococci could be found in the air passages of healthy cattle. Semmer was trying to bring some clarity and order into the mess of numerous bacteria which people had erroneously reported to be the cause of rinderpest.

Semmer criticized Mechnikov, pointing out that at the time of the latter's investigation, rinderpest had broken out in the cities surrounding his research station. Semmer rightfully contended that Mechnikov's experimental animals were therefore exposed to natural contagion, and thus no experimentally inoculated bacteria could be held responsible for any cases of disease which might subsequently develop. Mechnikov had been criticized unjustifiably by many people regarding his theory of phagocytosis, but the criticism Semmer leveled at him was warranted.

Had Semmer merely maintained a discreet silence, as did all of the other misguided etiologists, the passage of time would have served to obscure everyone's mistakes within a few years. But Semmer was not content to hide behind a wall of silence. It tells us much about his character to know that his honesty compelled him to withdraw his previously published claims in public print. Today this may not sound like much, but at that time a European professor was a respected figure—a symbol of academic authority, not to say infallibility—and most professors would have considered it detrimental to their image to make such an admission, even privately. To make it in a German journal, and thus in effect to an international audience, required considerable courage and no little humility. A man of integrity, Semmer obviously had plenty of courage to go with it. One looks in vain for similarly candid public expressions of error in the lives of Semmer's contemporaries. Although he did not discover the cause of rinderpest, Semmer was in good company—Robert Koch, sent by the British government to South Africa in 1895 for this specific purpose was not able to discover it either.

In one of the obituaries written of him, Semmer's successor, Waldmann, pointed out that Semmer's life was made miserable by petty intrigues, not further specified.[510] Because he was writing in imperial Russia, it was no wonder that Waldmann was not more specific, since his criticism would have had to have been directed at the same imperial government responsible for the trouble. Semmer himself, however, had shed light on some aspects of his harassment while he was still alive, in the paper discussed above.[518] He was a strong adherent of vaccination for rinderpest—a minority view opposed by a group of powerful bureaucrats in St. Petersburg, who recommended eradication of the disease by slaughter. He pointed out with considerable logic that the methods which were effective in Central Europe would not work in the steppes of Russia.

He related an incredible series of hindrances that were put in the way of his field experiments in the south of Russia. Even though Count Orlov gave a grant of 60,000 rubles to support research on rinderpest vaccination, Semmer was obstructed by the intrigues of officials of the Russian government. The amazing and disgraceful details read like a page out of one of Dostoevsky's novels—almost inconceivable from our (American) viewpoint—the folly, the stupidity, the pettiness on an epic scale are overwhelming merely to read about. Semmer points out that certain government officials did not want to bring rinderpest under control in the Russian Empire, since this would have put them out of a job. He writes sarcastically and very bitterly about the veterinary administration of the government and the "so-called Veterinary Committee" which consists only to a minor extent of veterinarians. He says that many of its members have spent their whole lives sitting at a desk and know nothing of practical requirements. Four hundred years and 500,000 rubles would be needed to solve the rinderpest vaccination matter in the Institute for Experimental Medicine in St. Petersburg. The same solution could be had in two to three years for 2,000 rubles in the field station at Poltava. Here we have one of the first examples of a competent and dedicated scientist railing against the curse which has not yet been lifted—the stupidities of desk-bound bureaucrats.

Semmer ends his article with a bitter tirade—a vivid rendition of the conditions in the Institute of Experimental Medicine. He makes it quite clear that the department of epizootiology was starved for funds and received no moral support in lieu of money. It is not apparent to me why Semmer left Dorpat to assume this unpleasant St. Petersburg job; he must have been promised opportunities that were not fulfilled. He points out that other members of the Institute, such as the chief of the chemistry department, received 7,000 rubles a year and that he, himself, after 30 years of service to the state got only 4,000 rubles. He is also bitter that he was cheated out of his removal allowance when he transferred in the state's service from Dorpat to St. Petersburg, although it was customary for the state to pay such an allowance. This dismal picture shows that regardless of the reputation that the Institute for Experimental Medicine later acquired, neither it nor the Russian government had the wit to value a man like Semmer, who was considered an outstanding scientist by the whole of the international fraternity of veterinary science. It gives the lie to Unterberger's or Jessen's or Ravich's claims[605] at the International Veterinary Congress in Vienna in 1865[444] that the Russian government valued its veterinary scientists.* Or perhaps Semmer was a victim of the

*Even then there was a "party line," and those who wished to remain in the government's good graces knew how to follow it at home and propagate it abroad.

fact that the Institute for Experimental Medicine was under the Ministry of Health and that the ministry responsible for animal health (the Ministry of Internal Affairs) had no say in the Institute's affairs. The fact that the Ministry of Internal Affairs decided to start its own veterinary laboratory shortly thereafter would support this speculation.

Evidence of the backbiting to which Semmer was subjected all of his life can be found early in his career, in comments in volume 1, number 1, of the *Arkhiv Veterinarnykh Nauk,* by its editor, Ravich.[477] The latter's scientific criticism may have been partly justified, but his vindictive attitude and biting tone were not, and represents in my view abuse of the editorial privilege. Especially so when directed by an established professor at the prestigious Military-Medical Academy, Director of its Veterinary Division, and an influential member of the government in a powerful ministry, at a young and struggling prosector—a rank lower than lecturer in this rank-conscious country. On the other hand, just two years later, Semmer was elected an honorary member of the St. Petersburg Veterinary Society, a group founded and run until his death by Ravich, so his tirade may not have been motivated by personal malice, but perhaps only by overzealous defense of his own views against the differing views of Semmer.

To an extent, Semmer's problems reflected those of anyone of intellectual ability in Russia at that time. In an age and under a regime where ability to intrigue counted for much, whereas merit and a sincere desire to serve the best interests of the state counted for little, a man like Semmer was bound to come to grief. The responsible veterinary officials in the capital were busy preparing the ground so that the next epizootic could break out unhindered, just as the responsible military ones were preparing the armed forces for what was to be their next defeat—at this particular time by Japan. One disaster or another was always in the offing.

Semmer also suffered because of his personal attributes—he was honest, he was outspoken, and he was a member of a minority nationality in an empire ruled by Russians. His French obituary,[627] written, I believe, by his friend Vladimirov (but disguised by transliterated French initials*), makes it clear that he was the butt of national prejudice because of his "origine livonienne" (Livonian, that is, Latvian, origin). Semmer was indeed a giant persecuted by pygmies.

Semmer's successor in the chair of pathology was Johann Waldmann (1856–1922), who graduated from the Dorpat Veterinary Institute in 1880 (Fig. 10). After a period in private practice he returned to his alma mater as a prosector in anatomy in 1884 and later switched to pathology. Waldmann got his M.V.Sc. in 1892 from Dorpat with the dissertation, carried out under Semmer, *Statistika i Kazuistika Vskrytii Trupov Loshadei, Proizvedennykh v Yurevskom Veterinarnom Institute s 1874 po 1892* (Statistics and Case Reports of Autopsies on Cadavers of Horses Carried Out in the Yurev Veterinary Institute from 1874 to 1892).

*While I don't know who the author of his French obituary[627] is, my suspicion falls on his friend and longtime associate Dr. A. Vladimirov; the initials "A. W." which sign it could represent the French transliteration of this name. The fact that Semmer is not mentioned in the *Russkii Biograficheskii Slovar* may also be because of the Russian chauvinistic jealousy over Semmer's Livonian origin related by "A. W." Although Semmer was not a Baltic German, he was probably a victim of the dislike felt by many Russians for all of the Baltic peoples. Graham[187] (p. 20) relates that as late as 1880, Russians proposed for membership in the Imperial Academy of Sciences of St. Petersburg were still being "blackballed" by its Baltic German members. This engendered understandable bitterness on the part of excluded Russians, especially when such outstanding men as the chemist Mendeleev were kept out. I doubt whether these feelings had yet been dispelled by 1918, when the volume of the above dictionary that would have carried Semmer's biography was published. Thus, it may have been a predominantly Slavophil feeling rather than an antiveterinary one that prevailed at the Institute for Experimental Medicine and resulted in the difficulties Semmer encountered.

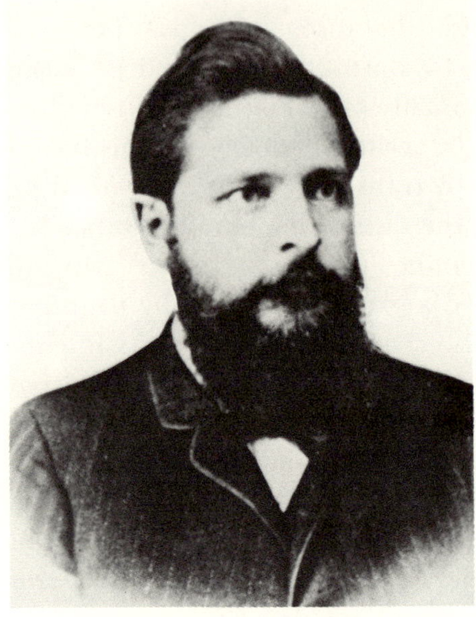

Figure 10. Johann Waldmann.

Upon Semmer's departure in 1892 for St. Petersburg, Waldmann took over the teaching of pathology, having previously spent five years as assistant in this department. He was sent abroad for study in 1894, but I do not know to which country. Waldmann taught meat hygiene and veterinary jurisprudence in addition to pathology. In comparison with Semmer's 175 publications, the half dozen or so put out by Waldmann are meager, and I do not believe that he influenced the development of veterinary pathology in Western Europe. Nor did he serve on the editorial board of German veterinary journals as Semmer did, although for many years, Waldmann contributed abstracts of Russian literature to the *Zeitschrift für Tiermedizin* and to the *Jahresbericht der Veterinärmedizin.* Though he was eclipsed by both his predecessors, we must remember that he stepped into the shoes of a great man, and one, moreover, whose career had unfolded during the blossoming of both pathology and bacteriology and was therefore "a hard act to follow."

As we have seen, the first teachers of pathology (Brauell and Semmer) at the Dorpat Veterinary Institute made a respectable contribution to veterinary pathology as a scientific discipline. Some of this is considered in more detail in Chapter 11. Under Waldmann, a sufficient number of autopsies were conducted at the Institute (Table 1) to provide the undergraduate veterinary students with adequate exposure to the practical as well as the theoretical aspects of pathology. By comparison, for example, the annual reports of the New York State Veterinary College list no autopsies whatsoever for the same years, although numerous clinical cases are tabulated. It was not until 1916 that V. A. Moore, dean of the New York State Veterinary College, was able to report with respect to autopsies: "A room for this purpose has been equipped and all fatal cases are carefully examined."[362] At most other American veterinary colleges, such a room had not yet been built by 1916, and the teaching of pathology was considerably behind that in Dorpat.

Waldmann's biographical album of Dorpat alumni, published with Negotin in 1898, is a valuable historical docu-

Table 1. Autopsies at Dorpat Veterinary Institute

	1905	1907	1908	1909	1910	1912	1913	1914
Horses	36	40	36	28	35	53	48	56
Cattle		14	10	15	17	11	16	7
Pigs	19	30	13	25	12	13	12	7
Dogs	40	63	71	39	40	52	59	39
Chickens	17		21	28	13	7	2	6
Sheep	3	4	2	6	2	2	3	4
Cats	4	4	5			8	5	4
Other								2
Total	149	203	168	150	141	164	159	125

Data from *Zhurnal Nauchnoi i Prakticheskoi Vet. Med. izd. Yurev. Vet. Inst. 1:* 36, 1907; *2:* 29, 1909; *3:* 30, 1909; *4:* 31, 1910; *5:* 31, 1911; *7:* 29, 1913; *8:* 28, 1914; *9:* 35, 1916.

ment, unique in Russian veterinary annals.[609] (Ivanovskii[217] had published a list of the St. Petersburg alumni, but it gave only their names and year of graduation.) Perhaps Waldmann's greatest claim to fame in the context of our survey of Russian veterinary pathology is that he encouraged and educated N. D. Ball (see Chapter 7), who did his M.V.Sc. dissertation in Waldmann's department.

Shortly after the turn of the century, Professor Waldmann had working for him as assistant Dr. Ernsts Paukuls (1872–1940), who graduated from Dorpat cum laude in 1889 and obtained his M.V.Sc. in 1901. He then studied at the University of Bern, obtaining the Doctor of Veterinary Medicine degree in 1903. From 1901 he was an assistant in the pathology department at the Dorpat Veterinary Institute and reached the rank of professor in 1917. When this Institute became a faculty of the University of Tartu in 1919, Paukuls received the chair of general pathology and therapy and held this for a year and a half. He then went to the newly founded veterinary school in Riga, Latvia, as its first dean.

Of the 19 publications which Tehver[589] lists as having been written by Paukuls between 1901 and 1916, about 10 are in the realm of pathology, dealing either with neoplasia or malformations; two additional ones deal with histology. Because of the chaotic conditions consequent upon the breaking up of the fringes of the Russian Empire, Paukuls' career changed abruptly when he was in his forties. Nevertheless, the works Tehver cited indicate that he made several modest but useful contributions to veterinary pathology.

By the time Estonia gained her independence after World War I, the Dorpat faculty members of Russian nationality had already returned to Russia, to Saratov, whence the library was also evacuated. Paukuls went thereafter to his native Latvia. Waldmann remained with the Dorpat school after it became the veterinary faculty of the University of Tartu. He died in that city on April 18, 1922.

His successor, Michael Hobmaier, was a German, well trained by Kitt in Munich. Besides a thorough grounding in pathology, he brought to his Estonian students a precise and meticulous autopsy technique that was the marvel of those who beheld it. He taught in Tartu until the end of the period covered by this book, but since Estonia was then free of Russian domination, I shall not deal with these years here.

4 Veterinary Pathology in St. Petersburg

Long whiskers cannot take the place of brains.
—Russian proverb

The Military-Medical Academy

In St. Petersburg (then the capital of the country), veterinary education began on June 17, 1808, in a veterinary division of the Military Medical Academy (Figs. 11 and 12), whose name was changed shortly thereafter to the Medico-Chirurgical Academy.*[570] Although it was under the aegis of the Minister of Internal Affairs, the reason for existence of the school continued to be primarily the training of physicians (and pharmacists) for the army. As far as I can tell, the Academy received the most financial support and was the finest of the medical schools in the Russian Empire. Vucinich[624] explains that in the late 1840s the Academy raided all four of the universities of Russia for the purpose of taking their best men for itself. The result was an academically very strong faculty, which by the end of the nineteenth century had included at one time or another such internationally renowned men as Pirogov, Botkin, Sechenov, and Pavlov. Other well-educated and very capable physicians, who either lent support to or participated actively in the veterinary pro-

*It was changed back to its former name in 1881 and was taken over by the Ministry of War.[626]

gram were the anatomist and histologist Feodor N. Zavarykin and the pathologist M. M. Rudnev, of whom more will be mentioned later. In no other educational institution in the world was the veterinary faculty associated under one roof with physicians of such ability and distinction,* and the future would seem to have augured well for it. And, in fact, veterinary education did get off to a fine start and reached a very high niveau. (Figure 13 shows a student of this period.) Unfortunately, however, the fruitful collaboration of medical and veterinary scientists which ensued was not destined to endure.

The first veterinary teacher was Professor I. D. Knigin,[171] a Russian; the government had first offered the job to Delabare Blaine, a famous London veterinarian, who declined it.[560] Pathology was not taught in the veterinary division of the Academy in the first half of the nineteenth century. Shortly after midcentury, pathology was taught by Professor Joseph Ippolitovich Ravich (1822–1875), who is regarded by Pinus[417] as having played the leading role in the development of veterinary pathology in Russia in the second half of the nineteenth century (Fig. 14). Born in Slutsk, Belorussia, Ravich was a remarkable man, who, according to his Russian eulogists, did not learn to read and write until he was 25 and burned himself out trying to make up for lost time later.[651] His German obituary,[9] however, states that after being edu-

*I have learned much about the Academy from a large (centenary) commemorative book written by Ivanovskii in 1898, a mine of information.[217] The extent of people's interest in the history of medicine can perhaps be gauged from the fact that when I found it in the Library of Congress in 1974, its pages were still uncut!

Figure 11 (following page). Bird's-eye view of St. Petersburg in the late nineteenth century. The Military-Medical Academy is at the lower left (arrow). Other landmarks are: The Hermitage (12), Equestrian statue of Peter the Great (15), School of Equitation (21), Nevsky Prospect (25), Hay Market (31), The Citadel (43), Academy of Sciences (51).

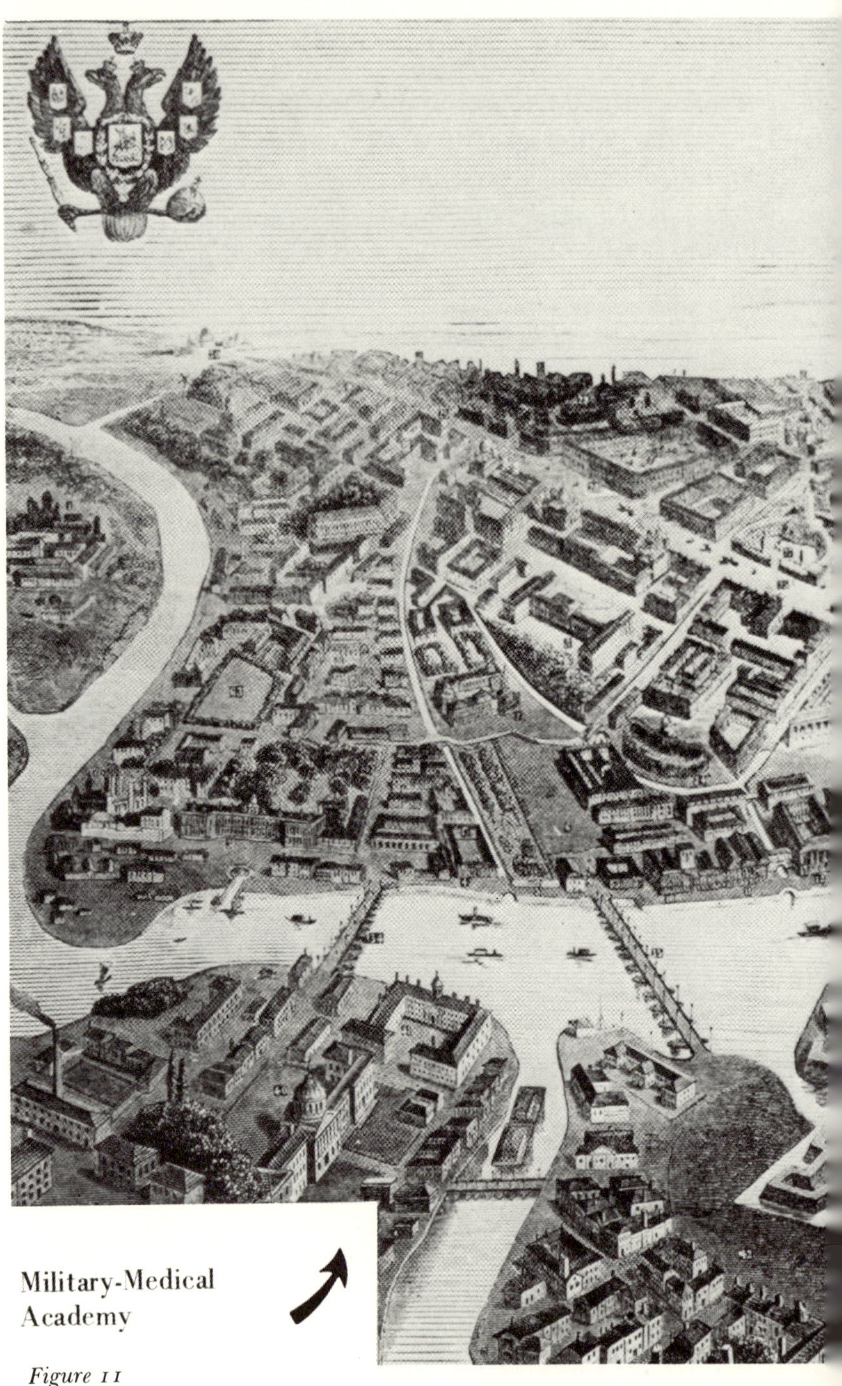

Figure 11

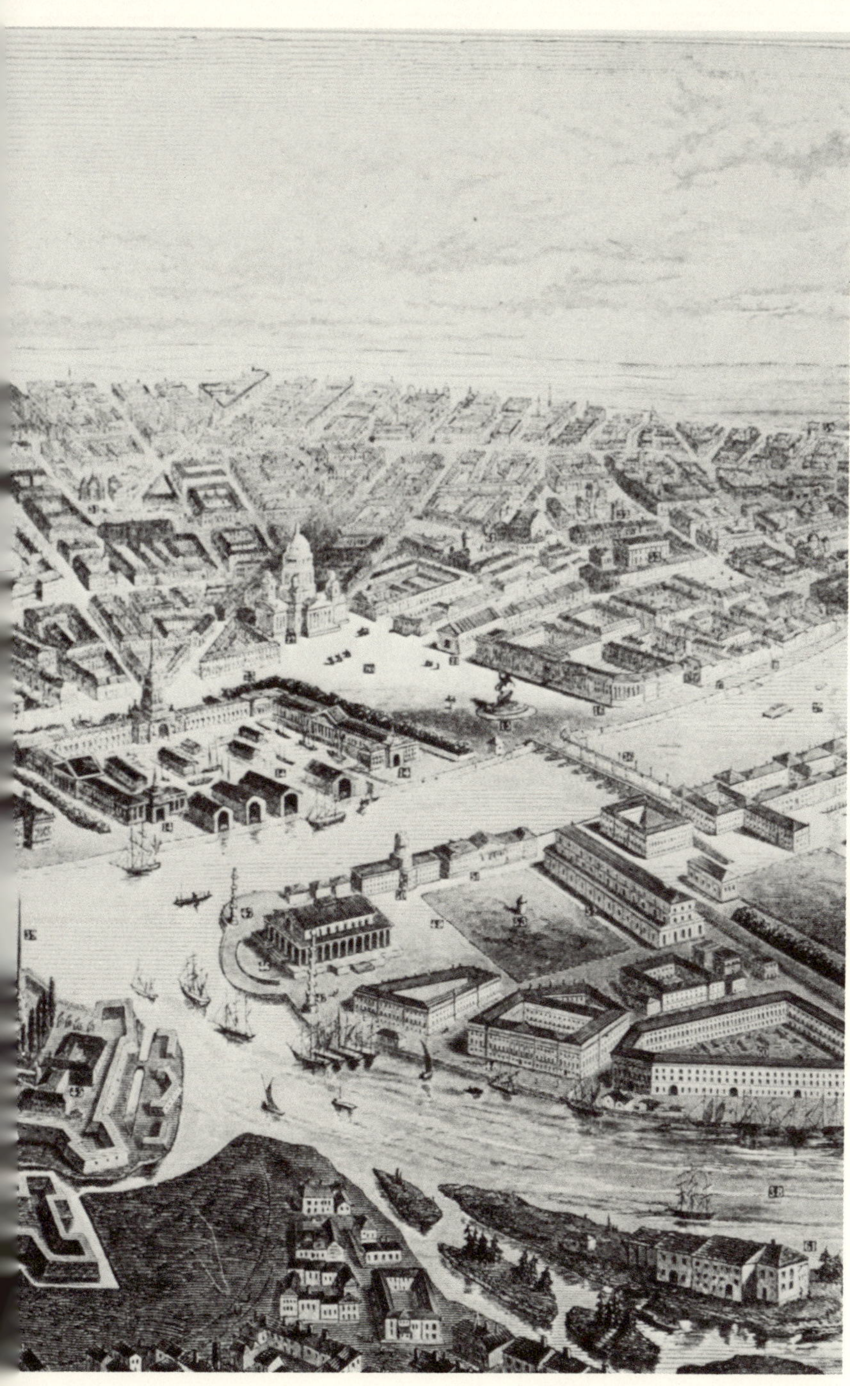

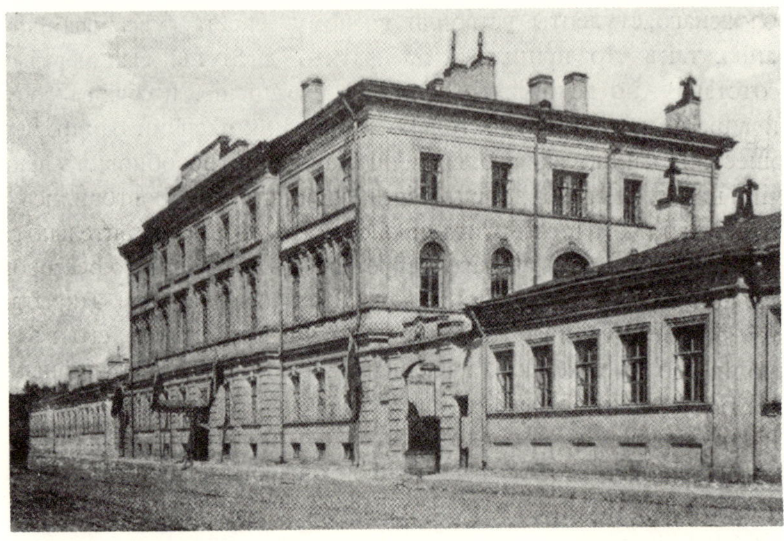

Figure 12. Buildings of the veterinary division of the Military-Medical Academy of St. Petersburg, around 1880.

cated in local schools and by a private tutor, he was sent to Germany in 1841 to prepare himself for the study of medicine, that is, he was literate at the age of 19. Since I have no access to any original documents, I am not able to reconcile the discrepancy between these two versions of Ravich's early education.* Whatever he may have done to prepare for it, Ravich entered the veterinary division of the Medico-Chirurgical Academy in 1846 and graduated as a veterinarian in 1850.[11]

From 1850, Ravich served for three years as regimental veterinary surgeon in various cavalry formations and returned to the Academy to study for his Master of Veterinary Science degree. This study, however, was interrupted by the Crimean War, in which he served from 1854 with the

*Henry James once said that "a historian is a person who wants more documents than he can really use," but he was surely not alluding to any historian writing about Russia!

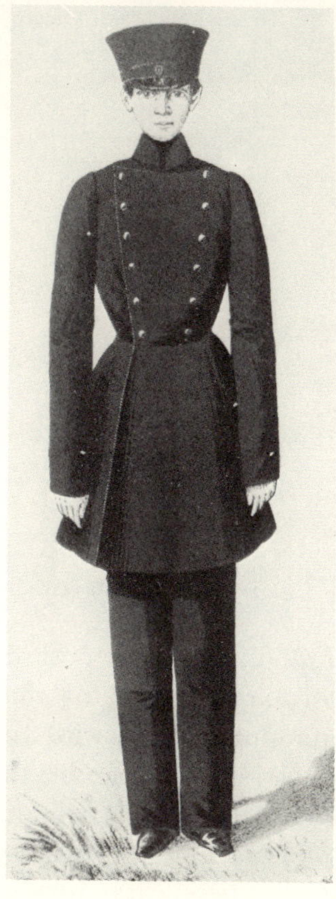

Figure 13. Student in the uniform of the veterinary division of the Military-Medical Academy of St. Petersburg.

cavalry, rising by 1858 to corps veterinary surgeon.[286] During this time, he completed his M.V.Sc. at Dorpat in 1856, when the German language—and through it German culture and influence—still reigned supreme in that city.[526]* I have not seen his dissertation, but from its date I assume that Brauell was his mentor.

*His dissertation *Razsuzhdeniya o razpoznavanii revmaticheskikh boleznei loshadei* (Reflections on the Diagnosis of Rheumatic Diseases of Horses), 1856, was written in Russian, the first one in this language to be accepted at the Dorpat Veterinary Institute. All the subsequent M.V.Sc. dissertations at Dorpat were in German until 1884.

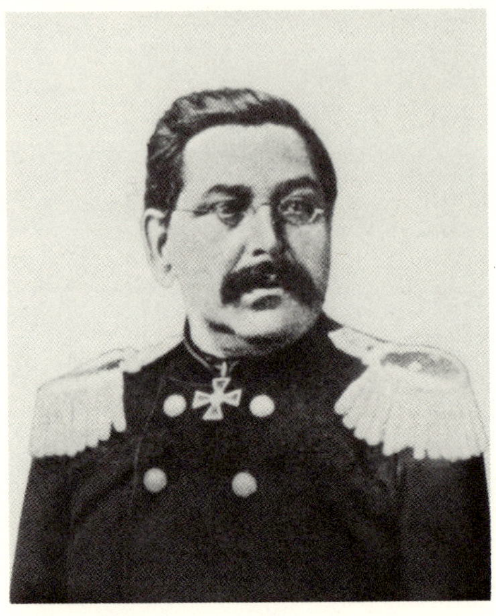

Figure 14. Joseph I. Ravich.

In 1859 he was the winner of a competition for the post of Privat-Dozent (lecturer) in the veterinary division of the Academy.[125] He took up his academic duties there with an inaugural lecture entitled "O sushchnosti i patologicheskikh izmeneniyakh sapa u loshadei" (The essence and pathologic changes of glanders in horses).[286] To prepare him for teaching, Ravich was then sent abroad for over two years, during which he studied physiology with Claude Bernard in Paris† and pathology in Berlin with Virchow (who, incidentally, was born just one year before Ravich).

In 1860 he published a small book *Obshchaya Zoopatologiya* (General Zoopathology, see Fig. 15) dealing with infectious diseases of domestic animals. His paper on the pathogenesis of glanders,[436] which he published at the end of his stay with Virchow, shows how clearly he was able to think about

†During this time the renowned physiologist I. M. Sechenov (1829–1905) was also on leave from his post in the Medico-Chirurgical Academy to study with Bernard.

ОБЩАЯ

ЗООПАТОЛОГІЯ

ИЛИ

СОВРЕМЕННОЕ УЧЕНІЕ О БОЛѢЗНЯХЪ ДОМАШНИХЪ ЖИВОТНЫХЪ.

ЧАСТЬ I.

ИЗМѢНЕНІЯ КРОВИ, ЛИМФЫ, ОТДѢЛЕНІЙ И ПИТАНІЯ.

СОЧИНЕНІЕ
МАГИСТРА ВЕТЕРИНАРНЫХЪ НАУКЪ
ІОСИФА **РАВИЧА.**

САНКТПЕТЕРБУРГЪ.
ВЪ ТИПОГРАФІИ МАВРИКІЯ ОСИПОВИЧА ВОЛЬФА.
1860.

Figure 15. Title page of Ravich's book "General Zoopathology."

pathogenesis and how critically he saw through fallacious explanations of the disease.* He himself was fallible, however, as when he took to task those who claimed that the nodules of "pearl disease" were tubercles.[435] Ravich was interested in histology as well as in pathology, and two of his papers dealt with strictly morphologic research.[437,438] In one of these, on the growth of the hoof, he went out of his way to acknowledge the contributions of Brauell and showed that he was able to distinguish useful contributions and show respect for their author, even when he disagreed with some of his conclusions.

Ravich became a specialist in epizootiology, and in 1864 he was appointed head of the veterinary division of the Academy, where he also taught physiology, histology, general pathology, and pathologic anatomy. Certainly there was no better trained veterinarian heading a veterinary college anywhere in the world at that time. Also in 1864, he published an important work, "Noveishie patologicheskoi anatomii chumy krupnogo rogatogo skota" (Latest investigations of the pathological anatomy of cattle plague) in the *Voenno-Meditsinskii Zhurnal* (Military Medical Journal) *89* (Sect. IV): 1-62; *90* (Sect. IV): 1-27. Ravich published the same work in German later that year, both in a veterinary journal and as a separate small book.[439] In 1961, Pinus alluded to this as one of the classical studies on rinderpest, and I agree with him. It has been overlooked in the West during the twentieth century, even though it was cited extensively in the British Royal Commission's report on cattle plague in

*Ravich praised Virchow's efforts to shed light on this aspect of comparative pathology (glanders), but 92 years later, Koropov[265] (p. 72) claimed that Ravich took "a critical approach to Virchow's cellular theory, pointing out its one-sidedness and its disregard of the role of the nervous system." There are reasons to doubt Koropov's veracity in view of the praise mentioned above, Koropov's failure to document his contention, and the statement of Ravich's eulogists lauding him because he introduced Virchow's cellular theory to Russia's veterinarians[651] (see Appendix I).

1886.[8] For example, the third report stated: "The Russian pathologist, Ravich, has already described with great accuracy some of these congestive phenomena."

Ravich founded the journal *Arkhiv Veterinarnykh Nauk* in 1871 and edited it until he died.[393] It became the best veterinary journal in the country and remained so until its demise in 1917; all of the contemporary veterinary pathologists mentioned in this book published in it.

In 1875, a few days before he died, he published the book *Rukovodstvo k Izucheniyu Obshchey Patologii Domashnikh Zhivotnykh* (Manual for the Study of the General Pathology of Domestic Animals). His death was a heavy blow to Russian veterinary medicine and was considered a loss to veterinary medicine at large by his German eulogist.[9] Ravich had become known abroad through his publications in German, both work published originally in German and Russian work republished shortly thereafter in German. He also became known through representing his country at international veterinary congresses in 1865 and 1867 and the international meetings on the control of rinderpest convened in Vienna in 1872 and 1875.[365]

Measured by any of several yardsticks—percentage of population who could read and write, miles of paved roads or of railway trackage—nineteenth-century Russia was a backward country in comparison to the United Kingdom or the United States. Though it may seem paradoxical, the few veterinary pathologists working in Russia—such men as Semmer or Ravich—were incomparably better educated than their English-speaking contemporaries. Nowhere is this better demonstrated than in the amusing spectacle made by Professor James Simonds* of London at the International Veterinary Congress in Zurich in 1867.[648]

*Royal Veterinary College, London, President of the Royal College of Veterinary Surgeons, Chief Veterinary Advisor to the Privy Council.

Simonds attended the meeting as representative of Her Britannic Majesty's government, but was unable to comprehend a word of the discussions being held there. He had been to Europe a decade earlier to study rinderpest, accompanied by an interpreter.[560] This time he came alone and was obliged to sit dumbly by while a kind colleague gave the delegates the gist of his speech in German, beginning with an apology for his understanding neither it nor French! Simonds continued his passive participation when, a bit later, Ravich, taking on several adversaries simultaneously, adroitly parried arguments from French, German, and Russian delegates, alternating from fluent German to elegant French and back again, his intellect and erudition sparkling forth in both languages. The proceedings of this congress are revealing in that they show Ravich at his best, which was the equal of anyone in European veterinary medicine at that time. And the esteem in which he was held likewise emerges from these proceedings—Professor Zangger, the chairman, stated at one point that Ravich, who had already spoken, requested permission to speak again but the rules did not permit him to do so unless the delegates wished to waive them. The assembly rose to its feet to indicate that Ravich should be given the floor.

Ravich did considerable work on the pathology of rinderpest and also on its prophylaxis. His account of traveling 28 days from St. Petersburg to a rinderpest research station reminds us that travel in Russia with hardly any railroads or paved roads—conveniences we take for granted—was not easy in his day. His later allusion to being repeatedly bitten by flies in traveling through the woods adds another dimension to Russian travel! In a day when we ride in air-conditioned (or heated) vehicles on smooth roads, cushioned by pneumatic tires, steel springs, hydraulic shock absorbers, and foam rubber upholstery, it is hard to envision limping for days in a steel-tired, wooden-wheeled, unsprung carriage over a pair of rough ruts through insect-infested woods.

These were the conditions that prevailed in Ravich's day and for many years thereafter. Travel in the winter may have been less bumpy, but it was hardly less exacting (see Fig. 63).

After arrival at his field research station, Ravich conducted experimental work on the value of vaccination in preventing rinderpest. Unfortunately, he reached the wrong conclusion—that such immunization was not effective in protecting against the disease—and, as a consequence of his recommendation, the research station was shut down.

Pinus[471] states that from 1869 the veterinary students at the Medico-Chirurgical Academy were taught pathology along with the medical students by Professor M. M. Rudnev, a medical pathologist, and Rudnev himself confirms this information.[451] There is also evidence that the pathology department of the veterinary division was directed, from the time of Ravich's death in 1875 until it closed in 1883, by Professor A. A. Raevskii, a veterinarian. The year 1869 was six years before Ravich's death, and I do not know why the veterinary students should have been taught pathology by Rudnev. One can speculate that as director of the veterinary division of the Academy, member of the Veterinary Committee in the government, representative of Russia to international bodies for epizootic disease control, and editor of the country's leading veterinary journal, Ravich's duties did not leave time for him to teach pathology in addition to his four other subjects during the last six years of his life. Unfortunately, I lack access to the primary historical documents that would enable me to clarify this question. Similarly, I do not know who taught pathology to the veterinary students during the time between Ravich's death in 1875 and Rudnev's death in 1878—whether Rudnev, Raevskii, or both. Some accounts attribute the teaching to one man and some to the other. Probably both of them did. Since I cannot unravel their interrelationships, I must resort to merely recounting the activities of each.

Arkady A. Raevskii (1848-1916) was born in Voronezh

and obtained his school education there (Fig. 16). In 1866 he graduated from the veterinary division of th Medico-Chirurgical Academy with distinction, recognized by a gold medal. From 1871 to 1872 he worked in the department of anatomy under the noted histologist Professor F. Zavarykin, doing research on the histology of the hoof. Raevskii was awarded the degree M.V.Sc. for this work, and one of the outstanding illustrations from his dissertation[429] is depicted in Figure 17.

In 1875, after working abroad for two years (location not specified by Kalugin[223]), Raevskii was appointed adjunct professor in the veterinary division of the Academy, heading the department of general zoopathology, pathologic zootomy, and epizootiology. He lectured on these subjects to both the veterinary and the medical students and in 1879 and 1881 was promoted to extraordinary professor and ordinary professor, respectively.[223] Raevskii was also interested in medicine; he took courses in medical science at the Academy

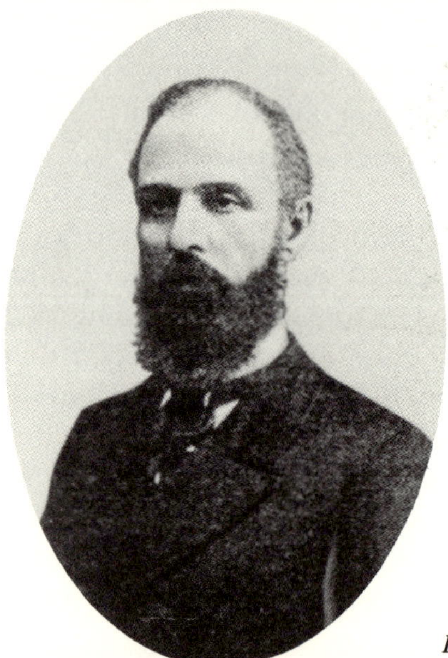

Figure 16. Arkady A. Raevskii.

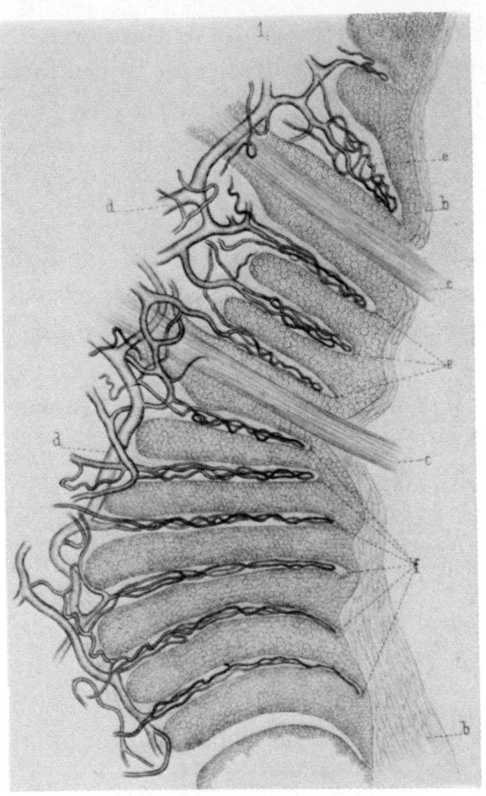

Figure 17. Illustration from Raevskii's thesis on histology of the hoof.

and obtained his diploma as a physician; in 1884 he was granted the degree Doctor of Medical Science.

Raevskii's interests gradually shifted to bacteriology, and in 1882 he was sent to Paris to work in the Pasteur Institute on anthrax. Upon his return from France, he organized a bacteriologic laboratory in the veterinary division of the Academy that was used both for research and to teach the subject to veterinary and medical students. In this laboratory also, graduate veterinarians or physicians could do experimental work in pathologic anatomy. For example, S. A. Ivanov published an M.V.Sc. dissertation on the lesions of rabies in the central nervous system.[215] Several people completed their dissertations under him, among them Uspensky on pulmonary glanders in the horse for the M.D. degree,[608] Kikiloff[245] on the development of tubercles in cattle, and Matsulevich on the neuropathology of canine distemper for the M.V.Sc.[342]; the latter two were published in German journals.[460]

After the closing of the veterinary division in 1883, Raevskii taught the course in epizootiology to the medical students until he left St. Petersburg to assume the directorship of the Kharkov Veterinary Institute two years later. From that time on he worked in bacteriology, and his career, which had begun in histology and moved to pathology, never returned to the latter discipline.

According to Kalugin,[223] Raevskii wrote a book on infectious diseases of animals in 1880 and one on pathologic anatomy of domestic animals in 1882. The latter book, *Patologicheskaya Anatomiya Domashnikh Zhivotnykh,* is mentioned in another historical paper by Magda[314] but apart from these two I have encountered no citation of it by anyone else, nor have I been able to find such a book. Kalugin and Magda are probably referring to the republication of an extended article with the above title which appeared in the *Arkhiv Veterinarnykh Nauk* in 1877 and 1878, a rather pedestrian compilation with no pretensions to originality. If so, they have gotten the year 1882 wrong—the same material was published as a monograph in the year 1879.[431] It is correctly cited by Ostapenko.[377] From the rarity of the citation of this book even in the Russian literature, one can assume that its influence on the development of veterinary pathology in Russia was probably negligible. Perhaps it was intended only as a teaching aid for Raevskii's own students. The extent of his total contributions to veterinary pathology in St. Petersburg remains to be determined; extensive information is available to me only on his subsequent activities in Kharkov, but by then he had left our discipline.

We return now to Professor Mikhail M. Rudnev (1837-

1878), who held the chair of pathology in the medical division of the Academy (Fig. 18). He had prepared himself for this post by spending the years 1863 to 1865 in Germany, mostly in Virchow's laboratory, but had worked also with other German pathologists. He returned to St. Petersburg well versed in the best of contemporary cellular pathology.[216] Rudnev was greatly interested in comparative pathology (for example, rabies[449] and trichinosos[132,448,450]) and particularly in comparative oncology.[529] He was the first to discover a case of human trichinosis in Russia, shortly after his return from Virchow's laboratory (see the final section of Chapter 11 for details).[282] It would be interesting to know whether Rudnev obtained an insight into and interest in comparative pathology from Virchow or from his contact with the veterinarians at the Military-Medical Academy; I have not been able to ascertain this.

Rudnev wrote in 1871[451]: "Im Jahre 1869 erhielt ich von

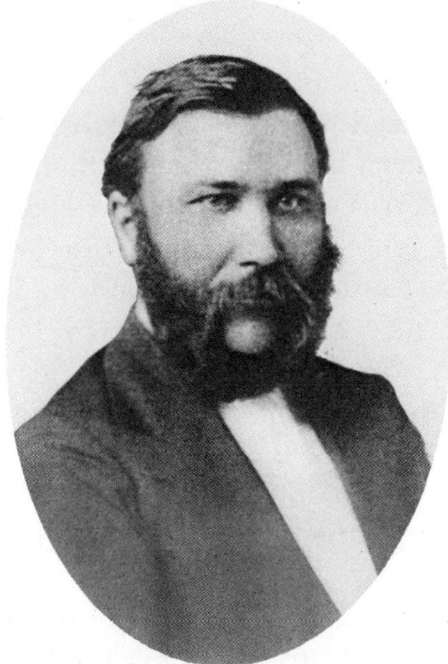

Figure 18. Mikhail M. Rudnev.

Seiten der Medicinisch-chirurgischen Academie zu St. Petersburg den Auftrag, die pathologische Anatomie der Thiere an hiesiger Thierarzneischule vorzutragen." (In the year 1869 I received the assignment from the Medico-Chirurgical Academy of St. Petersburg to lecture on pathologic anatomy of animals in the local veterinary school [the veterinary division of the Academy].) As pointed out previously, Rudnev got this assignment six years before Ravich's death, whether at his own request or at Ravich's would be interesting to know. The influence of Virchow on Rudnev's approach to teaching pathology is evident from his remark: "Es befand sich ein ziemlich bedeutendes Material zu praktischen Uebungen der Studirenden in meinen Händen." (There was a rather significant amount of material for the practical exercises of the students at my disposal.) Like his mentor, Virchow, Rudnev viewed his appointment as lecturer on pathologic anatomy not as a mere assignment to lecture, but as an opportunity to involve the students in the discipline of pathology by having them study pathologic material postmortem.

To point out that Rudnev was in this respect at least three-quarters of a century ahead of many teachers of veterinary pathology in the Western world is an obligation an honest historian cannot evade. An equal obligation is to point out that Rudnev's apparent ignorance of canine histology caused him to report what he considered to be lesions in the kidneys of rabid dogs. He was soon set straight by Bollinger,[113] another physician who was teaching veterinary pathology (in Munich), and thereafter he made no scientific blunders of which I am aware. On the topic of rabies, Kolesnikov's work, done in Rudnev's laboratory in 1875 and 1881, soon settled on the real seat of the lesions in the central nervous system.[254,258]

Rudnev's assistant Kolesnikov, a physician, followed up this line of work after Rudnev's death, obtaining his M.D.

degree with a dissertation on the histopathology of rabies in the dog.[259] Among other comparative interests, he had in 1877 published work on tuberculous mastitis in cattle, done in Virchow's laboratory in Berlin,[256] on melanotic tumors in white horses[255] and on intestinal anthrax in man.[261] He also taught in the veterinary division of the Academy.[217] I have not been able to find any further biographical details on him.

Rudnev's life was short—a mere 41 years—and his participation in the teaching and research of the veterinary division of the Academy was even shorter, spanning little more than a decade. But his influence in educating scientifically oriented veterinarians was considerable, despite the brevity of his allotted span on earth. For example, Lange, whom Rudnev mentions as his assistant in the veterinary division in 1871, later became director of the Kazan Veterinary Institute, a position from which he exercised great influence in turning out veterinarians of high caliber.

In 1872, Rudnev published a book *Rukovodstvo k ucheniyu Obshchei Patologii* (Guide to the Study of General Pathology).[230] That same year, he supervised the research work leading to the M.V.Sc. dissertation of Viktor E. Vorontsov (1844–1900), who became a leading Russian veterinary scientist and journalist (Fig. 19). The title was "Data on the Surgical Pathology of the Joints in Animals," and following completion of this work, Vorontsov was invited to remain on the faculty of the Academy as assistant professor of veterinary surgery.

He in turn, along with Rudnev, directed the research work for the M.V.Sc. degree of another Russian veterinarian, Mstislav A. Novinskii (1841–1914) (Fig. 20). Working with two mentors who had a lively interest in experimental pathology, Novinskii made the famous first successful transplantation of an animal neoplasm, the canine venereal tumor. His dissertation was printed in 1877, and the work

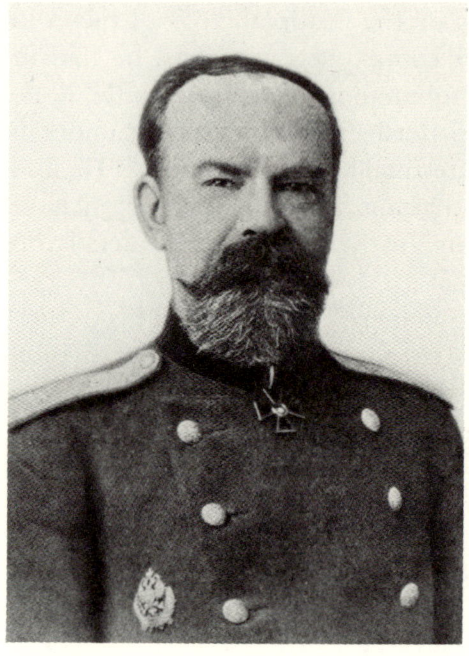

Figure 19. Viktor E. Vorontsov.

published in a German scientific journal the following year.[529,534] Thus, as Pinus claims, experimental oncology really began as a branch of science from the work of a Russian veterinarian, and, unlike many important advances in science, it can be traced unequivocally to the work of one man. In this case, Bishop Sheen's definition of history* does not apply, either to the Russians or to Americans!

Unfortunately, assignment to the army terminated Novinskii's research activities,[534] and with the cessation of veterinary instruction at the Academy in 1883, veterinary pathology, which had gotten off to such a fine start there, reached a dead end. One year before this happened, however, N. Kolesnikov, the physician assigned to the veterinary

*"History—the British never remember it; the Irish never forget it; the Russians never make it, and the Americans never learn from it."

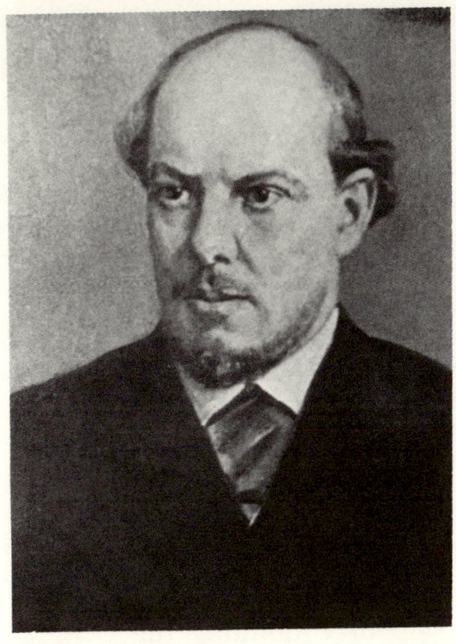

Figure 20. Mstislav M. Novinskii.

division, who had also worked under Rudnev's direction, published an excellent description of the histopathology of rabies in dogs—in German in *Virchos's Archiv.*[258]

Semmer[513] relates that the veterinary division of the Academy was closed by the Minister of War because the expenses it was causing were greater than those of the other veterinary schools in the empire. At its closing it was, next to Dorpat, scientifically the strongest school in the empire; because of the staff in the rest of the Academy, it was potentially the strongest. The minister did not care about this; he could get all the veterinarians he wanted for the army from the other three schools at no cost to his ministry. Throughout veterinary history one encounters examples of penny-wise, pound-foolish politicians—in England, in the United States, in Canada, and on the Continent—and Russia was no exception. During the almost two hundred years that St. Petersburg was the capital of Russia, all important government decisions could only be made there. Many were botched. When one considers what might have developed in Russian veterinary medicine, but particularly in veterinary pathology, had the veterinary division remained open, it becomes evident that none were botched worse than this one.*

Although the veterinary division was closed, it was not forgotten, and in 1898 the Kharkov Veterinary Institute dedicated the volume of its scientific proceedings to the Academy (by this time again called the Military-Medical Academy) on its one hundreth birthday. No doubt this was the work of Raevskii, who was then director of the Kharkov Veterinary Institute.

In 1901, consideration was given to reestablishing some veterinary activity at the Academy in the form of a chair of comparative pathology. Chernyak[149] relates that a commission composed of prominent physicians and veterinarians met to consider the question of continuing the chair of epizootiology at the Academy. This chair, filled by Professor Vorontsov, had remained as a vestige of the previous veterinary division until his death in 1900. The commission passed a resolution to create in its place a chair of comparative pathology.[12] Although Chernyak says nothing further regarding this resolution, it was implemented, and Nikolai N. Mari was appointed Professor of Comparative Pathology at the Academy in 1902.

Mari's inaugural address[336] shows signs of great humility: "I am the first representative in Russia of an independent chair of comparative pathology, and the novelty of this position makes me meditate deeply and weigh my strength. The

*In fairness to the minister, D. A. Milyutin, most of his other schemes for thrift led to great improvements in the efficiency of the army. There can be but few war ministers in any country who ever succeeded, as he did, in cutting almost one thousand men from the headquarters staff of the ministry and in reducing the paper work by 45 percent (Seton-Watson,[521], p. 386).

question whether my knowledge and teaching experience permit me to place the chair I occupy at the level on which it must stand by virtue of its position troubles me in spite of myself." He defined what comparative pathology should be, using examples from the realms of inflammation and neoplasia and leaning heavily on Mechnikov's work. The address shows that Mari had a broad intellectual sweep in scanning the horizon of pathology, but I have not been able to determine whether he contributed much to the discipline after taking up his appointment in 1902.

Mari remained at the Military-Medical Academy for fourteen years. During March and April of 1916, he served as acting chief of the Academy, the only veterinarian ever to be entrusted with its command.[278] He then left St. Petersburg to go to Novocherkassk (see Chapter 7). Whether the chair of comparative pathology he thus vacated was ever again filled, I do not know.

The Institute for Experimental Medicine

This Institute is best known because it was the scientific home of the famous physiologist, I. I. Pavlov. It was founded in 1890 by an endowment from Prince A. P. Oldenburgskii to give Russia "an advanced scientific-medical institute of an academic type." Its primary purpose as cited by Vucinich[626] was "to study the common contagious disease of men and animals and to search for scientific means of combating them." Semmer's account indicates that it soon drifted far afield from these goals, if, indeed it ever pursued them. Eventually the Institute was taken over by the government and was called the Imperial Institute for Experimental Medicine.

The first incumbent of the chair of epizootiology was C. Helmann (1848–1892), an 1872 graduate of the Dorpat Veterinary Institute. He was one of the founding members of the Institute for Experimental Medicine in 1890, and in 1891 published his discovery of mallein.[206] (Kalning of Dorpat independently made the same discovery that same year.[352] Discovery of this diagnostic material, used in an allergic test for glanders, has also been attributed to Babes, but my comparison of the respective publications indicates that the priority belongs to the two Russians.) Helmann died two years after his appointment and was succeeded, in 1892, by Eugen Semmer, who came from Dorpat to assume this post (Fig. 21).

Semmer held the appointment for three years before reaching retirement age. During this time, the budget of the chair of epizootiology was slashed and a promised building was given instead to another department. It is apparent from Semmer's description of the situation that the Director, S. Lukyanov, was totally unsympathetic either to the

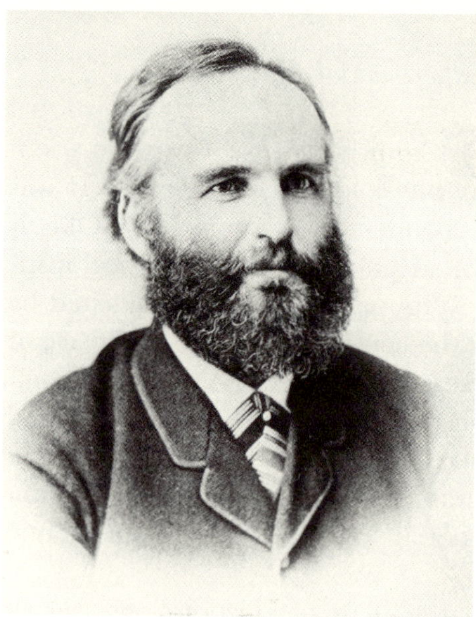

Figure 21. Eugen Semmer later in life than depicted in Figure 6.

Epizootiology Department itself, which he did not want in his Institute, or to Semmer personally.

In either event, and I do not know which one applies, poor Semmer's lot during his last three years of official service to the Russian Empire was not a happy one.[518] He relates, for instance, that the limitations imposed on him by inadequate space and money enable him to keep only half a dozen cattle at the Institute. At the rate at which he can replace them, he estimates sarcastically that it will take 400 *years* to work out the answers to development of a prophylactic rinderpest vaccine. Yet—and this he tells without rancor or bitterness, but it sounds like a page out of a Dostoevsky novel—his efforts to undertake field trials in the Ukraine were subverted (see also Chapter 11) by sinister forces, which he does not dare to name even in the relatively safe haven of a German journal.[518] Assisting Semmer in the work on rinderpest in the steppes of southern Russia was the veterinarian Mikhail G. Tartakovskii (Fig. 22).

Semmer was succeeded after his retirement in 1895 by A. A. Vladimirov (1862–1942) (Fig. 23). He graduated in medicine from Dorpat University in 1888 and specialized in

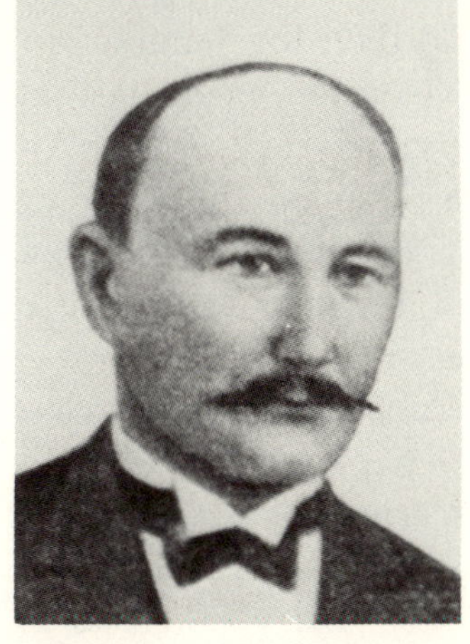

Figure 22. Mikhail G. Tartakovskii.

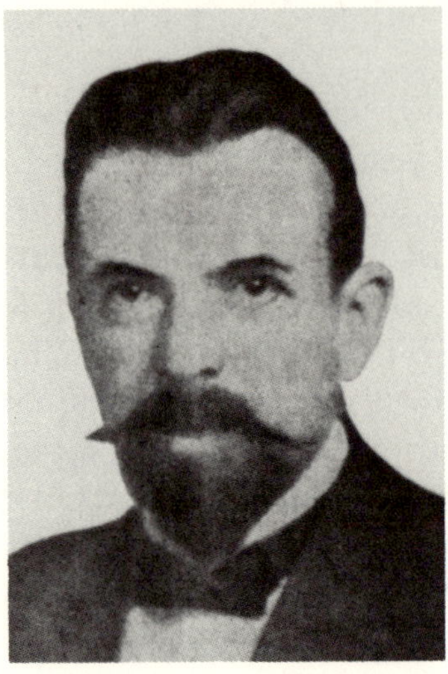

Figure 23. A. A. Vladimirov.

the newly emerged science of bacteriology, pursuing studies under Robert Koch. Vladimirov then was appointed assistant in the department of hygiene of the medical faculty of Dorpat University and also in the bacteriology department of the Dorpat Veterinary Institute. In 1891 he moved to St. Petersburg and became an assistant in the Department of Epizootiology of the Institute for Experimental Medicine; thus he worked first for Kalning and then for Semmer. In 1895 he was sent to France to study veterinary medicine and received the veterinary diploma that same year from the Alfort Veterinary School.[551] He then assumed the chair of epizootiology as Semmer's successor and held this position until World War I. Later (1918–1928) he directed the entire Institute for Experimental Medicine.[164]

Held in high regard in European bacteriologic circles, Vladimirov in 1913 contributed the chapter on glanders to the second edition of Kolle and Wassermann's *Handbuch der pathogenen Mikroorganismen.*[637] In 1914 he was a delegate of Russia to the Tenth International Veterinary Congress in London.

We return now to M. G. Tartakovskii (1867–1935), who also served under Semmer as an assistant in the epizootiology department and under Vladimirov as assistant head of the department. He was born in Poltava, Ukraine, studied veterinary medicine at the Kharkov Veterinary Institute, and graduated in 1890.[609] He passed his M.V.Sc. examination at the Dorpat Veterinary Institute in 1893, but did not submit a dissertation and get the degree until 1898.[576,589] He thus obtained his undergraduate instruction in pathology from Ostapenko and his postgraduate experience under Semmer, whom he joined in St. Petersburg as an assistant in 1893.

There are several articles by Tartakovskii in the early volumes of the *Arkhiv Biologicheskikh Nauk* dealing with the pathology of infectious diseases and beautifully illustrated.[572] During the period 1894 to 1900 he also abstracted Russian articles in German for the *Jahresbericht der Veterinärmedicin.*

Although Vladimirov, Tartakovskii's chief at the turn of the century, did not complain in print about the Institute's treatment of its epizootiology department, one may perhaps assume that Tartakovskii saw that it had little future. Thus, when a promising position became vacant elsewhere in St. Petersburg in 1902, he took it. We shall pick up the thread of his career again later.

After the turn of the century, most of the research work of the epizootiology department, as judged by several of its annual reports (in the Institute's journal, *Arkhiv Biologicheskikh Nauk*), was concerned with protozoology. Several of these reports between 1906 and 1913 mention that diagnostic pathology service was provided for the Petrograd Zoo; however, I have not found any scientific publications based on such pathologic material. In any event, the epizootiology department was not able to make its presence felt in satisfying the research requirements for disease control in Russia. Chernyak[150] states that this is understandable, but I think he means only to other Russians, versed in reading between the lines; he doesn't really give any reasons. These are given by Semmer in the critical article just mentioned and can be summed up in a few words: opposition from the director of the Institute and from its other departments, which competed with the epizootiology department for funds, and opposition from the veterinary directorate in the central government, which did not want anything of a practical scientific nature to be done outside of its control. Whether the epizootiology department survived these jealousies and hatreds beyond World War II have not been able to determine.

The Veterinary Laboratory, Ministry of Internal Affairs

Since the problems of epizootic diseases were not being solved at the Institute for Experimental Medicine, the Ministry of Internal Affairs, which was charged with the responsibility for control of such diseases, decided to set up its own laboratory in an attempt to cope with them. This was done in St. Petersburg in 1898, under the direction of Jan Gordziałkowski (1862–1944), a Polish bacteriologist, who had graduated as a veterinarian in Kharkov in 1888 and received an M.V.Sc. from Dorpat in 1896 (Fig. 24). He served but briefly and left this post in 1902 for one at the Military-Medical Academy.* While still an undergraduate, Gordziałkowski had worked in the pathology department of the Kharkov Veterinary Institute under A. P. Ostapenko and had published a lengthy paper on postmortem diagnosis.[184]

The second director was M. G. Tartakovskii, who held

*In 1919, Gordziałkowski succeeded in leaving Russia for the newly created state of Poland. He played a leading role in organized veterinary medicine, veterinary education, and veterinary publication in Poland in the ensuing two decades. Millak relates that he died during the Warsaw uprising in 1944 caused by the inhuman conditions of the occupation.[355]

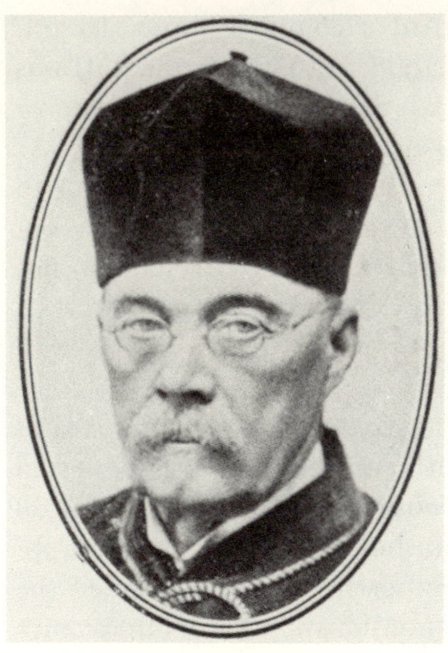

Figure 24. Jan Gordziałkowski.

the directorship from 1903 to 1908.[262] Tartakovskii was much more successful in getting money for the new Veterinary Laboratory from the Ministry of Internal Affairs than Semmer had been in getting it for his chair at the Institute for Experimental Medicine. Tartakovskii reported that the location of the first Veterinary Laboratory was unsuitable because on Kievskaya Street there was neither gas nor electricity; the laboratory was lit by kerosene; its operation was carried out on kerosene burners, resulting in poor quality of work. Furthermore, it was impossible to keep and dissect animals infected with glanders and anthrax in rooms with wooden floors, without running water or sewers, because the house was inhabited by other tenants! He therefore asked that the laboratory be moved to another location, and a house that had both gas and electricity was found on Arsenal Street.[150]

Five years later, the Director was successful in getting the ministry to spend a large sum of money (122,131 rubles, 81 kopeks) for the construction of a completely new laboratory.* This was completed in 1908; at that time the staff was expanded and a pathological department organized, of which Ivan I. Shukevich (Fig. 25) was appointed head.[150] As far as I can determine, this department existed from 1908 to 1911 only on paper, as Shukevich was immediately sent abroad for postgraduate study. (Tereshkov[591] states—contrary to Chernyak—that Shukevich was appointed head of the pathology department after his return home in mid-1911.)

Tartakovskii was one of the six delegates from Russia at the Eighth International Veterinary Congress in Budapest in 1905. He is listed in the proceedings of the ninth congress, in the Hague, in 1909, as the author of a paper on pleuropneumonia of horses; but whether he actually attended the congress I do not know. He is not shown in the group picture with the other Russians who attended (frontispiece). By 1909, Tartakovskii had been replaced as director of the Veterinary Laboratory (by I. M. Sadovskii), but I have not found out why. From 1909 to 1912 he was in charge of postgraduate courses on poultry husbandry and poultry diseases which he inaugurated at the Veterinary Laboratory.[556]

Ivan I. Shukevich (1869–1919) was born in Kharkov. His eulogist Romanovich, writing in 1922, emphasized that although of Polish descent on his father's side, Shukevich was to be considered a Russian, as he "had no knowledge of the Polish language"![446] Apparently the need to demonstrate that Russia owes nothing to people of other nationalities living within its thrall was already present early in the Bolshevik era.

Shukevich graduated from the Kharkov Veterinary Insti-

*Later, in 1919, when the Leningrad Veterinary Institute was founded, it occupied these same premises.[150]

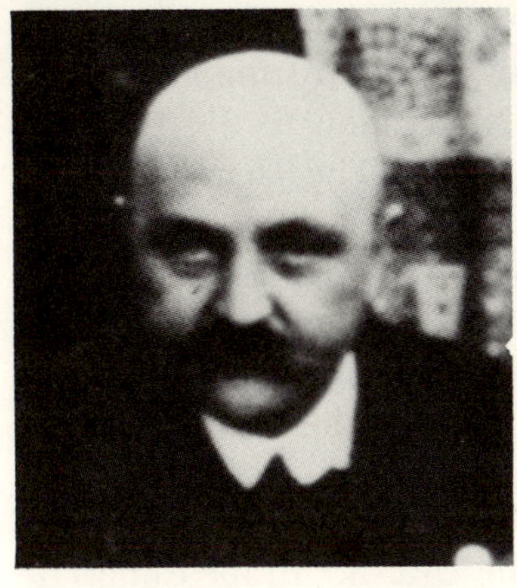

Figure 25. Ivan I. Shukevich.

tute during the time that Ostapenko was teaching pathology there. During the late 1890s he worked at meat inspection in the Moscow slaughterhouse, and at the turn of the century he worked also in the bacteriology department of the University of Moscow. Somewhat later, I judge about 1904, he worked at the Institute for Experimental Medicine in St. Petersburg, in the Department of Epizootiology, headed by A. A. Vladimirov. During his sojourn in Moscow, he was exposed to the teaching of Nikolai F. Melnikov-Razvedenkov (see p. 115), who was assistant professor of pathology in the medical faculty of the University. Although I have not been able to determine the extent of Melnikov-Razvedenkov's influence on Shukevich, it seems to have been considerable.[446]

Shukevich's earlier scientific publications were mostly bacteriologic in orientation; however, he pursued investigations in pathology during the same period. By 1905 he had already published a large work on actinomycosis[536] and reported on the amyloidosis in horses used for antiserum production.[537] He also examined the livers of 1,510 horses at the Moscow abattoir—a prodigious task—and found amyloidosis in 156 of them. He joined the Veterinary Laboratory in 1907, was sent abroad in 1908, and worked with Mechnikov* at the Pasteur Institute in Paris until 1911. He was a member of the Russian delegation to the Eleventh International Veterinary Congress at The Hague in 1909 (see frontispiece). Upon his return from the Pasteur Institute, he actively headed the pathology department of the Veterinary Laboratory.

In addition to working in the Veterinary Laboratory in St. Petersburg, Shukevich went on expeditions to investigate animal diseases in the far-flung corners of the empire. He reported on rinderpest in the Khirgiz Steppes[539] and on trypanosomiasis of camels† in the Urals.[542] In the camels he found also some cases of amyloidosis of the liver and spleen; his nicely illustrated account is the first modern scientific paper on the pathology of the camel.[543]

Pinus states that Shukevich has a leading place in the history of Russian veterinary pathologic anatomy and supports this contention by listing half a dozen important publications by him between the years 1910 and 1916.[417] His last work, on gastroenteritis of cattle, which appeared in 1926, was published posthumously. Romanovich says that Shukevich was an extremely meticulous scientist, who carried out his research work with *Nemietskoyu strohostyu*—German thoroughness!

Shukevich's most interesting paper, from the historical standpoint, is without a doubt his "Report on the activity of the pathologic anatomy department of the Veterinary Laboratory, Ministry of Internal Affairs, from July 1911 to

*Romanovich points out that although Shukevich was a nephew of Mechnikov's (on his mother's side), he never traded on this prestigious relationship.[446]

†In North America we tend to associate camels with nomads of the hot desert regions. However, camels grow thick winter coats and were economically very important animals in the Central Asian part of the Russian Empire.

January 1914."[541] In addition to its primary responsibilities for research, diagnosis, and preparation of biologic diagnostic and vaccine products, the Veterinary Laboratory also began around 1910 to provide education, that is, to offer refresher courses. These were designed to bring the latest scientific discoveries to the attention of veterinarians engaged in disease control, meat hygiene, or clinical practice. Shukevich and his colleagues Romanovich, Uranov, and Petrovsky jointly presented these courses. Shukevich's enthusiasm for pathology as a discipline and his zeal in conveying knowledge of this discipline to his colleagues emerge vividly from the lines of the above named article. I did not succeed in conveying the flavor in an attempt to paraphrase it and therefore elected to print a representative passage in translation:

> Since the time the Pathologic Anatomical Department commenced refresher courses in bacteriology, given twice a year in the Veterinary Laboratory, a short course in pathologic anatomy was added to it. The emphasis of the courses was on bacteriology, and only a small segment of time was devoted to pathologic anatomy, putting the latter in an unfavorable position. Because of this, the course on pathologic anatomy was not presented the way it should have been.
>
> Another obstacle was the absence of the necessary laboratory space for the autopsy of large animals and of accomodations for the reception and keeping of animals. Also, difficulty was experienced in the delivery of cadavers during the first two courses in the fall of 1912 and the spring of 1913.
>
> Out of concern for an assured supply of cadavers, the personnel of the department, from May 1913 on, took upon themselves the postmortem work at the city rendering plant. To our regret, the facilities of this plant were too small to conduct the courses with the students. This resulted in cutting the course in pathologic anatomy to a minimum.
>
> Our idea was to familiarize the students, during lectures, with the basic theoretical and practical aspects of the subject.

> Also, to impress on them the importance of familiarity with the microscopic aspects of the disease processes, since a knowledge of pathologic histology would put into their hands a tool to use in the difficult pathologic anatomical cases which they might encounter in their practice.
>
> This intention in presenting the courses stirred up opposition.
>
> (1) It was stated that for veterinary practitioners pathologic histology is a luxury of no practical use.
>
> (2) It was stated that the working conditions of veterinarians are such that they will not provide the scientific environment necessary to conduct histopathological investigations.
>
> We do not agree with these objections! We believe that familiarity with the basic characteristics of pathological development is necessary for each veterinarian and that this knowledge will not be unproductive. Each veterinarian should be able to look through a microscope and recognize the characteristics of those developments, a knowledge of which represents the basis of veterinary science. We should not forget that cellular pathology represents the foundation for scientific pathology and since the veterinarian is a scientist and should be one, he should possess clear and specific knowledge of the basic characteristics of pathological processes.
>
> In regard to the second objection, it seems that with a strong desire and persistence on the part of many veterinarians, conditions could be achieved which would permit the possibility for a simple histopathological investigation (equipment without microscope would be 50–75 rubles). Although there could be some difficulty, time for such necessary work could always be found.

Shukevich did not specify from whom the opposition came—presumably it was from someone inside the Ministry of Internal Affairs who was afraid that good education would cost money. However, a further reading of Shukevich's report indicates that he and his colleagues did succeed in imparting a considerable amount of information, and demonstrating much material, both gross and histologic, despite their lack of funds and facilities. Included in this instruction was teaching the students (the veterinarians taking the refresher courses) how to cut and stain their own microscopic sections. As Shukevich put it in setting forth further justification for involving veterinarians in pathologic anatomic and histologic diagnosis, "Such work, illuminated by scientific ideas, could to some extent *brighten up the harsh life of the Russian veterinarian*" (italics added).

In the same article, reporting the activities of his department, Shukevich et al. devoted considerable space to a description of their museum. He had begun work on this in 1911 and by 1914 had created a museum containing over 500 pathological specimens and over 100 parasitological ones. Representative specimens had been exhibited in St. Petersburg at the All-Russian Hygienic Exhibition and the Draft Horses Exhibition and in Kharkov at the Third All-Russian Veterinary Congress.

At the time of writing, in 1914, Shukevich considered that the initial purpose of the museum, a basic collection to serve as an educational resource for the refresher courses, had been fulfilled. He now envisioned something of wider scope, and again an indication of his vision is best presented in translation:

> Now we have a second task—how to organize in our department a larger museum of comparative pathology, where we could with some degree of accuracy demonstrate the processes of disease in humans and in animals.
>
> At the present time, such a museum does not exist in Russia. Its importance would be not only for the doctor or person with an interest in biological science, but also for any intelligent person. The best example of the likely success of such a museum is the attendance at our exhibit by nonveterinarians during the Third All-Russian Veterinary Congress.
>
> By creating such a museum in Russia, a land with such diverse fauna and such immense territory, containing regions with polar and with tropical climates, an unlimited variety of important scientific material could be collected. To our regret,

our departmental facilities at the present time are too congested, and available funds too limited to fulfill our plans. We must postpone these for a later time, and probably a much later time.

The last remark, made just prior to the outbreak of the World War, was unfortunately most prophetic. A man of vision, Shukevich was, alas, not destined to see his dream fulfilled. Perhaps it was partially fulfilled after his death by the Leningrad institution known during its brief existence as the Institute of Comparative Pathology, discussed later in this chapter. The museum created by Shukevich was eventually transferred to Moscow (see p. 169) when the whole of the Veterinary Laboratory was evacuated from Petrograd in 1918.* The new museum established there at the successor institution (the All-Union Institute for Experimental Veterinary Medicine) was named the Shukevich Memorial Museum, so that his role in creating it lives on. A few duplicate specimens were left behind for the newly formed Petrograd Veterinary-Zootechnical Institute, later to be known as the Leningrad Veterinary Institute.[43,114]

Shukevich had been active in bacteriology prior to his appointment to the Veterinary Laboratory, and with the outbreak of World War I he resumed activity in this field. I believe he did so because he was frustrated by the meager support for veterinary pathology, and saw in the war an impending health crisis in which his training would permit him to make an immediate contribution to his country's welfare.

*As mentioned above, specimens from this museum had already undergone a long journey—they were exhibited in Kharkov in 1913 at the Third All-Russian Veterinary Congress. Romanovich related that Melnikov-Razedenkov, who by this time was professor of pathology in the medical faculty of Kharkov University, came daily to admire these specimens![446] The latter's influence can still be detected in 1975—volume 5 of the *Veterinarnaya Entsiklopediya* has a color plate (p. 112) showing museum specimens prepared by the method of Melnikov-Razvedenkov.

In this judgment he was not mistaken. He worked for the Russian Red Cross in a mobile (railroad) bacteriological laboratory on gas gangrene and other problems of human infection.[591] In October, 1919, he contracted typhus and died in Tiflis, Georgia, falling victim to a disease that was to claim many others during the Civil War and the years immediately thereafter.* He was the only one of the historical figures in this book to die "with his boots on" in the cataclysm that engulfed Russia.

Even though he had temporarily left it, Shukevich's first love was veterinary pathology; his death was thus a grievous loss to this discipline in Russia. The enthusiasm he felt for veterinary pathology, the thoroughness with which he practiced it, and the aspirations he nurtured for its future in Russia were perhaps matched by N. D. Ball (see Chapter 9), but exceeded by no contemporary. Unfortunately, the times were not propitious for the fulfillment of these aspirations.

The Institute of Comparative Pathology

We have followed the career of Professor M. G. Tartakovskii through two institutions: the Institute for Experimental Medicine and the Veterinary Laboratory of the Ministry of Internal Affairs. I do not know what he did between the years 1912 and 1917. From the latter year until 1922, he directed the Central Agricultural Bacteriologic Laboratory in Petrograd.[262] According to Kolyakov, he organized the Institute of Comparative Pathology in Leningrad in 1923 and directed it until 1932. The work done here was on bovine pleuropneumonia and on diseases of poultry; Tar-

*General Drew writes that in Russia between 1917 and 1922 "more than 10 million cases are thought to have occurred in a population of 120 million, with a fatality rate exceeding 30%."[161]

takovskii had early shown an interest in the latter.[579,583] I have not been able to find any detailed information on the Institute of Comparative Pathology. except for the statement by Chernyak[150] that the Institute was on the former premises of the above-mentioned Veterinary Laboratory.

In 1930, Sir Frederick Hobday visited the U.S.S.R.[210] and reported on an Institute of Comparative Pathology in Leningrad, directed by Professor Tartakovskii. According to his account, it dealt with diseases of birds, fish, and insects. This Institute was also mentioned by Miessner, who visited it three years later and wrote that it had many laboratories and a large museum.[353] Pinus[417] wrote that the museum was unique in its selection and number of specimens, as well as in the quality of their preparation. The end of this Institute is not as easy to trace as its beginning; Chernyak[150] relates that the museum is now a part of the Leningrad Postgraduate Veterinary Institute.

According to one account, the latter was organized in 1937; its director, Cheredkov, reported two years later that it had a museum containing 4,000 preparations, but did not say what their source was.[134] Since it is highly unlikely that the Postgraduate Institute was able to prepare 4,000 specimens in two years, this probably means that the Institute of Comparative Pathology was absorbed by or converted to it sometime between 1933 and 1939; I have not determined which date. Nor can I reconcile two other accounts of the opening date of the Postgraduate Veterinary Institute. Writing in 1956, Lvov says that that year was the twenty-fifth anniversary of the Postgraduate Institute.[309] If this is true, it was founded in 1931, although Shifanovich gives 1930 as the year![533]

During the last year of his life. Tartakovskii was again engaged in research on pleuropneumonia. A serious research worker, his scientific output was marked by large research projects. His bibliography contains but few case reports. His major contributions to veterinary pathology were in hiring Shukevich while director of the Veterinary Laboratory and in building up the museum in the Institute of Comparative Pathology. Otherwise, I believe his influence on our discipline in Russia was small, particularly in comparison to that of his contemporaries, Ball and Bohl. It was enduring, however; the atlas of veterinary pathology compiled by Kokurichev in 1973 contained beautiful colored illustrations of many of Tartakovskii's specimens.[252]

5 Veterinary Pathology in Kharkov

The Kharkov Veterinary Institute

Veterinary education began in Kharkov in the University in 1805, the year of its founding, with a chair of veterinary science in the medical faculty. In 1851, this chair was expanded into a newly organized Kharkov Veterinary Institute, independent of the University. Even after it became an independent institution, however, the KVI maintained its ties with the University, inasmuch as instruction of the veterinary students in physiology, histology, chemistry, botany, zoology, and general pathology continued to be given there, the latter by Professor A. P. Reprev of the medical faculty.[529a] As the map (Fig. 26) shows, the KVI was in proximity to the University. During the late 1850s and 1860s, various departments were organized in the Kharkov Veterinary Institute; founding of the chair of pathologic anatomy followed in 1876. This chair was held for 33 years, from 1876 until 1909, by Professor Aleksandr P. Ostapenko (1852–1928).

A. P. Ostapenko (Fig. 27) was born in Zinkove, Poltava province, Ukraine, in the year 1852 (some accounts state 1854). He was educated in the classical high school in the town of Poltava and after graduation in 1872 enrolled in the Kharkov Veterinary Institute. He graduated as a veterinarian cum laude in 1876 and was asked to stay on for specialization and training as a lecturer on the faculty. What form this training took I have not been able to discover; in January of 1878 he submitted a dissertation "Ozone in relation to the animal organism" for his M.V.Sc. degree. After having taught in the newly organized department of pathologic anatomy for two years, he was named its head in 1878. Ostapenko was promoted through the various academic ranks to ordinary professor in 1891 and honored professor in 1903.

I have not been able to determine from whom—either at home or abroad—Ostapenko received any training. I can find no record of his ever having gone abroad, either to study or to attend one of the international veterinary congresses at which other veterinary pathologists from Russia were delegates. Certainly he would not have been trusted to go abroad during the ninth congress in 1909, the year he was dismissed. The allusion in his book on postmortem technique[377] to the equipment and installations in the autopsy room of the Berlin Veterinary College suggests that he had been there, but cannot be considered as evidence. Nor have I come across any indication of an association with the pathology department of the medical school at the nearby University of Kharkov. Thus I do not know whether Ostapenko was self-taught or whether he just appears so because of my inability to turn up the requisite information. As with Blumberg, there is no biographical sketch of Ostapenko in the multivolume Soviet *Veterinarnaya Entsiklopediya,* which does not make the historian's task any easier.* Whether this omission is an oversight or whether the editors considered Ostapenko too unimportant to merit a biography or too politically unpalatable to be mentioned one can only guess.

Whether or not he ever went abroad, Ostapenko was not

*He is mentioned, in passing, in a list of half a dozen names of veterinarians concerned with sanitary science in Volume 1 (p. 917), 1969, of this encyclopedia.

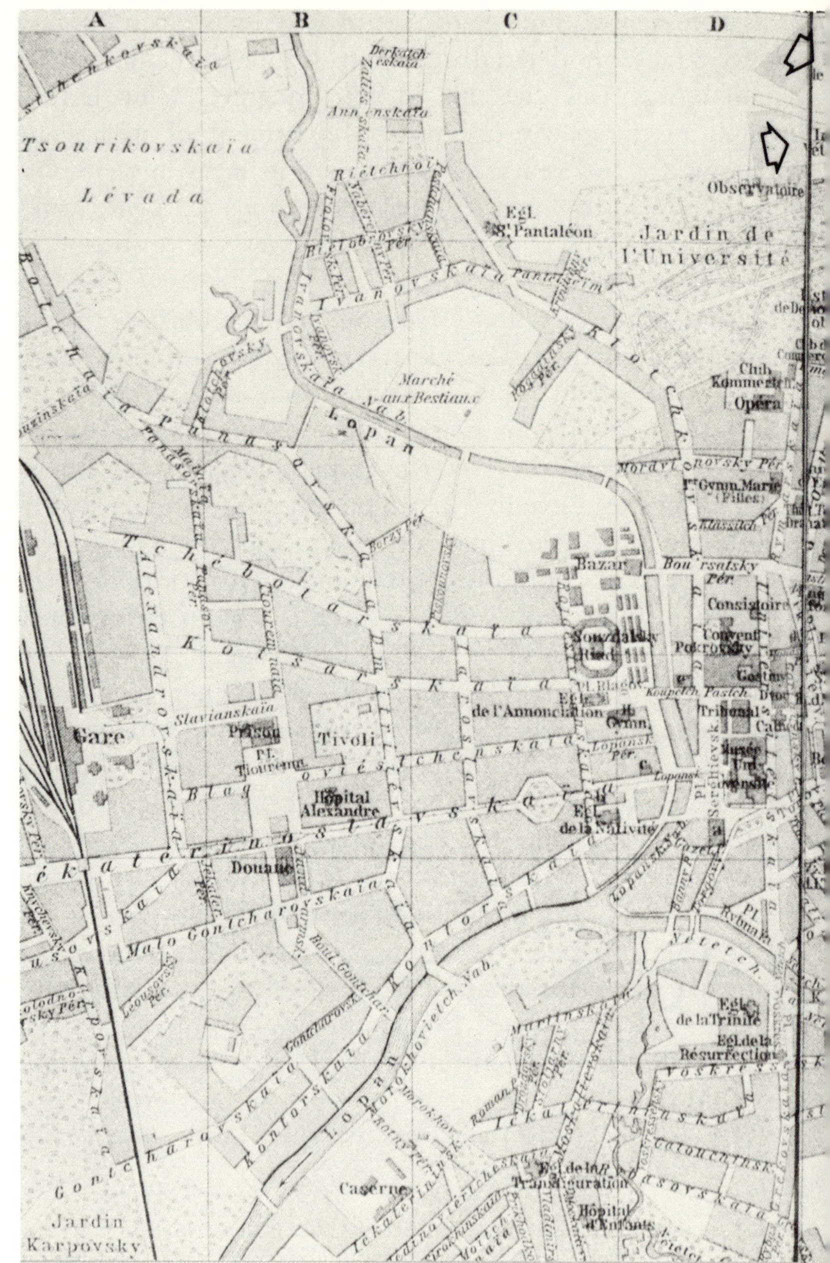

Figure 26. Map of the city of Kharkov about 1910. The locations of the Kharkov Veterinary Institute and the medical faculty of Kharkov University are indicated by arrows.

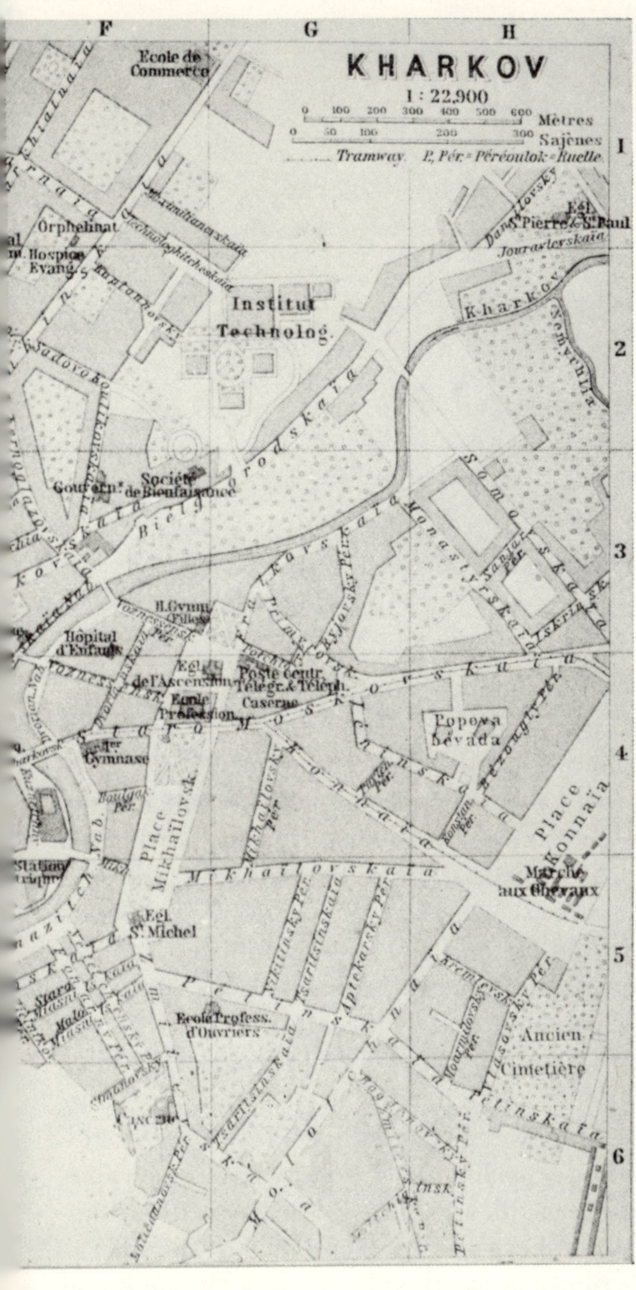
KHARKOV
1 : 22,900
Mètres
Sajènes
Tramway. P, Pér. = Péréoulok = Ruelle
F
G
H
1
2
3
4
5
6
Ecole de Commerce
Orphelinat
Institut Technolog.
Société de Bienfaisance
Hôpital d'Enfants
Ègl. de l'Ascension
Poste centr. Télégr. & Téléph.
Caserne
Ecole Profession.
Gymnase
Place Mikhaïlovsk.
Ègl. St. Michel
Ecole Profess. d'Ouvriers
Popova Lévada
Place Konnaïa
Marché aux Chevaux
Ancien Cimetière
Ègl. St. Pierre & St. Paul
Kharkov
Bielgorodskaïa
Monastyrskaïa
Mikhaïlovskaïa
Pétinskaïa

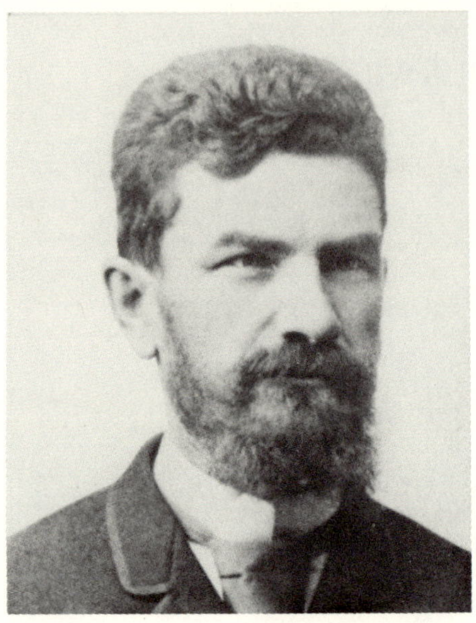

Figure 27. Aleksander P. Ostapenko.

unfamiliar with foreign languages; he translated books on meat inspection, veterinary obstetrics,[382] and microscopic examination of animal tissues from French, and Friedberger and Fröhner's "Clinical Diagnostic Methods" from German.[383] He wrote his first book, a small one, which seems to have been forgotten even in Russia, in 1882 shortly after he began his teaching career.[377] Entitled *Kratkoe Rukovodstvo k Patologo-Anatomicheskomu Vskrytiyu Trupov Domashnikh Zhivotnykh* (Short Manual on Pathologic-Anatomic Examination of the Cadaver of Domestic Animals) (Fig. 28), it is a book on autopsy technique and on the interpretation of gross lesions. Pinus,[417] who wrote on prerevolutionary veterinary pathology, does not mention it in his list of Ostapenko's publications, nor does Blumberg refer to it as a forerunner of his own book on autopsy technique.[73] Ostapenko's book antedates Blumberg's by a full 13 years, but it has neither illustrations, as does Blumberg's nor the seasoning of Blumberg's 25 years of experience at the time he wrote it. While it may

КРАТКОЕ РУКОВОДСТВО

КЪ

ПАТОЛОГО-АНАТОМИЧЕСКОМУ

ВСКРЫТІЮ ТРУПОВЪ

ДОМАШНИХЪ ЖИВОТНЫХЪ.

Доцента А. П. Остапенко.

ХАРЬКОВЪ.
Типо-Литографія Окружнаго Штаба.
1882.

Figure 28. Title page of Ostapenko's book "Pathologic-Anatomic Examination of Domestic Animals," one of the earliest in any language on this topic.

show that it is dangerous to rush prematurely into print, it shows more importantly that Ostapenko was serious about the teaching of his subject and prepared to put himself to trouble to do so. We will search in vain for any American or British veterinary pathologists who wrote any book on his discipline in 1882 or, for that matter, decades thereafter.

Papers on original observations, varying from case reports[374] to fairly large contributions,[379] began in 1882 with a report on teratological findings[376] and dealt with sarcoma in dogs,[378] urolithiasis,[381] hepatitis in horses, and lesions encountered in food animals at meat inspection.[386] Ostapenko also wrote a textbook *Rukovodstvo k Patologicheskoi Anatomii i Gistologii Domashnikh Zhivotnykh* (Manual of Pathologic Anatomy and Histology of Domestic Animals) in 1902.[384] This book was severely criticized by V. V. Bogdanovich[76] (whose qualifications to do so I have not determined), who compared it unfavorably with Mari's book, which is discussed on page 153. In essence, Bogdanovich complained that Ostapenko had produced a misleading, confusing, and outrageously overpriced potboiler. From looking at a microfilm of Ostapenko's book, I suspect that the criticism was justified, but I deplore its biting sarcasm and intemperate tone.

In October 1905, Professor Ostapenko was appointed Acting Director of the Kharkov Veterinary Institute, and in 1906 he was confirmed as Director and appointed a privy councillor of state. In 1905, Russia had been swept by considerable revolutionary activity, and the autocratic government was forced to respond in several ways, including creation of a parliament, the Duma. The government was also forced to void a restrictive statute of 1884; and the Provisional Regulation of August 1905 reestablished academic autonomy in the country's universities.[625] This news was received with enthusiasm by the academic community, and a period of relative peace and order prevailed for a couple of years in the various universities and higher educational institutions.* I believe that Ostapenko was known to be a liberal and that his appointment as director of the KVI was a consequence of the general peacemaking attitude forced on the imperial government by the prevailing social upheaval.

However, the tsarist Minister of Education, Alexander Schwarz, was a strong conservative—what the Communists would term a "reactionary"—and, as Seton-Watson describes him, out of sympathy with the educated class.[526] He embarked on a policy of gradual retreats from the liberal commitments to the universities.[625] In 1909, for example, he forbade the free attendance of women at university lectures, and also dismissed several university teachers who had socialist leanings. One of those who incurred his ire was Professor Ostapenko.

Ostapenko's career at the KVI was abruptly ended in 1909, when the Minister of Education ousted him from both his chair and the directorship of the Institute. The circumstances of this ouster emerge with something less than crystal clarity from the sources I have read, but, as nearly as I can tie them together, are as follows.† G. G. Villents, editor of the journal *Veterinarnaya Zhizn* (Veterinary Life) quotes an article from *Russkie Vedomosti* (Russian News), which cites the Kharkov newspaper *Utro* (Morning) as its source.[617] According to this account, Ostapenko was summoned to St. Petersburg and upbraided because he had formed an academic council

*Unlike those in the English-speaking countries, all were centrally directed by the national Ministry of Education. (The Military-Medical Academy was directed by the Minister of War.)

†Nosik,[372] dean of the Kharkov Veterinary Institute in 1952, merely says that Ostapenko was dismissed, but does not say why. The inference is that such dismissal was a common occurrence in those days. I think Nosik does not discuss it because the reason was somehow unpalatable or could not be discussed during the last Stalin years, being related to Ostapenko's Ukrainian nationalism.

to govern the Institute, which besides the professors included junior staff members and *even* students.* The minister asked him to dissolve the council, but Ostapenko refused. The minister then asked him to resign and was again refused, whereupon he dismissed him.†

Although out of favor with the imperial government, Ostapenko was not exiled to Siberia. On the contrary, he was even allowed to keep his rank of professor. We find him still thus designated in 1912, when he published a lengthy article on his activities in meat hygiene at the Kharkov Municipal Abattoir during the years 1908–1912; he is listed as head of the veterinary department of this institution.[386] He had been interested in meat hygiene prior to his dismissal, and according to Pinus[417] had started a museum at the KVI with pathological specimens from the abattoir. He had also inaugurated the course in meat hygiene at the KVI in the early 1900s. Thus, he merely switched from part-time to full-time work in meat hygiene after his dismissal from the KVI.

Three more fairly large papers by Ostapenko during the years 1915 and 1916 indicate that he remained at the Kharkov abattoir until just before the revolution of February 1917.[387,389] Two of these papers provide some amusing but puzzling insight into the situation at the Kharkov Veterinary Institute.[387,389] They begin with the description of canine

*The latter were particularly suspect in nineteenth- and early twentieth-century Russia as radical troublemakers, which they quite often were. Revolutionary unrest occurred at all four of the empire's veterinary schools in 1905.

†In an editorial comment in *Veterinarnaya Zhizn,* Villents expressed doubt about the veracity of the account—to do this in public print in tsarist Russia was an extraordinarily courageous act. Yet Villents and his journal are labeled "counterrevolutionary" by a 1968 writer in the *Veterinarnaya Entsiklopediya!* I do not know the basis for this label—perhaps Villents did not side with the Bolsheviks in 1917, being prescient enough to foresee that replacing one tyranny with another would not appreciably further the interests of the Russian people.

and feline cases of disease sent for autopsy to Ostapenko at the abattoir by his former clinical colleagues at the KVI. One can understand that the clinicians might have more faith in his ability as a pathologist than in that of his inexperienced replacement. But sending him material to autopsy and work up histologically must have been to some extent clandestine. Else why would the reports be hidden by being published with case reports of slaughtered cattle, under a title alluding only to the latter? Most fascinating of all, if this activity were dangerous or even merely risky, why point to it by publishing it?

Did Ostapenko enjoy living dangerously? Had he engendered such loyalty in his former colleagues that they were willing to do the same? Had he incurred the wrath of the Minister of Education only to be given a job by a rival minister? If the latter were the case, and he was not out of favor with the whole government, then some of my speculation regarding ostensible danger in associating with Ostapenko is, of course, groundless. These questions can probably be answered by access to the primary official documents of his case; without them they can only be raised.

To speculate just a bit further, one of the factors that may have led to Ostapenko's downfall at the KVI was sympathy for the movement for Ukrainian nationalism. Why otherwise would a man who was a victim of the Tsar's ministerial oppression be omitted from biographical treatment in both the centenary volume of the KVI Proceedings and in the *Veterinarnaya Entsiklopediya?* If his trouble merely came from being a Bolshevik or a liberal, one would expect that he would by now be rehabilitated as an honored historical figure. Ukrainian nationalism seems to be the only taint that would cause a man trouble under Tsar Nicholas II and still leave his name unmentionable 60 years later under the Communists. As just mentioned, however, his ability to retain his title and a good job means that he was treated extremely leniently, and his former colleagues' willingness to associate with him means that no opprobrium was attached to him, or not much. His case remains an enigma.

Ostapenko studied medicine sometime after his ouster, possible during the World War or the Civil War. He obtained his diploma as physician in 1920 from the medical faculty of Kharkov University. How he survived during those terrible years 1917–1921 I do not know. In May of 1927, the meeting of the Ukrainian Society of Pathologists was dedicated to the celebration of Ostapenko's fiftieth year of scientific and public activity.[411] At that time, Academician N. F. Melnikov-Razvedenkov, President of the Society, indicated that Ostapenko was head of the chemical-microscopical laboratory in the Ukrainian city of Debaltsevo (in the Don basin); it is not clear to me from the published proceedings whether Ostapenko was present at that meeting.[347] His trail fades out after 1927, but it is encouraging to know that he was still active at the age of 75. I have been informed that the records that might have shed light on his ultimate fate were destroyed during the German occupation of Kharkov in 1941–1942. Perhaps they were.

Apart from pathology, Ostapenko was interested also in history, and during the first All-Russian Congress of Veterinarians in 1903 he presented a paper on the history of veterinary medicine.[305] It is thus particularly ironical that neither the exact year of his birth nor the date, place, or circumstances of his death are known.

The chair of pathologic anatomy was held temporarily by Professor N. I. Petropavlovskii (18??–1925), who as Ostapenko's assistant had briefly described a few cases of tumors, malformations, and other lesions between 1898 and 1906.[399,403] He did not remain in this discipline but switched to clinical medicine. He headed the pathology laboratory during the years 1910–1912, when P. N. Krakht-Paleev, Ostapenko's actual successor, was abroad being trained for his new duties.

If one can judge by his work outside the purely descriptive

in pathology, it may have been well that Petropavlovskii left the discipline. In 1899 he reported a study of canine distemper, in which he reached the wrong conclusions regarding its bacterial etiology. This is forgivable, in the decade before the distemper virus was discovered. What I find hard to condone is his conclusion that the disease was similar to human bubonic plague. N. N. Mari[331] rejected Petropavlovskii's work, pointing out that his so-called distemper bacilli were nothing more than coliform bacilli and had nothing to do with causing distemper.

Also dating from this period is the work of a transient figure in pathology at the Kharkov Veterinary Institute, Aleksei M. Petrov. He worked in the pathology department between 1910 and about 1926, beginning while it was under the acting headship of Petropavlovskii. Petrov was interested in parasitic diseases and thus gravitated to doing his M.V.Sc. dissertation under Melnikov-Razvedenkov in the nearby medical faculty.[407] Petrov then worked as prosector under Khrakht-Paleev and taught meat hygiene as well as pathology during the several years that the former subject was under the pathology department. Sometime in the mid-1920s, meat hygiene was elevated to the status of an independent discipline at the KVI, and Petrov was appointed to the chair that was thus created. In 1930 he wrote a textbook called *Kurs Myasovedeniya* (Course in Meat Hygiene).

During the meeting of the Ukrainian Society of Pathologists held in May 1927, and dedicated to Professor Ostapenko, Petrov delivered the major biographical address, entitled "Fifty years of scientific and social activity of Professor A. P. Ostapenko."[411] He mentioned that Ostapenko was responsible for organizing the veterinary sanitary service (i.e., meat inspection) for the city of Kharkov. In a paper honoring Ostapenko, Petrov lauded him for his inspiring lectures, in which he censured bacteriologists for reducing all causes of diseases to bacterial infection. Petrov pointed out that current advances in biological science were passing veterinary medicine by, and attributed this to a dearth of veterinarians who thought like scientists and an excess of *feldsher* (veterinary assistant) influence which verged on quackery.[410a] Since the editor of the journal where this appeared was K. G. Martin, himself originally a *feldsher,* the latter statement was disputed in an editorial footnote. The Soviet government was training the sort of veterinarians it wanted, and one wonders how long Petrov survived this criticism of its efforts.

Petrov was not in pathology long enough to make a large impact on this discipline. Nevertheless, his work on the hepatic lesions of distomiasis in cattle and man remains a useful contribution to comparative pathology.[404,409] Like much that was published in Russian, it is unknown and uncited in contemporary Western books on human or veterinary pathology.

The autopsy statistics for the Kharkov Veterinary Institute for the years 1910–1912 make interesting reading (see Table 2). There is an increasing number of autopsies, with an astonishing percentage (over 50 percent) of dogs. The relatively high number of horses is understandable in an urban center, in a day when they provided the motive power for most forms of transport. I do not understand, however, why so few cattle are represented in the autopsy population in an agricultural country like the Ukraine. What is more, the statistics for the years 1924–1927 show a similar high proportion of dogs and almost no cattle. Perhaps in those latter years the hunger that prevailed resulted in no sick cattle being "wasted" in autopsy rooms? Whatever the reason for the statistics, it is clear that Ostapenko's abattoir material was vital for the teaching of pathology; the autopsies, would have exposed the students to little else but dogs and horses.

For almost four decades, from 1912 to 1949, the chair of pathology at the KVI was held by Professor Petr N. Krakht-Paleev (1873–1949), an 1896 graduate of the Kharkov Vet-

Table 2. Autopsies at Kharkov Veterinary Institute

	1909	1910	1911	1912	1917–21	1923	1924–25	1925–26	1926–27
Horses	35	13	34	68	148		34	42	23
Swine		7	6				19	4	2
Cattle	2	5	9	3			1	2	4
Sheep				1					
Goats			1	1			5	5	3
Dogs	31	93	74	113	72		150	98	84
Cats	4	2	3	17			16	6	12
Other	9	10	30	9	40		3	12	25
Total	81	130	157	212	260	62*	228	169	154

*The breakdown into species is not given in the report.

Data from *Sbornik Trudov Kharkov. Vet. Inst. 9*(4): 72–73, 1910; *12*(1): 150, 1914; and *Zbirnik Prats Kharkiv. Vet. Inst. 15*(1): 43–44, 1929.

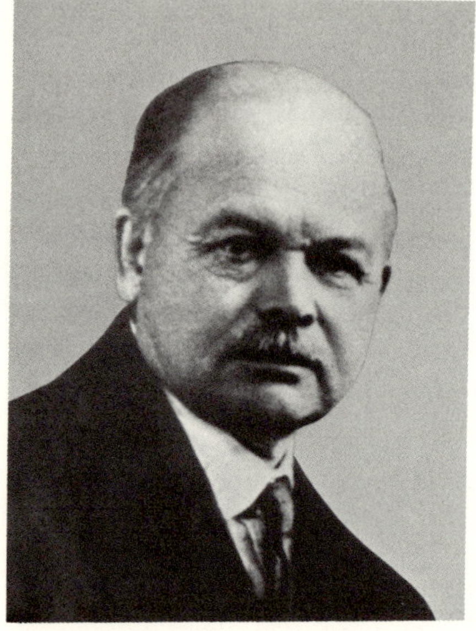

Figure 29. Petr N. Krakht-Paleev.

erinary Institute (Fig. 29). Like Ball and Bohl, he was exceedingly well trained as a veterinary pathologist. He began his academic career in his alma mater, teaching anatomy from 1896 until 1912. In 1905 he published an atlas of anatomy of domestic animals. He attended lectures in medicine while teaching veterinary anatomy and in 1907 graduated from the medical faculty of Kharkov University. During this time, he would have taken the pathology courses under N. F. Melnikov-Razvedenkov.

In 1910, the year after Ostapenko's dismissal, the Institute decided to groom Krakht-Paleev for the chair of pathology, and he was sent abroad to work with Schütz in Berlin.* In

*Not all Russian veterinarians who studied pathology abroad were pathologists—some were clinicians, who were using this means to advance their understanding of basic disease processes. Thus, in 1911–1912, N. I. Samodelkin, a veterinarian on the staff of the KVI, was working in Berne, under the well-known Professor Guillebeau (see *Semester Verzeichnis der Berner Hochschule, Sommer-Semester 1911*, p. 34, and *1912*, p. 36). Samodelkin published the results of this work first in a German journal and later in

1911 he moved to Dresden to study with the famous Ernst Joest, and he published a paper in a German journal on the anatomy and pathologic anatomy of the canine prostate based on work done during this sojourn.[269] He also worked with Joest on the histopathology of the tuberculous udder in the cow, which they published jointly.[221] Apparently unknown to them—or at least not cited by them—was the fact that the first substantial work on the subject had been carried out by another Russian, Kolesnikov, also working in Germany, in Virchow's laboratory, some 35 years previously.[256]

After leaving Dresden, Krakht-Paleev spent a semester with Theodor Kitt in Munich before returning to assume his duties as a pathologist in Kharkov. His exposure to the leaders of German veterinary pathology was now complete. In the "Collected Papers of the Kharkov Veterinary Institute" for 1914 we find a certificate (Fig. 30, translated below) of his Dresden sojourn, attested to by Professor Joest.[16] Apparently there was sufficient pride in this accomplishment to motivate its publication! Krakht-Paleev also spent part of his study time abroad in Austria and Belgium, although he did not stay in these countries long enough to undertake studies leading to publication.

> I herewith certify to Dr. Kracht-Paleeff that he worked in the Institute reporting to me during the period January 5, 1911, to January 13, 1912 (with the exception of the time from August 1 to October 1). Apart from that he audited the lectures on pathologic anatomy, the pathologic-anatomic demon-

---

Russian.[455,456] In 1926, Samodelkin, as rector of the Kharkov Veterinary Institute, appeared on a list of academic notables who sent greetings to the Kazan Veterinary Institute on its fiftieth anniversary.[18] When Nöller visited Kharkov in 1929, Samodelkin was professor of surgery there,[371] and he is mentioned in that capacity in the official publication of the KVI for that year. He must have run afoul of Stalin's murderous secret police in the 1930s, since papers on the history of the KVI and also on the history of Soviet veterinary surgery published during the 1950s fail to indicate that he ever existed! (See Appendix III for details.)

— 64 —

и съ операціями, производившимися при затруднительныхъ родахъ. Кромѣ того, Николай Ивановичъ въ Вѣнской школѣ посѣщалъ еще одну клинику, которая предназначена исключительно для рогатаго скота. Въ эту клинику принимается рогатый скотъ съ наружными, внутренними и инфекціонными заболѣваніями.

Въ концѣ отчета Николай Ивановичъ, на основаніи своихъ наблюденій, сдѣлалъ общую оцѣнку и сравненіе постановки преподаванія хирургической группы предметовъ въ ветеринарныхъ школахъ Германіи, Австріи и Швейцаріи съ таковой же въ нашихъ институтахъ.

На основаніи этой оцѣнки и сравненія, по мнѣнію Николая Ивановича, приходится сдѣлать заключеніе не въ пользу нашихъ Институтовъ.

Лицъ, излагающихъ хирургическую группу предметовъ, въ заграничныхъ школахъ больше, чѣмъ въ нашихъ; вспомогательный учебный персоналъ (приватъ-доценты и ассистенты) вполнѣ достаточенъ, по 2—3 ассистента при каждой клиникѣ; времени на изложеніе хирургическихъ предметовъ и на клиническое преподаваніе затрачивается больше; клиники устроены и оборудованы такъ, что совершенно обезпечиваютъ нормальную продуктивность работы какъ преподавательскаго персонала, такъ и студентовъ; въ клиникахъ студенты принимаютъ болѣе активное участіе при лѣченіи больныхъ животныхъ, чѣмъ у насъ, вслѣдствіе отсутствія фельдшерскихъ учениковъ и, наконецъ, какъ особенность заграничныхъ школъ,—это выѣзды профессоровъ со студентами для посѣщенія больныхъ животныхъ на мѣстахъ. Такіе выѣзды пріучаютъ студентовъ оказывать лѣчебную помощь при той обстановкѣ, въ какой имъ придется работать по окончаніи школы. Заканчивая отзывъ, я находилъ бы желательнымъ напечатать и этотъ послѣдній отчетъ Николая Ивановича о его научной заграничной дѣятельности въ „Сборникѣ Трудовъ Харьковскаго Ветеринарнаго Института“, подобно тому, какъ это сдѣлано и съ предшествующими отчетами“.

Опредѣлено: Отчетъ доцента Н. И. Самодѣлкина и отзывъ профессора М. А. Мальцева напечатать въ отчетѣ по Институту за текущій 1912 годъ.

21. Отзывъ профессора E. Joest'а о занятіяхъ прозектора П. Н. Крахтъ-Палѣева въ патологическомъ институтѣ Дрезденской высшей ветеринарной школы, слѣдующаго содержанія:

„Herrn Hofrat Dr. Kracht-Paleeff bescheinige ich hiermit, dass er in der Zeit vom 5 Januar 1911 bis 13 Januar 1912 (mit Ausnahme

— 65 —

der Zeit vom 1. August bis 1. Oktober) in dem mir unterstellten Institut gearbeitet hat. Er hat ausserdem die Vorlesungen über pathologische Anatomie, die patholog. anatom. Demonstrationen und Sektionen besucht. Während der Zeit seines Aufenthaltes im Institut hat Herr Dr. Kracht-Paleeff als besondere wissenschaftliche Aufgabe vom Unterzeichneten begonnene Untersuchungen über die Histogenese der Eutertuberkulose fortgesetzt und wird die Ergebnisse gemeinsam mit mir demnächst veröffentlichen. Herr Dr. Kracht-Paleeff hat die ihm übertragenen Untersuchungen mit Fleiss und sehr gutem technischen Geschick ausgeführt und stets ein lebhaftes Interesse für pathologische Anatomie bekundet. Medizinalrat Prof. Dr. E. Joest, Direktor des Pathologischen Institutes der Tierärztlichen Hochschule.

По заслушаніи этого отзыва, доложено на справку, что самая работа г. Крахтъ-Палѣева, подъ заглавіемъ: „Untersuchungen über die Frühstadien der Milchdrüsentuberkulose des Rindes“,—напечатана въ Zeitschrift für Infektionskrankheiten, parasitäre Krankheiten und Hygiene der Haustiere (zwölfter Band, 4 Heft. 1912) и въ концѣ отчетнаго года въ отдѣльныхъ оттискахъ получена дирекціей Института.

Опредѣлено: Принять къ свѣдѣнію.

Отчетъ о заграничной командировкѣ прозектора П. Н. Крахтъ-Палѣева.

(Съ января 1912 г. по 1-е іюня 1912 г.).

Закончивъ въ началѣ января 1912 г. работу „Untersuchungen über die Frühstadien der Milchdrüsentuberkulose des Rindes“ у профессора Joest'а въ Дрезденѣ, я поѣхалъ въ Лейпцигъ къ профессору Шпальтегольцу для ознакомленія со способомъ приготовленія просвѣчивающихъ препаратовъ (übersichtige Präparate), которые на Дрезденской гигіенической выставкѣ невольно останавливали на себѣ вниманіе. Познакомившись съ работою и осмотрѣвъ подробно музей со множествомъ очень цѣнныхъ препаратовъ, я выѣхалъ въ Мюнхенъ.

Баварская Королевская Высшая Ветеринарная Школа основана въ Мюнхенѣ въ 1790 г. Находится въ министерствѣ „für Kirchen und Schulangelegenheiten“. Профессоровъ въ школѣ—10 ординарныхъ, 3 экстраординарныхъ, 34 ассистента. Студентовъ—до 300, семестровъ—7.

Институтъ расположенъ вблизи Университета. Отъ вокзала можно доѣхать № 12 трамвая до Университета и, идя по напра-

Figure 30. Pages from the annual report of the Kharkov Veterinary Institute, with certificate attested to by Ernst Joest.

strations and the autopsies. During the time of his stay in the Institute, Dr. Kracht-Paleeff continued, as a special scientific project, the investigations begun by the undersigned on the histogenesis of tuberculosis of the udder; he will shortly publish the results together with me. Dr. Kracht-Paleeff carried out the investigations assigned to him with drive and very good technical skill, and always showed a lively interest in pathologic anatomy. Medical Councillor Prof. Dr. E. Joest, Director of the Pathological Institute, Veterinary College of Dresden.

In 1918 he submitted a dissertation on the anatomy of the mesenteric artery in domestic animals to the Kharkov Veterinary Institute for the degree M.V.Sc. In 1937 he was awarded the degree D.V.Sc., as were apparently all of the holders of the M.V.Sc. up until that time.

From 1912 until 1949, a period of 37 years, Krakht-Paleev headed the department of pathology, with the rank of professor from 1917. As a scientist trained in both medicine and veterinary medicine, he also taught courses in epidemiology in the Kharkov Medical Institute and in the Kharkov Institute for Postgraduate Medical Education for eight years. He was a member of the Ukrainian Society of Pathologists, attended meetings at least from 1928,[316] and gave a paper on actinomycosis at one of its meetings in 1936.[178]

His major research interests were in tuberculosis and granulomatous infections, such as actinomycosis.[276] He did not publish very much despite a long academic career; of 14 publications of which I am aware, 4 are in the realm of anatomy and the rest in pathology.[274] Krakht-Paleev deserves great credit for bringing out his two-volume work[275] on pathology of domestic animals during the extremely difficult early 1930s, when heads were rolling all over the Ukraine (see Appendix III). The tenacity of purpose and perseverance necessary to complete such a project under those circumstances can only be marveled at.

When one reads in his report of 1929 that in the preceding decade conditions of work were—by Western standards—impossible, one is filled with tremendous admiration for the perseverance of this man.[274] To have had the courage to carry on during the disasters that engulfed the Ukraine on an epic scale in the 1920s and 1930s was to have had quite remarkable fortitude. During parts of the years 1919-1921, the clinics and laboratories of the Kharkov Veterinary Institute were requisitioned—at times by the Germans and at others by the White Russians—for use as a military veterinary hospital. During the early 1920s, because of lack of fuel, lectures and autopsies were sometimes conducted in rooms with temperatures below 0°C. There was no protective clothing available and often no running water, so that autopsies could not be done adequately and certainly not safely. After one was done there was no facility for washing up. One winter the cold in the underheated buildings was so intense that the museum jars froze and burst, ruining several thousand specimens that Ostapenko, Petropavlovskii, and Krakht-Paleev had laboriously prepared over a 40-year period.* One's mind boggles trying to imagine the feelings of someone who is watching his museum specimens freezing and is helpless to do anything to save them. Perhaps the effort to keep himself and his students from freezing took Krakht-Paleev's mind off his other troubles.

By 1929, Krakht-Paleev, with Petrov's help[372] had replaced some of the ruined specimens with 500 new ones, but not all were permanent preparations. What a futile gesture to try to judge the productivity or the effectiveness of such a teacher by the usual criteria of autopsy statistics or bibliography. Especially when superimposed on all of these troubles the

*Conditions such as these prevailed not only in Kharkov; during the winter of 1920-1921 there was no piped-in drinking water in Petrograd because the cold had burst the pipes.[395]

Kharkov faculty (like that of the other veterinary schools) was obliged to squander its energies for several years on fatuous pedagogical experiments, designed by ignorant Leninist party hacks to turn out more veterinarians in less time.† This was done at the same time that admission requirements were lowered![360,642] By the time the disastrous effects of graduating poorly educated veterinarians became evident,* Krakht-Paleev and his colleagues had lost half a decade during which they might have accomplished the rebuilding of their shattered laboratories.

In the volume commemorating the one hundredth anniversary of the Kharkov Veterinary Institute, Nosik, the dean of the school, mentioned that Krakht-Paleev had written a two-volume book on veterinary pathology.[372] He gave no bibliographic data, however, despite its mention in a 21-page paper on the history of the Institute discussing almost everything else in considerable detail. Koropov (who had already written two history books[264,265]), writing two years later,[266] likewise mentioned Krakht-Paleev's book in passing and committed the same error of omission in citing its title. When I finally succeeded in tracing the publication,† I discovered that it was in the Ukrainian language (Fig. 31). The Russian literature just cited on the history of the Kharkov Institute[266,372] implies that Krakht-Paleev's book is written in Russian, thus creating an impression that Ukrainian culture

†Although this particular experiment was abandoned about 1930, not until the 1950s was there to be a general diminution of what Brown has termed "the cruel farce of sacrificing present generations for a hypothetical future."[126]

*I believe that some of the so-called refresher courses given during the late 1920s and early 1930s were actually intended to add the missing curricular ingredients which the poorly trained veterinarians had not received. Krakht-Paleev was involved in at least one course of this kind in 1929.[32]

†Not easy, as it was omitted from the Soviet bibliographic compilation *Knizhnaya Letopis* in 1932 and 1933. Another "oversight"?

П. Н. КРАХТ-ПАЛЄЄВ

ПРОФЕСОР ХАРКІВСЬКОГО ВЕТЕРИНАРНОГО ІНСТИТУТУ

ОСНОВИ ПАТОЛОГІЧНОЇ
АНАТОМІЇ
СВІЙСЬКИХ ТВАРИН І ПТАХІВ

ЧАСТИНА ПЕРША

ПАТОЛОГІЧНА АНАТОМІЯ ОРГАНІВ
ТРАВЛЕННЯ І ЧЕРЕВНИХ ОРГАНІВ

Науково-методологічний сектор НКО УСРР дозволив до вжитку, як підручник для сільсько-господарських ВИШ'ів (віза № 483 в 1/X 1931 р.)

ДЕРЖСІЛЬГОСПВИДАВ
ХАРКІВ 1932 КИЇВ

Figure 31. Title page of volume 1 of Krakht-Paleev's book "Fundamentals of Pathologic Anatomy of Farm Animals and Birds."

did not exist in the 1930s. The illustration of its title page should help to set the record straight!

The two volumes are of modest compass, illustrated mostly by photographs of specimens from Krakht-Paleev's own museum; a few pictures are borrowed from K. H. Bohl in Kazan or from German books. Krakht-Paleev's book is not as replete with information as Nieberle and Cohrs' textbook of veterinary pathology, which had been published in Germany a year earlier, in 1931. On the other hand, it contains more useful information than its two contemporaries in the English language: Runnels' *Animal Pathology* and Gaiger and Davies' *Pathology and Bacteriology.* Its small page size, modest number of pages, and, above all, the abominable paper, of a quality unknown in Western books, make it clear that severe restraints were imposed on Krakht-Paleev's publication.

I have no direct evidence that the omissions cited above are an attempt to make us forget Ukrainian publications, but Ziman's recent indication that Soviet scientists are ordered not to cite previously published work by dissident scientists is at least food for thought.[650] The fact that Krakht-Paleev's successor was (1) Russian, and (2) active enough in politics to be a deputy to the Supreme Soviet[372] leads me to suspect that the Soviet government has deliberately drawn a veil over Professor Krakht-Paleev.* This veil begins with the absence of an obituary in *Veterinariya,* the national veterinary journal, and includes as its last layer the third volume, with the letter K, of the *Veterinarnaya Entsiklopediya* (1972), which makes no mention of him, although replete with biographies of people whose contributions to veterinary medicine are of lesser significance.

Evidence that scientific publication in Ukrainian was new

*There is likewise no obituary of him in the Soviet specialist journal *Arkhiv Patologii.* Of course, there is little one could have said in an obituary during Stalin's last and most paranoid years. To report that a professor educated in Germany, who had written a book in the Ukrainian language, had just died might have offended him.

in that era is found in the first volume of Krakht-Paleev's book, which contains at the end a glossary of Ukrainian terms (Fig. 32). The authorities must have regretted almost at once their decision to let this book appear—the first volume was published in a print run of 6,000 copies, but the second one, the following year, in a run of only 3,070 copies. Alternative causes may have been administrative bungling in the incompetent publishing bureaucracy or a shortage of paper—both volumes are printed on abominably poor paper. Ukrainian was never popular either with the Tsars or with their Bolshevik successors (see Appendix III).

Krakht-Paleev appears to have encouraged others to publish without putting his name on their work; examples are several papers by his assistant Pustovar during the decade 1929–1939. Pustovar also published a small book on veterinary pathology in the Ukrainian language.[428] Thus, his department was active enough and, had Krakht-Paleev followed a practice common in Western Europe, his bibliography could have been much longer. It is to his credit that it was not. Pustovar did not later get the chair of pathology; Krakht-Paleev was succeeded after his death in 1949 by a Russian woman pathologist, Nadezhda Tolstova-Pariiskaya. In 1964, Pustovar was still a lecturer in her department.

Krakht-Paleev's best-known pupil, and to my knowledge the only one who made a lasting mark on our specialty, was F. N. Ponomarenko(Fig. 33), who was his assistant during the years (1926–1931). He thereupon became professor of pathology at the Kiev Veterinary Institute and—beyond the period covered here—made noteworthy contributions to veterinary pathology, several published in German journals. Apart from Pustovar and Ponomarenko, I am not aware of any pathologist who was trained by Ostapenko or Krakht-Paleev and remained in the discipline; they did not start a "school" as did Semmer, Ball, and Bohl. In this respect, the Veterinary Institute in Kharkov does not rank in importance

СЛОВНИК УКРАЇНСЬКИХ ТЕРМІНІВ

Амоній - магнезій - фосфат — фосфорно-кислая магнезія.
Аміяк—аммиак.
Аміяк-фосфат—фосфорный аммиак
Арсен—мышьяк.
Ацетатова кислота—уксусная кислота.

Барвні речовини—красящие вещества.
Барвник—красящее вещество.
Безбарвний—бесцветный.
Бешиха—рожа.
Бісмут—висмут.
Блискавично—молниеносно.
Блювання—рвота.
Борлакова залоза—щитовидная железа.
Бородавчастий—бородавчатый.
Бочкувата форма—бочкообразная форма.
Брага—барда.
Брамник—привратник (пилярус).
Брижастий—складчатый.
Брила—глыба.
Бруднобрунатний—грязно-коричневый.
Брунатножовтий—коричнево-желтый.

Вагітність—беременность.
Вада—порок.
Валькуватий—валикообразный.
Вбирання—поглощение.
Веретенуватість—веретенообразность.
Вершок—верхушка (легких—верхівка).
Вершкуватий—сметанообразный.
Взаємне тертя—взаимное трение.
Вивідний протік—выводящий проток.
Вигин—изогнутость.
Виплив—истечение.
Випинання—выпячивание.
Виродливий—уродливый.
Виразкуватість—израненность.
Виравка—рана.
Висівкуватий—отрубевидный.
Виснаженість—истощение.
Виснажна хороба—изнуряющая болезнь.
Війка—ресница.
Вгодованість—откормленность.
Відпірність—сопротивляемость.
Відплив—отток.
Відриг—отрыжка.
Відростень—отросток.
Відхідник—задний проход.
Вічко—отверстие в решете, в сотах.
Внутрішньожильний—внутреннесосудистый.
Внутрічасточковий—внутридольчатый.
Водень-сульфід—сероводород.
Воло—зоб.
Воротяна вена—воротная вена.
Впровадження—втискивание.
Вуглеводани—углеводы.
Втручання—вмешательство.
Вузина—перешеек.

Гаман—кошель.
Головогольчатий—иглоголовый.
Горбистий—бугристый.
Грубина—толща (кожи).
Грушувата форма—грушевидная форма

Ґедзь—овод.
Ґила—грыжа.
Ґилявий—имеющий грыжу.
Ґляґ—сычуг.
Ґроно—гроздь, кисть.
Ґудзюватий—пуговчатый.
Ґума—резина.

Дванадцятипала кишка—двенадцатиперстная кишка.
Дворотка водяна—двуустка водяная.
Довгаста форма—овальная форма.
Догірно—восходящим порядком.
Додільно—низходящим порядком.
Доплив—приток.
Дочірні клітини—дочерние клетки.
Драглистий—студенистый.
Драглистонабресковий—студенисто-отечный.
Дуплина—полость.
Духопровід—воздухопроводящие пути.
Дучка—альвеола.

Жила—кровоносный сосуд.
Жовтобрунатний—желтокоричневый.
Жовтавий—желтоватый.
Жовтяниця—желтуха.
Жовчевий міхур—желчный пузырь.
Жуйні тварини—жвачные животные.

147

Figure 32. Glossary of Ukrainian terms (on the left) and their Russian equivalents (on the right), from Krakht-Paleev's book on veterinary pathology.

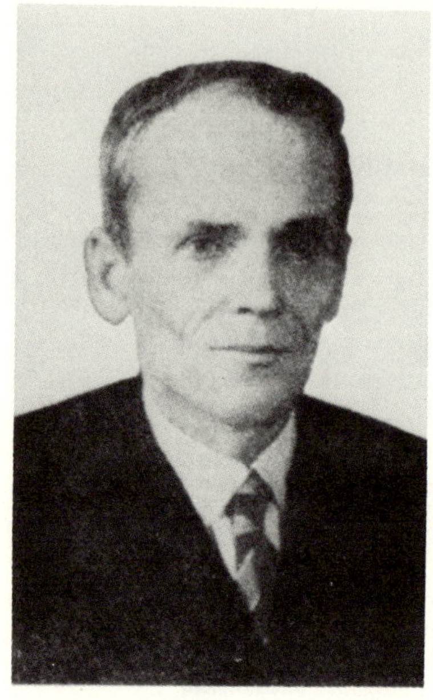

Figure 33. F. N. Ponomarenko.

with those in Dorpat and Kazan as a source of scientific influence on veterinary pathology in Russia.

During the period encompassed by this book, 1860 to 1930, the veterinary school in Kharkov seems never to have attained the stature of the ones in Dorpat and Kazan. K. Maehl, a Danish veterinarian who spent many years working in Russia and attended the All-Russian Veterinary Congress in Kharkov in 1913, wrote in derogatory terms about the disorder and filth in the clinics and the dissatisfaction* regarding the teaching staff.[313] Professor W. Nöller, of Berlin, who visited the KVI in 1929, however, spoke of it as being well equipped and the pathology department particularly so—it had either improved remarkably in the intervening sixteen years or was being viewed by a more sympathetic and charitable reporter.[371]

*It is not clear whether he meant that the students were dissatisfied with the staff or whether the veterinarians who attended the congress found them lacking in professional quality.

Faculty of Medicine, Kharkov University

Nikolai F. Melnikov-Razvedenkov (1866–1937) was a physician with lifelong comparative interests and a friend of veterinary pathology (Fig. 34). He is an important and interesting figure in Russian comparative pathology, who taught pathology in the medical faculty of Moscow University from 1889 to 1901. He left that post to assume the chair of pathology in Kharkov University, which he held until 1919.[1,15] In that year, during the chaos of the Civil War, he went to Ekaterinodar (now known as Krasnodar) and organized a new medical school there,[17] returning to his post in Kharkov in 1926.[23]

During the late 1890s, while he was still at Moscow, Melnikov-Razvedenkov autopsied two patients affected with echinococcosis and became interested in working out some of the then obscure aspects of the disease. He gathered human and abattoir material from Russia, Austria, Germany, and Switzerland, assembling it all in a large collection in Ernst

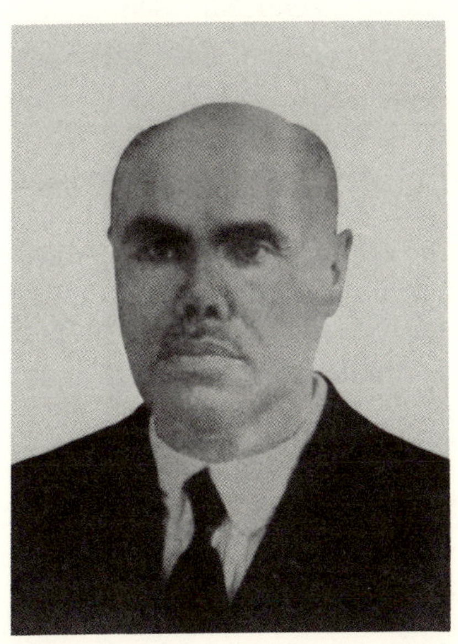

Figure 34. Nikolai F. Melnikov-Razvedenkov.

Ziegler's laboratory in Freiburg im Breisgau. Here he spent two years (1898–1900) working on the histopathology and pathogenesis of the disease. The resulting monograph published as a supplement in Ziegler's *Beiträge der path. Anat.* in 1901* is a complete, thorough, and beautifully illustrated work, which considerably advanced our knowledge of echinococcosis. Strangely enough, it is hardly ever referred to in most contemporary books on human or veterinary pathology today. The knowledge has entered the public domain, but the contributor of this knowledge has received little recognition in the West.[344]

Melnikov-Razvedenkov's breadth of thinking becomes evident in the introduction to his monograph on echinococcosis, where he states that the disease is of interest to pathologists in medical and veterinary institutions. He alluded to veterinary medicine again on the same page and further on in the monograph devoted a chapter to echinococcosis in animals. In the course of gathering his pathologic material, he had met Ostertag, of the Berlin Veterinary College, Kitt of the Munich Veterinary School, and Bollinger, Kitt's predecessor there. He thus became acquainted with several of the leading figures in veterinary as well as human pathology.[31]

This acquaintanceship gave Melnikov-Razvedenkov a breadth of outlook that seems never to have deserted him. I have already mentioned that he had an influence on Ivan I. Shukevich, at least in teaching him museum technique, but probably in imparting enthusiasm for pathology as well. Melnikov-Razvedenkov had published a method for the preservation of pathological specimens in 1899 that is still in

*Also published in German as a separate book and in 1902 in Russian as a book. A translation of the German title reads: "Studies on Echinococcus alveolaris"; of the Russian title: "A study of alveolar (multilocular) echinococcosis in man and in animals." I have compared both books and their contents are the same.

use in the Soviet Union today (*Veterinarnaya Entsiklopediya* 5: 112, 1975). Shukevich was a contemporary of his in the bacteriology laboratory of the medical school at Moscow University in the late 1890s. By the time the third All-Russian Congress of Veterinarians met in Kharkov in 1913, Melnikov-Razvedenkov had been teaching in that city for over a decade. Romanovich writes that Melnikov-Razvedenkov came to this congress daily to admire the specimens Shukevich had brought from St. Petersburg for exhibition.[446] He was interested not only in the specimens themselves, but in the fact that a protégé of his had learned his lessons so well.

Not long after Melnikov-Razvedenkov's arrival in Kharkov, the veterinary pathologist A. M. Petrov, who was an assistant in the Kharkov Veterinary Institute, conducted research with him on the comparative pathology of distomiasis in man and animals.[405,407]* And, as already mentioned, P. N. Krakht-Paleev studied human pathology under Melnikov-Razvedenkov.

Melnikov-Razvedenkov helped to organize the first All-Union Congress of Pathologists, held in Kiev in 1927. His report[346] emphasizes that many veterinary specimens exhibited there were of considerable comparative interest. He mentioned attendance also by veterinary pathologists, who "were very welcome guests."

The following year, Melnikov-Razvedenkov, who had organized the Ukrainian Society of Pathologists, reported that he had dedicated one of its meetings to A. P. Ostapenko, recalling that he was a veterinary as well as a medical pathologist.[347] By this time, Ostapenko had been out of veterinary pathology for quite a few years, but Melnikov-Razvendenkov was also a medical historian by avocation; hav-

*Melnikov-Razvedenkov's interest in comparative pathology was in the tradition set by his predecessor in the Kharkov medical faculty, Professor W. Krylov (see Chapter 11).

ing been present in Kharkov during Ostapenko's dismissal in 1909, he was not likely to forget the event, nor to let the victim sink into oblivion.

The proximity of the veterinary and medical schools in Kharkov (see map, Fig. 26) and Melnikov-Razvedenkov's comparative interests makes it almost certain that there was more contact between him and the veterinary faculty than I have brought to light. The obituaries and other biographical material that I have read on him, however, [1,17,23] do not mention even the little that I have found. I have devoted space to him here to fill this gap, and to identify a Russian comparative pathologist about whom there is indubitably more to be discovered.

The interest in comparative pathology in the medical school in Kharkov began with Professor Krylov, Melnikov-Razvedenkov's predecessor in the chair of pathology. His work on trichinosis is discussed in Chapter 11.

Faculty of Science, Kharkov University

Certainly the most distinguished alumnus of this institution during the nineteenth century was Ilya I. Mechnikov (1845-1916), the discoverer of phagocytosis and Nobel Laureate of 1908. A plaque in the Kharkov Veterinary Institute (Fig. 35) states that Mechnikov worked there in the laboratory of Professor Shcholkov from 1862 to 1864. What he actually did there to merit this citation I do not know, and it is not clearly stated in Koropov's historical book that illustrates the plaque (p. 103).[265] In fact, a few pages further on (p. 137), Koropov writes that Mechnikov worked in the botany department of the KVI in 1860—not the years given above.

Mechnikov does not allude to the KVI in his autobiography. Various biographers all relate that he attended the

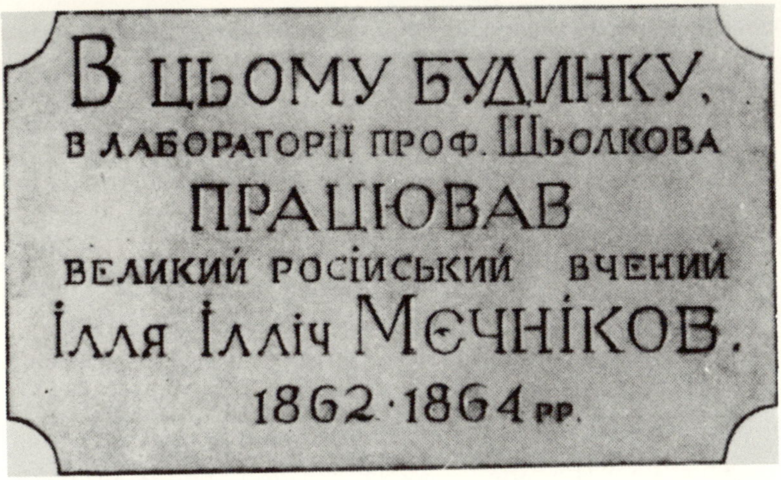

Figure 35. Memorial plaque in the main building of the Kharkov Veterinary Institute, illustrated in Koropov's book "History of Veterinary Medicine in the USSR." The inscription, in Ukrainian, reads: "In this building, in the laboratory of Professor Shcholkov, worked the great Russian scholar Illya Illich Mechnikov, 1862–1864."

University of Kharkov during the years 1862–1864; none, including the *Veterinarnaya Entsiklopediya,* 1973, make any mention of the Kharkov Veterinary Institute. As one can see from the map (Fig. 26), the Medical Institute and the Veterinary Institute were both close to the main University campus. Although their proximity permitted facile contact between students of each, the fact remains that the KVI was not a part of the University during the years in question.

Nosik[372] (p. 12) states that Mechnikov worked between 1860 and 1862 in the botany department of the KVI, and Kolyakov[262] says that Mechnikov learned microscopy there. In an earlier history, published in 1949, Koropov[264] (p. 93) also states that Mechnikov worked in the botany department of the KVI in 1860, that is, when he was 15 years old! However, four pages earlier in the same article,[372] Nosik lists botany among the basic science subjects that were taught to the KVI students *at the University*! Koropov[264] says that the KVI had a botany department in the 1860s, headed by Professor L. O. Pavlovich, but this is refuted by Nosik, who states (p. 5), that the KVI had no botany department even as late as 1873.

To add to the confusion, the Professor Shcholkov named in the plaque is not alluded to in Koropov's book nor in any historical article I have read on the Kharkov Veterinary Institute. A Professor Tschelkoff is mentioned by Olga Mechnikov in her biography[351] and a Professor Schtelkow by A. Berg in his biography;[53] however, both of them stress that this man was a *physiologist* and that he was at the *University.** Whether he lectured to the veterinary students or not, to claim him for the KVI is rewriting history. As I have shown elsewhere (Appendix III), Koropov is a practiced rewrite man. In the case of the picture (Fig. 35), he seems to be playing a more passive role and is merely depicting a plaque cast by some other manipulator. But Koropov's garbled statements which I have cited and also those of Nosik go further. Anyone can make a mistake and write 1860 when he means 1862, but to create a nonexistent botany department de novo is another matter.

Even at the University, which he did attend, Mechnikov found but little inspiration. His wife writes of the professors (p. 40): "Officials rather than scientists, they were content with ancient methods, and lectured without practical work from obsolete and ill-chosen manuals. A few of them drank, others neglected their work.... With the exception of Tschelkoff, his teachers had no decisive influence on his career, and his two years at the University formed but a colourless episode in his life."

Perhaps the plaque and the above four citations indicate a Soviet desire to lay claim to the fame of an internationally renowned scientist. If so, then this is not a purely Soviet

*The history book on the first century of the University of Kharkov also confirms this; by our system of transliteration the name is Professor I. P. Shchelkov.[373]

trait—Mechnikov was lionized by the tsarist government *after* he had won the Nobel prize. But he had to leave Russia to acquire his fame; i.e., to obtain the opportunity to work in a climate of freedom (see remarks by Olga Mechnikov, p. 228). Mechnikov was hounded out of Russia by several circumstances, of which only two will be mentioned here. Revo* writes[442] that the Odessa Medical Society forced the closing of his bacteriological laboratory on the grounds that his experimental work on fowl cholera would somehow result in an outbreak of cholera in human beings! The Society was motivated partly by jealousy and partly by ignorant fear. Robinson[443] points out that "just as many a French physician flung his M.D. into the face of Pasteur, telling him to earn a medical degree before he presumed to teach doctors, so various members of the medical fraternity of Russia balked at being under the direction of a layman like Mechnikov." Mechnikov also undertook some research work on rinderpest, which likewise led to harassment, this time from the veterinary profession, whose resentment he incurred.[397]

Knowing all of the above, it seems ironical to find him listed as an honorary member of the Educational Council of the KVI in 1912 (*Sbornik Trudov Kharkov. Vet. Inst. 11:* 4, 1912), with the names of several internationally respected figures in veterinary medicine from France, Germany, Italy, and Switzerland. Of course by 1912 he was already acclaimed outside of Russia. If Mechnikov, the great Russian comparative pathologist, played any role in the Kharkov Veterinary Institute more active than the honorary one of being so listed, its precise nature requires elucidation.

Figure 36 reminds us that veterinary pathology in Kharkov

*The *Zapiski Kiivskoho Veterinarno-Zootekhnichnoho Institutu,* in which Revo published his biographical note on Mechnikov, was one of a few short-lived (1924–1926) veterinary journals permitted to be published in the Ukrainian language, before Stalin consolidated his grip on the Kremlin and then on the Ukraine (see Appendix III).

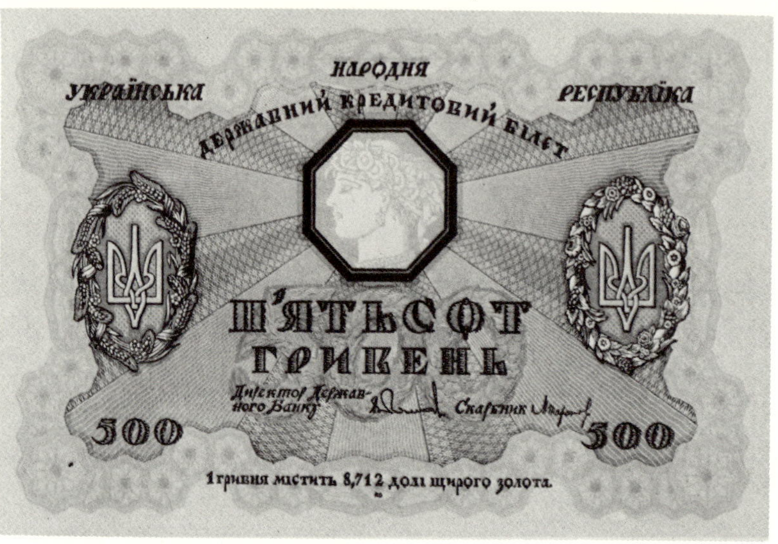

Figure 36. Banknote for 500 Hryven, issued by the short-lived independent Ukrainian Republic in 1921.

evolved under several regimes, one of which is all but forgotten today.

6 The Kazan Veterinary Institute

You cannot write in the chimney with charcoal.
—Russian proverb

In writing about the nineteenth century, the historian Seton-Watson relates that "the city of Kazan on the Volga was an important centre of Russian culture, the seat of a flourishing Russian university since 1805, but it was also the centre of a flourishing Tatar counter-culture, which more than held its own against Russian pressures."[527] Veterinary medicine was first taught in Kazan by one or two teachers, there being a chair for this subject at the local university occupied between 1841 and 1848 by Friedrich Brauell. The subsequently created veterinary school, the Kazan Veterinary Institute (Fig. 37), was authorized in 1873, and its opening ceremony took place on August 22, 1874.

The reasons for the placement of two veterinary schools in Kharkov and St. Petersburg may seem self-evident, since many large cities in Europe had such schools within their confines at that time. The reason for the establishment of two other schools in Dorpat and Kazan is less obvious. The University of Dorpat was intended by the imperial government to serve as a source of supply of faculty members for the other universities it intended to found.[434] Dorpat University was regarded as the cream of the academic institutions within the Russian Empire, and the decision to expand

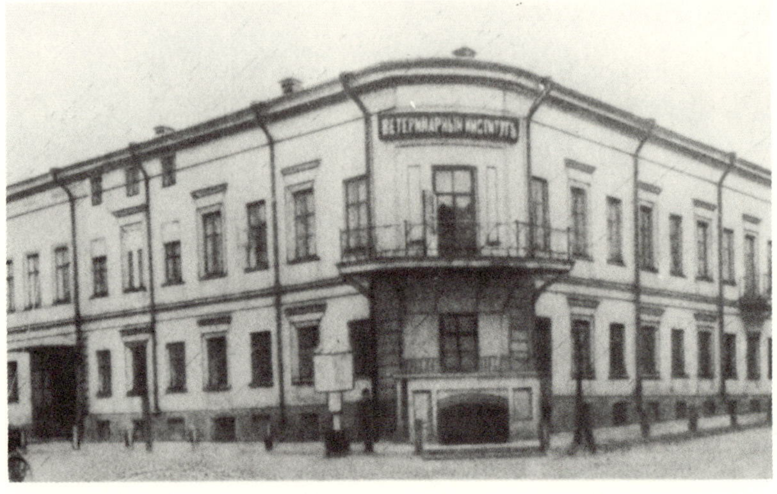

Figure 37. The Kazan Veterinary Institute at the turn of the century.

its chair of veterinary science into a teaching institute was a logical one.

Studentsov and Sabin explain why a veterinary school was organized in Kazan:[570] "The reasons for the establishment of the new veterinary institute specifically in Kazan were that a main route for the movement of commercial herds from Asia into Europe ran through that province, and that a veterinary institute in that territory was to serve as a veterinary sanitation cordon and as a watch point on the route between Asia and Europe. Another consideration was that the Kazan University was deemed to have great scientific vigor and large educational accommodations and was capable of offering the new institute the help it needed."*

*The Kazan Veterinary Institute was destined later to become the most important of the veterinary schools in Russia, particularly during the last decade covered by this book, 1920–1930. During this time, the cities of Tartu (Dorpat) and Warsaw were no longer in Russian hands, and the new veterinary schools in Moscow and Leningrad were still in their formative years. Arndt, writing in 1928 about the schools then extant, judged the one

Constantin Blumberg (1850–1897), the first teacher of veterinary pathology in Kazan, was an Estonian, born in Dorpat, Estonia, and graduated from the Dorpat Veterinary Institute in 1871 (Fig. 38). His dissertation for the M.V.Sc., done under Semmer's supervision, was entitled *Ueber den Bau des Amphistoma conicum* (On the Structure of Amphistoma conicum) and published in German. Following four years as provincial veterinarian in Voronezh, he returned to Dorpat as a lecturer in the clinics, but served only one year. According to Semmer,[513] Blumberg left the Dorpat Veterinary Institute in 1876 because of a dispute with the director, F. Unterberger, and with A. A. Saburov, the Curator of the Dorpat Educational District.*

While I do not know the nature of the dispute, one possibility may be that, following the death of Professor A. Unterberger, Blumberg was overloaded with too many responsibilities and duties, as alluded to by Chernogorov.[135] Or it may have been his sharp criticism of Director F. Unterberger's book on the Estonian horse.[604] This paper, in which F. Unterberger is attacked on several scores, appeared in print just after Blumberg had left Dorpat for Kazan.[55] If, however, the criticism of Unterberger's professional judgment and ability contained therein was a published version of what Blumberg had been expressing verbally, then one needs little imagination to see how it would have incurred the director's enmity. I derive further evidence that Blumberg did not hold F. Unterberger in very high esteem from the fact that in this paper he refers to him only by surname, or as

---

in Kazan to be "by common consent" the school providing the best veterinary education.[29]

*The jurist A. A. Saburov became Curator of Dorpat University and of the Dorpat Educational District in 1875. He was considered a liberal and in 1880 was appointed Minister of Education in the imperial cabinet with the special assignment to mollify or satisfy the numerous Russian students with radical leanings.[433]

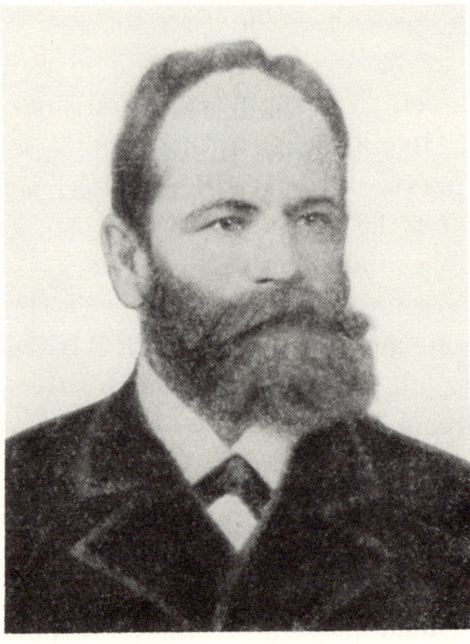

Figure 38. Constantin Blumberg.

"Director" Unterberger, whereas he refers to Unterberger's predecessor as "my unforgettable, highly honored teacher, Professor Jessen." In the same article, he also speaks of "my highly honored teacher, Professor Brauell."

Blumberg joined the faculty of the newly founded Kazan Veterinary Institute in 1876 as its first teacher of pathology.[10] He familiarized himself with human and veterinary pathology during study leaves in Germany in 1878 and 1887. On the latter, undertaken at his own expense, he worked in and reported on the institutes of Rudolf Virchow and Robert Koch as well as the Berlin Veterinary College.[67] Blumberg built a new autopsy room at Kazan, and it is apparent from his published description of it that he had spent considerable time studying others in Germany and elsewhere on the Continent.[60] His speech at its opening ceremony showed his interest in and knowledge of the history of both human pathology and veterinary medicine.[58]

In 1883 he published a tabulation of the diagnoses of the

325 autopsies he had conducted between 1876 and 1882.[59] While this average of about 50 autopsies per year may seem like a rather light load, we must remember that during these initial years he had no place to conduct them, as he so vividly describes.[60] The severity of the Russian winter must often have precluded outdoor autopsies for considerable periods. We would look in vain for an American, British, or Canadian veterinary school in which 50 autopsies per year were being conducted, either in the 1870s, or, for that matter, several decades thereafter. Blumberg described nine of the tabulated cases in detail, including brief mention of histologic examination. It is interesting to note that his examination included the central nervous system, something long neglected by veterinary pathologists the world over for decades in the nineteenth century and later. Under Blumberg, pathology in Kazan thus got off to a good start from the inception of the Veterinary Institute, despite the fact that he had to wait almost seven years before he could obtain an autopsy room.*

Blumberg's bibliography, while not extensive, contains some useful contributions.† He republished much of his work that first appeared in Russian in German journals, probably because only thereby could he reach an interna-

*The enthusiasm and accomplishments of Blumberg in spite of these adverse circumstances are commendable; he may have derived inspiration and moral support from the example of some of the scientists at the nearby University of Kazan. Magoun et al. write, in recounting the accomplishments of Russian chemistry at mid-century, "There was a popular saying among the chemists of that day, usually applied to Kazan, that the worse the laboratory, the better the research done in it. The rooms were so poorly ventilated that it was impossible to stay in them for long during experiments, and the chemists had to make frequent dashes out into the fresh air, often into the rain or snow."[315]

†His paper on the Estonian horse[55] shows that he was familiar with Estonian poetry as well as with other aspects of Estonian culture, at that time just coming to the forefront as part of the emerging national consciousness.

tional audience. In fact, if one sought recognition as a scientist, there was hardly a Russian audience of any consequence to be reached—Semmer[513] mentions 1,425 veterinarians in a nation of 100,000,000 people, with 35,000,000 cattle, 65,000,000 sheep, and 20,000,000 horses in 1886. Like Ravich and Semmer, Blumberg was active in domestic veterinary journalism and strove to bring the knowledge of veterinary science that was being developed in Western Europe to his Russian colleagues. Along with Semmer (and Gordiev of Kharkov), he founded the journal *Veterinarnyi Vestnik* in 1882 and helped edit it until 1883. The journal carried about 75 percent foreign abstracts and the rest original material. The selection of articles was predominantly scientifically rather than clinically oriented. The appearance of this journal was warmly greeted by Professor J. Csokor, of Vienna, who reviewed the first volume in an Austrian journal.[155]

Both Chernogorov,[135] who reviewed Blumberg's activity after 25 years of service to the Kazan Veterinary Institute, and his successor Bohl,[110] writing later with a perspective of 40 years, agree that he rendered great service to the Institute, which he served on two occasions as acting director. Yet, strangely, Blumberg is ignored in the Soviet *Veterinarnaya Entsiklopediya,*[552] in which there is no biographical article on him. His name appears, as if by chance, only under the entry of the *Veterinarnyi Vestnik.*

I do not know whether the omission is an oversight,* because Blumberg is not considered important, or whether he is looked at askance by whoever is determining the party line in the encyclopedia. A brief biography of him does appear in a recent Soviet publication on the history of medical and veterinary parasitology,[132] which may indicate that he was

*Perhaps his bare mention under the *Veterinarnyi Vestnik* is the real oversight! Censors must surely have the same problems in achieving consistency as more honestly motivated editors.

not currently in disfavor and that his omission from the encyclopedia is inadvertent. On the other hand, the book just referred to was published in Belorussia in 1965, and the volume containing the letter B in the veterinary encyclopedia in Moscow in 1968, during which interval the party line may have changed.

During the 1870s, the question of the transmissibility of tuberculosis had not been settled, despite many positive experiments (beginning with Villemin's in 1865) which showed that it was infectious rather than hereditary. The reason for the unsettled nature of the question was that many negative results had also been obtained and published by numerous investigators. As will be recalled, Virchow was one of the leading skeptics. Blumberg contributed to our store of knowledge by infecting a number of sheep, which he fed with pathological lung tissue from human beings who had died of tuberculosis. He found tuberculous lesions in the animals when he killed them and concluded that his findings supported the ones of Villemin, who had first contended that the disease was transmissible by inoculation.[56] Blumberg also established in this experiment that the human material was infectious for lower animals. Only a scant three years were to elapse between Blumberg's publication in 1879 and Koch's discovery of the tubercle bacillus in 1882; in the meantime, Blumberg was on the right track and following in the tradition of careful experimentation established by his mentor Semmer at his alma mater.

In 1887, Blumberg spent some time studying in Koch's institute, so that Blumberg's results in sheep must have been known to Koch—as indeed similar results obtained by others. Nevertheless, as an example that even great men may err, Koch challenged the transmissibility of human tuberculosis to lower animals by announcing at the Tuberculosis Congress in London in 1901 that human tuberculosis *could not be transmitted to cattle.* Blumberg thus has the distinction of having established a fact (the transmissibility of human tuberculosis to lower animals, albeit not to cattle), which Koch challenged but which time soon proved to be nevertheless a fact.

Two points are of further interest in Blumberg's tuberculosis paper. First, Blumberg obtained the human material from A. V. Petrov (1837–1885), professor of pathology in the medical faculty of Kazan University. This evidence of helpful cooperation between the medical and the veterinary pathologists in Kazan is an early example of collaboration in comparative pathology.* Such interest was also shown a couple of decades later by Nikolai M. Lyubimov, Petrov's successor (see below). Second, Blumberg examined the central nervous system in the autopsies of the sheep, indicating an unusual degree of thoroughness for a veterinary postmortem examination in that day or indeed 50 years later. Whether he learned this thoroughness from Semmer, who had published on cerebral lesions in horses back in 1871, or from his visits to German institutions, I do not know, but the thoroughness of Blumberg's autopsy technique is noteworthy, particularly for that era.

According to Chernogorov, Blumberg was the first to introduce laboratory work in pathologic histology to veterinary students in Russia.[135] Until then, pathology had been taught by lectures and autopsy demonstrations.

Blumberg published as much on parasitology as he did on pathology and started a collection of parasites that was still being studied in Kazan in the mid-1920s.[232] At a time when the anatomical structures of the cestodes were first being recognized and many descriptions were erroneous, Blum-

*This collaboration, or at least mutual interest, was again discernible in 1961, when Ippolyt Davydovsky, the dean of pathologists in the Soviet Union, gave the keynote address at the Second All-Union Conference of Veterinary Pathologists.[156]

berg's good fixation and sharp observation led to an original description of lasting value. This received the tribute of two of the leaing contemporary parasitologists in Germany, Küchenmeister and Zürn.[285] In one of his parasitological papers,[57] we find amusing evidence that despite Bohl's and Chernogorov's descriptions of him as a very kindly individual, he could, when aroused, give a good account of himself, at least in print. After taking to task the blurred illustrations of an author who had criticized his staining technique for cestodes, Blumberg fired a withering salvo that can be savored fully only in its original German, although its spirit emerges partially in translation as well:

> Zum Schluss will ich noch bemerken, dass die citirte Erstlingsarbeit H. Kahane's durch etwas mehr Bescheidenheit kaum viel an ihrem Werthe eingebüsst hätte.

> In conclusion, I would like to remark that had the cited first work of this author been characterized by somewhat more modesty, it would hardly have diminished any of its value.

Blumberg's book on autopsy technique, *Sektsionnaya Tekhnika,*[73] was published in Russian in 1895, and was still cited in twentieth-century Russian literature as a lasting and valuable contribution.[417] Viewed by contemporary standards, it still seems to be one. It is a well-organized and beautifully illustrated volume of a production standard that has not again been reached by any Russian book on veterinary pathology during the twentieth century.

Blumberg laid considerable emphasis on meticulous autopsy technique, as witness not only the writing of his book, but of the 1883 article already mentioned. He was an admirer of Karl Rokitansky and quoted him in his book. He pointed out that accurate postmortem diagnosis was the only basis on which Russia could hope to control its devastating epizootics. His was not the earliest book on autopsy technique, being preceded by Ostapenko's in 1882, but his was the earliest book in veterinary literature that emphasized the importance of careful and systematic dissection and careful recording of lesions at postmortem examination. A review in the *Arkhiv Veterinarnykh Nauk* of St. Petersburg drew favorable attention to the book, pointing out that it was based not only on the author's 25 years of experience, but also on his knowledge of the foreign literature.[561] It was also reviewed favorably in the *Oesterreichische Monatsschrift für Thierheilkunde.*[248]

There cannot be many copies of *Sektsionnaya Tekhnika* still in existence. I have therefore reproduced some of the plates from Blumberg's book (obtained on loan by courtesy of the National Library of Medicine) on the endpapers of this book, so as to make them accessible to a wider audience than could otherwise see the originals. They serve to remind us also that rubber gloves were not invented until the twentieth century, making the postmortem examination of a glandered horse, for example, a hazardous operation that sometimes took the life of the veterinarian performing it.

Blumberg's career was cut short by death (following a surgical operation) in 1897 during a scientific visit in Berlin, at the early age of 47 years, but not before he had selected his successor.* This was the 25-year-old Karl H. Bohl, one of his Kazan graduates of 1895, whom he had appointed as prosector the previous year. Bohl dominated Russian veterinary pathology for 60 years, mostly by virtue of his superior ability and education, but partly because of his longevity (1871–1959). His teaching and research efforts and his output of books and papers never flagged over this prodigious span of time, during which his activity continued almost unabated well into his ninth decade.

Karl H. Bohl (Fig. 39) was born in St. Petersburg in 1871,

*Blumberg was apparently not well known abroad. I have found no obituary of him in any German or Austrian journal, either the ones he published in or others.

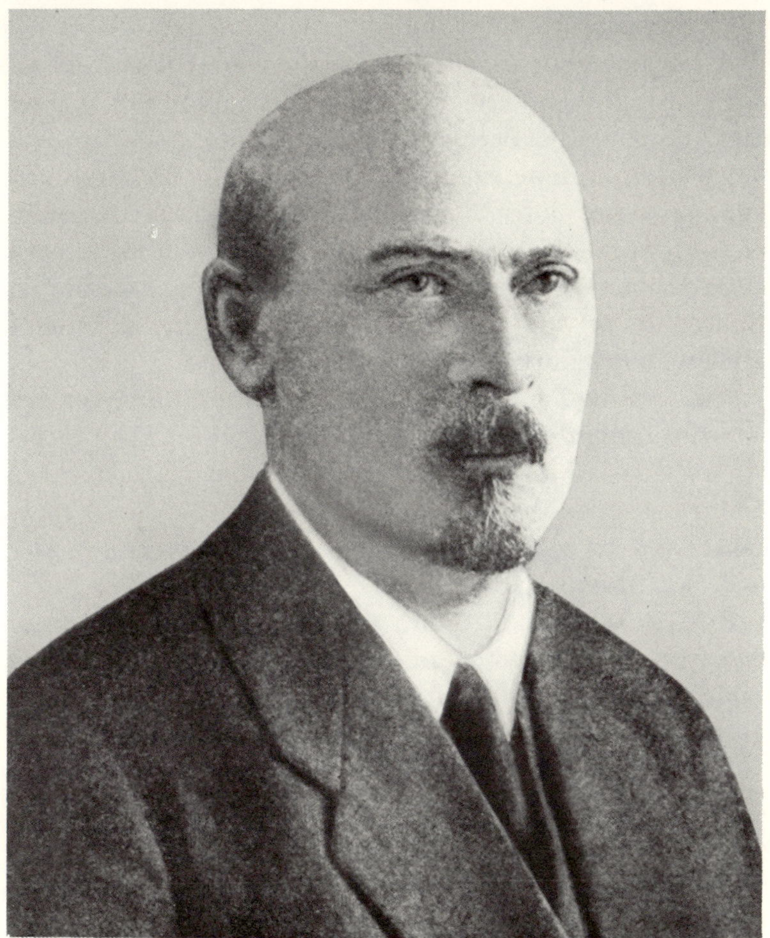

Figure 39. Karl H. Bohl in the mid-1920s.

the son of a German carpenter.[616] During the nineteenth century, Russian cities were full of Dutch, German or Swiss craftsmen, many of them working on projects directed by the French or Italian architects whom the various tsars favored and therefore imported. Presumably, Karl's father, Heinrich K. Bohl, was one of these craftsmen. During Karl's childhood, the family moved to Kazan, and he received his elementary education in that city at the Kazan Academy.[22]

Viktorov relates that the family was large and hardworking, the latter being an attribute which the young Karl Bohl acquired as a child and never lost. In describing Bohl's career after 35 years of service on the Kazan faculty, Viktorov mentioned inexhaustible energy as one of his chief characteristics. An anonymous biographer relates that as a young man—presumably during his college days—Bohl experienced financial difficulties and earned a living by tutoring children in private homes and by helping in his father's cabinetmaking workshop.[20]

After graduating with distinction from the Kazan Veterinary Institute in 1895, Bohl spent a few months as a practicing veterinarian. He then returned to his alma mater as a junior teacher in the histology department, but soon (1896) transferred to pathology and worked as prosector under Professor Blumberg.

After Blumberg's death in 1897, Bohl was given charge of the pathology department of the Kazan Veterinary Institute. While working to build it up, he began to study lesions in the central nervous system; this was to remain a lifelong interest. He did a master's thesis (1899) on the neuropathology of canine distemper under Lyubimov,* the pathologist at the Medical School of Kazan University, who was himself a pupil of Recklinghausen's.[641] Bohl also began to assemble specimens for what was later to become a very large and useful teaching museum.

*Professor Nikolai Lyubimov (1852–1906), like his colleague Rudnev in St. Petersburg and his predecessor Petrov in Kazan, already mentioned, had more than a passing interest in veterinary pathology.[345] He also directed the work for a Master of Veterinary Science of the veterinarians Polovinkin on canary pox[423,424] and Karaulov on plague.[231] This interest in comparative pathology still exists in Kazan; G. Nepryakin, the professor of human pathology in 1966, alluded to these two works as well as Bohl's contributions in recounting the history of the past hundred years of his chair.[364]

Bohl was subsequently sent to study abroad on several occasions, under men who represented the cream of German human and veterinary pathology—Virchow, Schütz, Kitt, and Joest. It does not depreciate Bohl's own attainments to point out that no veterinary pathologist in any country ever had the privilege of instruction and stimulation by such a stellar array of talent and genius. Curiously, Bohl's German training, at least the portion of it provided by Virchow, freely acknowledged at his fortieth anniversary celebration[110,452] and in his more recent biography,[593] was in 1961 apparently repudiated by himself.*

Bohl was promoted (fairly rapidly for those days) from lecturer to extraordinary professor to ordinary professor, reaching the latter rank in 1905. Before the outbreak of World War I, he had completed writing his first book—to which I will return later—and his students had the benefit of an exceedingly well-prepared teacher. Figure 40 shows a group of them, in uniform as was the dictate in those days, listening to a lecture demonstration shortly after the turn of the century. There was also a goodly amount of autopsy material, and the total, while not large by some standards, was sufficient for teaching gross pathology (see Table 3). Even in the war year 1916 Bohl reported on 33 new preparations that were added to the museum. On the basis of this material and his knowledge of the literature, Bohl published his first book, "Principles of Pathologic Anatomy of Domestic Animals," between 1912 and 1914 (Fig. 41).[99]

*The third (posthumous) edition of his latest textbook[111] is marred by senseless tirades against Virchow, most likely contributed by his editor, N. A. Naletov. One finds it hard to imagine an 88-year-old pathologist either believing such nonsense or—even in Russia—fearing officialdom enough at this advanced age to turn on his long dead mentor. It is easier to imagine that since Bohl himself was dead, he was helpless to reject words being attributed to him. For further discussion of the anti-Virchow era, see Appendix I.

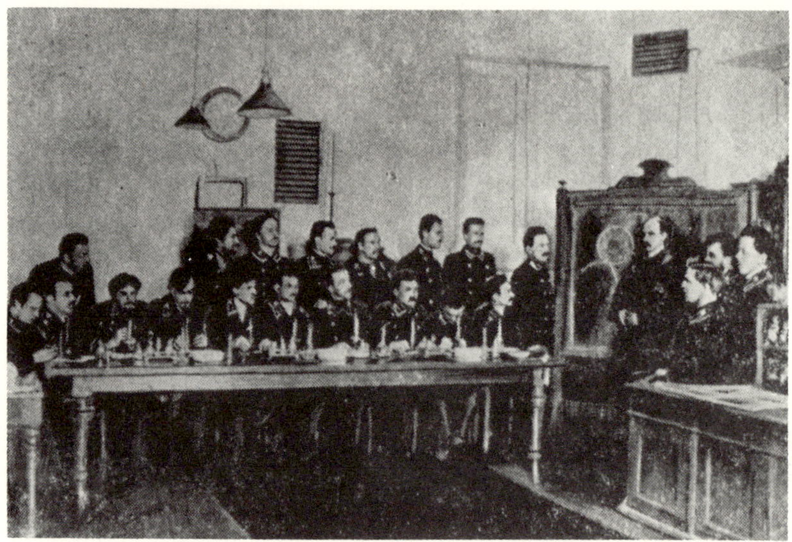

Figure 40. Professor Bohl in the classroom with veterinary students.

During the first few years of the twentieth century, Bohl had N. A. Soshestvenskii (1876–1941) as assistant in his department in Kazan. He wrote a book on pathologic histology during this time, which appeared over a two-year period in the 1913 and 1914 proceedings of the Kazan Veterinary Insti-

Table 3. Autopsies at Kazan Veterinary Institute

	1899	1904	1916
Horses	59	74	53
Cattle	30	33	53
Pigs	4	4	20
Dogs	27	31	89
Cats	4	6	6
Goats		10	5
Sheep		1	
Chickens	8	54	43
Rabbits		5	

Data from *Uchen. Zap. Kazan. Vet. Inst. 17:* 83-84, 1900; *22:* 378-381, 1905; *34:* 125-126, 1917.

К. Г. Боль

Профессоръ Казанскаго Ветеринарнаго Института.

ОСНОВЫ
ПАТОЛОГИЧЕСКОЙ АНАТОМІИ
ДОМАШНИХЪ ЖИВОТНЫХЪ.

ВЫПУСКЪ I-й.

Патологія кровеносной и лимфатической системы, кроветворныхъ органовъ, крови и железъ внутренней секреціи.

Съ 9 рис. въ текстѣ.

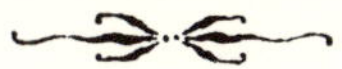

КАЗАНЬ.
Типографія Д. М. Гранъ, Б. Проломная.
1913.

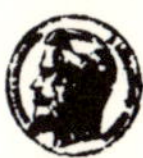

Figure 41. Title page of Bohl's first book, "Principles of Pathologic Anatomy of Domestic Animals."

tute.[567] He also published a few reports of interesting autopsy cases in 1913,[566] but thereafter left pathology for the fields of parasitology and pharmacology. His successor as Bohl's assistant, I. V. Smirnov, published a brief paper on actinomycosis in swine in 1918[558] and was the first of Bohl's assistants to complete his training in the postwar period. He worked on the nasal lesions of glanders in the group that formed the nucleus of what became the Bohl school of veterinary pathologists.[559] I have not been able to trace Smirnov beyond 1926 and do not know if he remained in the field of veterinary pathology.

In 1919 the whole of the Kazan Veterinary Institute was placed under Bohl's direction. He expanded it considerably during the two decades that it remained there and did likewise with the pathology department, of which he retained the chair. He also helped his colleague Viktorov to found the Siberian Veterinary Institute in Omsk in 1918 and gave lectures there between 1918 and 1921 under conditions of unbelievable political and social upheaval.[615]*

In 1924 the Kazan Veterinary Institute celebrated its fiftieth anniversary, and among the several representatives who sent greetings from German veterinary schools were the anatomist Ellenberger and one of Bohl's mentors, the pathologist Ernst Joest, under whom he had studied before World War I.[18] I have found no mention of this anniversary in the Western veterinary press, except a two-line footnote in a scientific paper by Bohl in the *Deutsche tierärztliche Wochenschrift.*[94]

In 1924, together with Ball and several other veterinary scientists, Bohl joined the original editorial board that launched the national veterinary journal, *Veterinariya.*[203]

Having been trained (by Lyubimov and Virchow) also in

*Conditions were bad in Kazan itself. During the winter of 1919–1920 the temperature in the lecture rooms at the KVI seldom exceeded 6°C.[183]

human pathology,[111] K. H. Bohl was pressed into service for a few years (1921–1924) to teach the course in pathology in the medical faculty of Kazan University[364,365] and to hold the chair of pathology at the Kazan Institute for Postgraduate Medical Education (1922–1930) simultaneously with his own at the KVI.[452] In so doing he tided his country over a period—during the years immediately following the Civil War—when medical teachers were in woefully short supply. To my knowledge, this decade of successful activity by a veterinarian in medical education is unique in medical history.* Appreciative comments were expressed for his help both in the 1930s[247,616] and at the centenary of the medical faculty in 1965.[365]

One can try to get some insight into what kind of a man Bohl was, but one is accorded little information from perusing his scientific publications. Occasionally, a rare glimpse may be had from a chance encounter with a biographical publication. Thus, the personal affection and esteem which Bohl engendered among his students has perhaps been best expressed by A. M. Klementeva, who taught as an assistant lecturer at the Institute for Postgraduate Medicine in Kazan.[247] Writing in the volume of collected papers published in honor of his thirty-fifty anniversary as a teacher, she described him as "direct and open, free of affectation, with the philosophic serenity of a true biologist, calmly accepting setbacks, limitations, and personal shortcomings." And, indeed, nothing less could have sufficed during those troubled times. The Institute for Postgraduate Medicine was created during

*There have been other examples of veterinarians working in medical appointments such as Krakht-Paleev at Kharkov University, but he had taken a medical diploma after qualifying as a veterinarian. In the United States, Fred Boerner, V.M.D., worked at the University of Pennsylvania Hospital, 1920–1960, and in Australia, Lionel Bull, B.V.Sc., at the Adelaide Hospital, 1925–1935. However, these two neither held the top job in the medical discipline they were teaching, nor did they simultaneously hold a chair in a veterinary school.

the Civil War, when starvation and epidemics were exacting a fearful toll,* and at first it had neither its own dissecting room nor a laboratory. Bohl triumphed over all of this, as an article in the local medical journal, likewise celebrating his thirty-fifth anniversary as a teacher, also attests.[516]

As far as I can tell from articles listing him as department head, Bohl served in four other capacities simultaneously with his appointment at the Kazan Veterinary Institute. As already mentioned, he lectured in pathology at the newly founded veterinary faculty of the Omsk Agricultural Academy during the years 1919 to 1921. He was acting chairman of the pathology department at the Moscow Veterinary Institute from approximately 1928 (the year his son Boris began work there) until 1932, when his son was appointed to the chair. Bohl also acted as head of the pathology department at the Leningrad Veterinary Institute following Ball's death in 1930 until Chernyak was appointed to this chair in 1933. Kokurichev's paper on spavin of horses identifies Bohl as the head of the Leningrad chair of pathology.[250] From 1937, Bohl directed the Kazan Veterinary Scientific Research Institute (Anonymous,[22] p. 66) (Fig. 42). In 1938 the Institute was named in Bohl's honor.[279]

When he died ("in harness") in 1959, Bohl was understandably renowned throughout the Soviet veterinary world, on which he had exerted a profound influence longer than anyone else. He was almost totally unknown abroad, however, where except for about a dozen papers in German, his work was unavailable (and hence unknown) to those who could not read Russian. Despite his German parentage, his

*Paul Scheffer,[466] who reported from Moscow for the newspaper *Berliner Tageblatt,* mentions (p. 86) the decree in 1921 stopping railway traffic for six months to the "hunger areas" because of the typhus which existed there. These areas were essentially isolated so that the people in them could either starve or die of typhus. Professor Holzmann, former rector of the Kazan Veterinary Institute, did the latter.

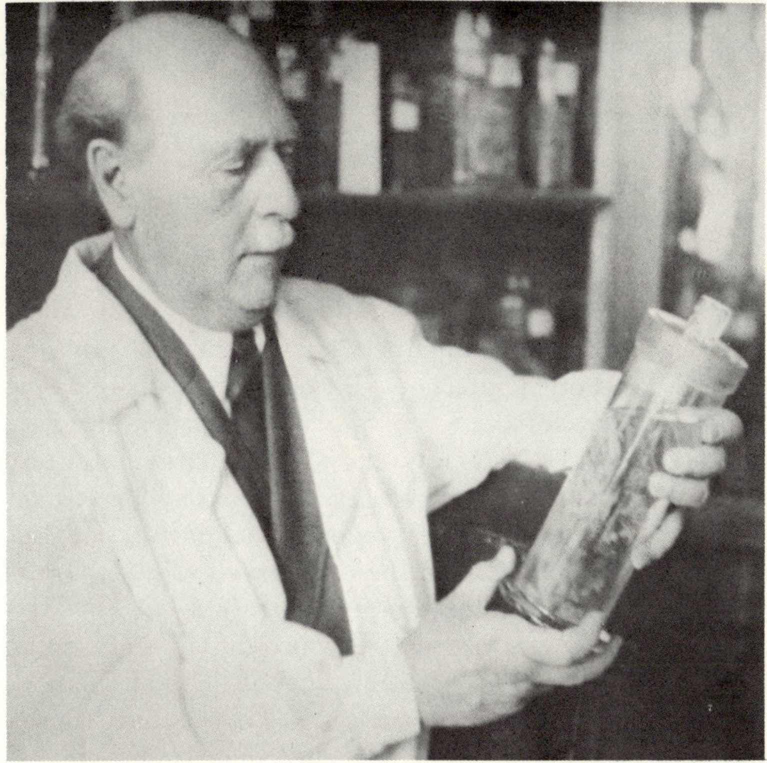

Figure 42. K. H. Bohl in the museum of his institute, circa 1950.

training in Germany, his fondness for things German, and the trend of other Russian veterinarians (including his son and his student Almeev) to do so, Bohl published little in German journals. Although most of his work was abstracted in the German *Jahresbericht der Veterinärmedizin,* this did not suffice to give him the universal recognition claimed by his eulogists.[593]* As a matter of fact, his early important work on

*I have been unable to find any notice of Bohl's death in any non-Russian journal except the *Monatshefte für Veterinärmedizin,* Leipzig. Even in that journal he was eulogized not by a German but by a Russian, his pupil Almeev.[5] He may have outlived his fame, however; most of the

the neuropathology of canine distemper has lain unread since 1899 in the few libraries that have it in the Western world. Yet, as I have written elsewhere, it is the most thorough of the few original works on the neural lesions available before 1900![460] Likewise, his visits to Germany seem to have been forgotten, if one can judge by the fact that none of the three leading West German journals carried his obituary.

Bohl and his students made important contributions to the pathology of canine distemper, equine encephalomyelitis, glanders, and other infectious diseases. His textbooks were standard works for the teaching of veterinary pathology in Russia and the U.S.S.R. for almost three-quarters of a century. The first, *Osnovy Patologicheskoi Anatomii Domashnikh Zhivotnykh*[99] (Principles of Pathologic Anatomy of Domestic Animals), was published in the early 1900s (1912–1915) in separate chapters in the *Ucheniya Zapiski Kazanskago Veterinarnago Instituta.* It reached a second edition in 1925 as an independent book with a slightly altered title increasing its scope to domestic mammals and birds. Revised third, fourth, and fifth editions appeared in 1930, 1933, and 1938. He replaced this with a larger book, written in conjunction with his son and other collaborators, *Osnovy Patologicheskoi Anatomii Selskokhozyaistvennykh Zhivotnykh*[111] (Principles of Pathologic Anatomy of Farm Animals) in 1950. This reached a second edition in 1954 and a third (posthumous) one in 1961, the latter in Chinese and Polish translations.[183]

Bohl devoted considerable effort to research work on glanders. According to Vereschchagin,[613] glanders was constantly present in Kazan and environs, but the severest out-

famous Europeans who attended the 150-year celebration at Hanover with him in 1928, and who might therefore have known him, died before he did. There was thus hardly anyone left who might have written his obituary.

break occurred in the Tartar Republic after the First World War.

Traveling somehow (rail? road?), despite the shattered transportation system, between Omsk and Kazan, Bohl soon realized the havoc glanders was causing and the vital importance of understanding its pathogenesis. In the early 1920s, he set to work on the disease personally, and in addition he formed a small team from among his assistants, to whom he assigned special aspects of the problem. The team comprised his son Boris (pulmonary glanders), B. G. Ivanov (lesions in the lymph nodes), and I. V. Smirnov (nasal glanders). I have summarized their work briefly in the chapter on glanders. As stated there, I have not arrived at an appraisal of whether Bohl's group did the most important or the most original work vis-à-vis Ball's group in Leningrad or Eberbeck's in Germany.

In the late 1920s, Bohl first observed a new disease of the central nervous system in horses in the southeastern portions of the Soviet Union. In 1931 another outbreak occurred in the northern Caucasus. The consensus among veterinary scientists was that the disease was a forage poisoning; but Bohl, who had studied the brains of affected horses histologically, insisted that it had to be a viral infection. He was familiar with the appearance of viral inflammation in the brain—with canine distemper from his own work more than a quarter of a century earlier and with Borna encephalitis from his knowledge of the German literature and probably of sections received from German colleagues, some of which are illustrated in his book. He was thus on firm ground in contending that a filterable virus had to be involved in the etiology of the mysterious equine disease. Within the space of a couple of years, several Russian veterinary scientists had proved that Bohl was right by isolating the virus responsible for Russian equine encephalomyelitis.

Bohl maintained his contacts with German veterinary science after the Revolution by making visits to Germany. In October 1927, he attended a large conference on diseases of breeding animals in Jena.[634] He was accompanied by his son Boris, who was at the time in training as a junior pathologist in Kazan. The following year, Bohl again visited Germany, this time as the official delegate of the U.S.S.R. to the 150th anniversary celebration of the Hanover Veterinary College.[616] To my knowledge, this was the last time that he left Russia.

Bohl gave two brief speeches during these celebrations, the transcripts of which are reproduced in Figures 43 and 44 (translated below) from the published proceedings. The first was at the meeting of the Society of Friends of the Veterinary College of Hanover on June 13, 1928.

Prof. Dr. Bohl, Kazan, als Vertreter Rußlands:

Magnifizenz! Meine sehr geehrten Damen und Herren! Als Vorstand der Kazaner Tierärztlichen Hochschule habe ich den ehrenvollen Auftrag, die Tierärztliche Hochschule zu Hannover mit folgendem Wortlaut zu begrüßen:

Das Kazaner Staats-Veterinär-Institut sendet seinen Herrn Kollegen der Tierärztlichen Hochschule zu Hannover seine herzlichsten Glückwünsche zu dem Jahrestage ihres 150jährigen Bestehens. Der Vorstand, das gesamte Lehrpersonal nebst der Studentenschaft der Kazaner Hochschule sind von dem Wunsche beseelt, daß es der durch ihre hervorragenden Gelehrten und zahlreichen wissenschaftlichen Leistungen ruhmvoll bekannten Hannoverschen Tierärztlichen Hochschule beschieden sein möge, noch weitere Hunderte von Jahren zu Nutz und Frommen der gesamten Veterinärmedizin ihre fruchtbare Tätigkeit entfalten zu können.

Figure 43. Facsimile of K. H. Bohl's speech in Hanover in 1928.

Prof. Dr. Bohl, Kazan, as representative of Russia:

Magnificence! Very honored ladies and gentlemen! As head of the Kazan Veterinary College I am charged with the honor of greeting the Veterinary College of Hanover in the following words:

The Kazan State Veterinary Institute sends its colleagues at the Veterinary College of Hanover its heartiest best wishes on the jubilee date of the 150th year of its existence. The director, the whole of the teaching staff as well as the student body of the Kazan College are imbued with the wish that the Hanover Veterinary College, known for its outstanding scholars and innumerable scientific accomplishments, may continue for more hundreds of years to develop its fruitful activity for the benefit and profit of all of veterinary medicine.

The second speech was given as part of the formal academic celebration on June 14, 1928.

Professor Dr. Bohl, Kazan, für die Hochschulen Rußlands:

Werte Versammlung! Mir ist die ehrenvolle Aufgabe zuteil geworden, die Tierärztliche Hochschule zu Hannover vom Volkskommissar für Landwirtschaft und vom Vorstand des Veterinärwesens und der Tierärztlichen Hochschulen der U. d. S. S. R. zu begrüßen. Die Wissenschaft ist international; sie erkennt keine Grenzen, und dennoch treibt jedes Land, jedes Volk die Wissenschaft nach seinem Geiste. Wir drüben hegen eine besondere Neigung zu dem, was hier auf deutschem Boden in den deutschen Hochschulen geleistet wird. Eine Mehrzahl von uns sind Schüler deutscher Hochschulen gewesen, und das ist auch der Grund dafür, warum uns heute die Jubilarin so nahesteht.

Es möge der Tierärztlichen Hochschule in Hannover, die 150 Jahre hindurch zur Entwicklung der Wissenschaft so viel beigetragen hat, vergönnt sein, in der Zukunft noch viel mehr für diese Entwicklung zu tun!

Figure 44. Facsimile of K. H. Bohl's second address in Hanover in 1928.

Professor Dr. Bohl, Kazan, for the universities of Russia:

Esteemed assembly! I have been allotted the honored obligation, of greeting the Veterinary College of Hanover on behalf of the People's Commissar of Agriculture, the Head of the Veterinary Directorate, and the veterinary colleges of the U.S.S.R. Science is international; it recognizes no borders, but nevertheless each land and each people pursues science according to its spirit. We over there [i.e. in Russia] cherish a particular inclination to that which is accomplished on German soil and in German universities. A majority of us have been students in German universities, which is the reason we feel such an affinity for the celebrating institution today.

May it be granted to the Veterinary College of Hanover, which has contributed so much to the development of science throughout a period of 150 years, to accomplish even more of this development in the future!

One wonders how much of his sentiment for Germany expressed in these words was motivated by his ancestry and how much by his acquired taste for things German, resulting from his earlier study trips. In view of his words, his survival during the purges of the 1930s becomes even more remarkable, in fact, little short of incredible. Here is a man with seemingly all of the taints necessary to mark him for destruction—not only the taint of having studied abroad, but worse, he has maintained his foreign contacts and expresses admiration for a foreign culture, far beyond what is called for by the courtesies of his official visit.

If the words reproduced above had become known in Russia during the worst of the excesses of the mid-1930s, Bohl might well have gotten into trouble. No matter how pleasant a man or how useful he was, there would have been somebody seeking to curry favor for himself by denouncing him to the secret police. But, Bohl's visit was barely known in Russia—I have found no mention of it in the veterinary press—and the German jubilee volume in which his speeches were printed consists of some 400 pages of Gothic script, not conducive to easy reading. Nor did this volume receive wide circulation outside of Germany. Bohl was probably smart enought not to circulate copies of his speeces in Kazan and to make sure that the German jubilee volume either did not get onto the shelves of the library at the Kazan Veterinary Institute or disappeared from them when prudence so dictated (about 1933 or 1934).

Both Bohl and Krakht-Paleev (the two people in our chronicle whose careers extend beyond 1930) survived the horrible deportations and killings in the U.S.S.R. ordered in the 1930s by Stalin. Even a modicum of curiosity leads one to wonder, *how?* I do not know, but it seems to me that only those worldly enough to have developed political skills could survive. I construe Bohl's renaming of the Kazan Veterinary Institute in honor of N. E. Bauman* as evidence of such skills. His endearing personal qualities did no harm, however. Bohl's opting to remain in his post in Kazan rather than seeking a more prestigious one in Leningrad or Moscow may also be evidence of political skill. Did he realize that it might prove dangerous to be too close to the seat of power, or did he merely prefer to live in Kazan?

The noted historian Ulam[603] discourages me from speculating by saying: "When we look for criteria by which certain people were spared, we are on very uncertain grounds." Possibly someone realized Bohl and Krakht-Paleev were important to agriculture? Of the two, Bohl, at least, was the acknowledged top man in his country in his scientific discipline, and this position probably conferred a measure of protection, since he might have been considered indispensable. Perhaps they survived because they kept a low profile? Or because even Stalin, paranoid as he was, and his secret police, ruthless as they were, could not kill everybody.

Of Krakht-Paleev's political life I know nothing. Bohl

*N. E. Bauman, a professional revolutionary, active in the Bolshevik party, was born in Kazan, the son of a German carpenter. He graduated in 1895 from the Kazan Veterinary Institute, which was later named after him. A close associate of Lenin's in founding the underground revolutionary newspaper *Iskra,* Bauman was in and out of prison several times between 1897 and 1905, sometimes escaping and sometimes being released. The "Great Soviet Encyclopedia" says that he was brutally killed in Moscow by an agent of the secret police during a demonstration in 1905, and that 300,000 people turned out for his funeral.[26] Bauman has been accorded the status of a hero in the Soviet pantheon, and articles praising him seem to pop up constantly in Soviet veterinary literature, not unlike weeds in a neglected garden. It is hard to leaf through the veterinary journals of any decade since 1920 without encountering several such panegyrics. S. A. Gryuner (see p. 179) seems to have been the first to have burdened a veterinary journal with praise of this unsavory-looking anarchist.[199]

joined the Communist party early—during the Civil War—and may have adroitly arranged just the proper amount of party participation to survive. He was a member of the Kazan City Council; as such, he would have had access to the party hierarchy, even if only at the lower echelons. But as a municipal politician, who was—I assume—unambitious for higher office, he would not have been considered a threat even by the most suspicious party hack. The above is speculation, of course; but if one reflects on the vicissitudes Bohl surmounted during the Revolution and Civil War and his commitment to things German, the conclusion that he had a sure instinct for survival becomes well-nigh inescapable. Finally, one must remember that throughout the Soviet years, applied scientists were generally treated with respect, and in the case of leading ones,* whose labors were obviously enhancing the national welfare or the national image, with kid gloves. Bohl was in the respect category, and to a lesser but apparently sufficient extent, so was Krakht-Paleev.

It is a remarkable sensation, after having become acquainted with Bohl's career piecemeal, in individual episodes of his life, to then scan it rapidly as a whole from beginning to the end. One obtains an impression of sheer scale; almost 65 years in professional life and almost all of them lived at or near the highest peaks of academic responsibility and endeavor. The variety and the comprehensiveness of the experience crammed into one human life span has no counterpart in American veterinary pathology, nor, to my knowledge, in British or German either. This unparalled con-

*One of international renown, I. Pavlov, was even able to criticize the regime with impunity and continue to receive its support. Stalin is reputed to have said, when he saw Pavlov crossing himself, "There he goes again—a slave to his reflexes."[302] However, I know of no other scientist who was treated so indulgently. In 1928, Russian scientists suffered the indignity of having their Academy of Science packed with enough Bolshevik ignoramuses to destroy it in all but name.[187]

tinuity of useful effort built upon a base of solid training is unique, as is Bohl's continued production of textbooks over a 48-year period, although Cohrs' publication from 1931 to 1973 almost equals it. But, to reiterate what Viktorov[616] wrote in 1931, Bohl had "inexhaustible energy"—a necessary prerequisite for the career he achieved.

Some of the pathologists whom Bohl trained became leading figures in Soviet veterinary pathology.[597] Chief among these were his son Boris, K. Vertinskii, B. Ivanov, K. Almeev, E. Zuikova, and N. Tolstova-Pariiskaya—the latter two, the first female veterinary pathologists in the world.* However, in the period covered by this chronicle, that is, up to the year 1930, these people were either still in training in Bohl's laboratory or had only just completed it. A description of their achievements thus falls outside the scope of this book, even though, because of his longevity, I have continued the account of Bohl himself until his death in 1959.

One seeks in vain for an American counterpart of Bohl in the decade 1920–1930. We were able to feed the starving Russians during the famines of this decade, but our country was not able to recognize or willing to support veterinary pathology in any manner even remotely comparable to that of the impoverished recipients of our charity. As a result, veterinary pathology in the United States languished during this period, and in the United Kingdom even more so, while it flourished in Russia, particularly in Kazan under Bohl.

*The third one was also a Russian, N. A. Borodulina, of the Saratov Veterinary Institute.[595]

7 The Warsaw Veterinary Institute

> There was a moaning in the village. The cavalry, trampling the crops, was changing horses. In exchange for their tired hacks, the troopers were confiscating draft horses. Nobody was to blame. There can be no army without horses.
>
> —Isaac Babel, *The Remount Officer*

Bohl was not alone, however, in shaping Russian veterinary pathology. The teaching of veterinary medicine in Moscow and St. Petersburg, abandoned, respectively, in the mid- and late nineteenth century, was destined to arise again in the 1920s, and a national veterinary research institute would be founded. In all three of these ventures, as well as in the veterinary diagnostic and research laboratories of the largely horse-transported Red Army, Nikolai D. Ball, a Dorpat graduate of slight build but towering stature, was the key figure. He began his career as a teacher of pathology in Warsaw. Before relating Ball's activities, it is necessary to sketch in some information on veterinary instruction in that city.

By the last decade of the nineteenth century, with the veterinary schools in Moscow and St. Petersburg closed, the Warsaw Veterinary Institute was the oldest veterinary school in the Russian Empire.[334] It had been founded in 1848 and had continued in operation through many vicissitudes, including forced Russianization in 1865, to graduate several hundred veterinarians, most of them Poles.

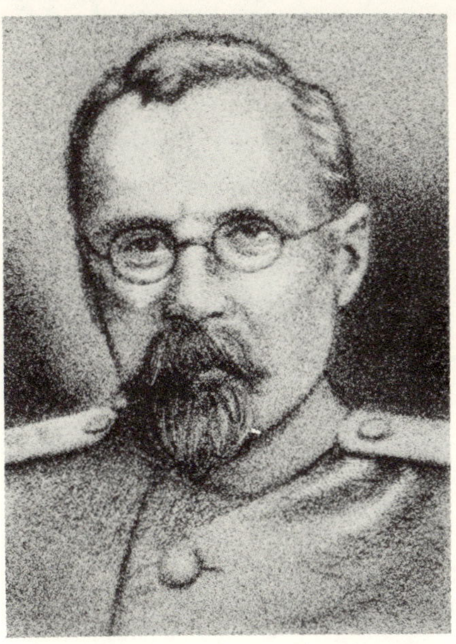

Figure 45. Nikolai N. Mari.

In 1891, Nikolai N. Mari (1858–1921) was appointed as the first full-time teacher of general pathology and pathologic anatomy at the Warsaw Veterinary Institute (Fig. 45). These subjects had been taught part-time before that by P. Seifman. Mari was the son of an Italian architectural engineer, L. A. Mari, who had emigrated to Russia at the invitation of its government.* N. N. Mari graduated cum laude from the Kazan Veterinary Institute in 1881 and worked as a district veterinarian in that area, chiefly in rinderpest control.[277]

Mari also studied part-time in the laboratories of physiology and histology of Kazan University during 1883 and 1884. In 1888 he passed his examination for the M.V.Sc. degree at the Kazan Veterinary Institute and then submitted

*As we have already seen, French and Italian architects played a considerable role in shaping the face of eighteenth- and nineteenth-century Russia.

his dissertation, which he was not permitted to defend for political reasons. As the Soviet historian Krapivner charmingly puts it, he submitted his dissertation in 1888 "at a time when the Tsar's satraps were hunting down all the opposition in the country."[278] For some reason, Mari was considered a suspicious personality in the eyes of what Krapivner terms two "reactionary officials," Lange, Director of the Institute, and Maslennikov, Curator of the Kazan Educational District. Granting him the M.V.Sc. would have given him the license to teach, and they felt that Mari would exert an undesirable influence on the students.

He thereupon went to Moscow and was employed for about three years in the Moscow city slaughterhouse, applying the principles of the newly emerging science of meat hygiene and developing it himself as well. In 1891 he obtained his M.V.Sc. from the Kharkov Veterinary Institute, with a dissertation on actinomycosis,* and being thus qualified to teach, he went to Warsaw.

Millak[356] writes (in Polish) that during an era of suppression of Polish culture, Mari was the only Russian on the faculty of the Warsaw Veterinary Institute who treated the Poles decently.† During his tenure in Warsaw from 1891 to 1902, Mari wrote *Osnovy Patologicheskoi Anatomii Domashnikh Zhivotnykh* (Principles of Pathologic Anatomy of Domestic Animals), published in Warsaw in 1896–1898, one of the first Russian textbooks in this field.[330] He revised it in 1900, 1906, and 1913,[338] and followed it in 1913 with a book on meat

*Mari's dissertation on actinomycosis is listed by Petrov,[414] in his compilation of dissertations accepted by Russian universities, as Kazan, 1890, and not Kharkov, 1891. The discrepancy between Krapivner's account and this listing is one I cannot explain.

†There are numerous examples of how the Russians treated the Poles. Millak[354] mentions that when the Polish veterinarians in Warsaw began to publish the "Diaries of the Warsaw Veterinary Society," they were forced to publish a parallel edition in Russian, although the Society hardly had any Russian members.

inspection, the only Russian treatise on this subject, which was revised posthumously by Andreev in 1929.[339]
Mari (along with Nikolai P. Savvaitov) also translated Ostertag's famous book on meat hygiene into Russian and published it in two volumes in St. Petersburg in 1907 and 1908. Mari contributed articles on veterinary medicine and tuberculosis to the "Large Encyclopedia of Russian Agriculture, 1900–1912."[54]

The third edition of Mari's pathology book (Fig. 46), published in 1906, was reviewed by N. D. Ball, his successor in Warsaw, and met with a hostile reception.[37] He complained that, on the one hand, the book barely took cognizance of pathological histology, cornerstone of pathology, whereas, on the other, it overemphasized bacteriology, a discipline important enough to merit books of its own. Ball also complained that the book did not stand comparison with Kitt's veterinary pathology book in German.* Ball deplored that veterinarians who could not read German, and were therefore waiting to read a pathology book in Russian, had not been adequately served by Mari and must continue their wait.

I have been unable to get a look at the first two editions of Mari's book, which Ball says were better printed and reflected better the state of knowledge at the time they appeared. These first two editions were published privately by Mari while he was actively teaching veterinary pathology in Warsaw. He would therefore have had more control over the quality of the pictures, for instance, than in the third edition, published in St. Petersburg by a commercial publisher. While conducting autopsies (although I do not know how many he did), he would also have been closely in touch with reality as encountered in the autopsy room in the practical instruction

*Mari's book had but few illustrations, most of them borrowed—from Kitt, Johne, Ziegler, Neumann, Friedberger and Fröhner, and from a dozen other German and French authors.

Н. Н. Мари,

Профессоръ Императорской Военно-Медицинской Академіи.

ОСНОВЫ

ПАТОЛОГИЧЕСКОЙ АНАТОМІИ

домашнихъ животныхъ.

Патолого-анатомическая діагностика.

Для ветеринарныхъ врачей, врачей и студентовъ.

Съ 177 рис. въ текстѣ.

ИЗДАНІЕ ТРЕТЬЕ.

значительно исправленное и дополненное.

С.-ПЕТЕРБУРГЪ

Изданіе «Практической Ветеринаріи».

Нижегородская, 15.

1906.

Figure 46. Title page of the third edition of N. N. Mari's book "Principles of Pathologic Anatomy of Domestic Animals," published in St. Petersburg in 1906. The subtitle indicates that the book is for veterinarians, physicians, and students.

of veterinary students. Once Mari left Warsaw for St. Petersburg, this influence would no longer prevail; whatever instruction he gave on comparative pathology to the medical students in the Military-Medical Academy was merely lecturing.

Mari's preoccupation with bacteriology was understandable in a situation where most of the important diseases then recognized were infectious. Ball's criticism could have been leveled with equal fairness, for instance, at Gaiger and Davies' *Veterinary Pathology and Bacteriology,* which came out in Britain a quarter of a century later. Mari should have done what Kitt had done early in his career; separate his writings—obviously his daily work itself did not lend itself to such separation—into books on pathology and other books on bacteriology.

Another influence is visible in the third edition of Mari's book, the only one of the four I have seen. This is a Slavophil emphasis that perhaps is worthy of a few moments of reflection. His book is unusually thoroughly documented—bibliographic citations abound on almost every page, and many are also annotated in accompanying footnotes. These cited works are predominantly Western; Mari seems not to have overlooked anything of significance. However, he has also mined deeply in the Russian publications of the years 1885–1905, and citations of Russian works are very numerous.

Was he influenced by his exposure to the Poles for 10 years into a Slavophil attitude? Did his residence in the capital of Russia, with its extreme conservatism, conduce to this? Did his trouble with the authorities in 1888 lead him to try to become a conformist? Eventually, in 1916, the government would entrust him with the acting directorship of the prestigious Military-Medical Academy; was he already heading in this direction in 1906?

The Slavophil attitude is expressed overtly in the fourth

(1913) edition of his book, which I have not seen, but is clearly implied in Khomitskii's citation from its preface: "The reader will notice that special attention has been paid to our native literature. The times when books by Russian scientists and investigators could be ignored are past beyond all question."[241] As pointed out above, however, Mari had already begun to emphasize Russian work in his third edition in 1906. I can only raise questions regarding this fascinating man's efforts to educate his countrymen; I cannot answer them. Thus, it would be interesting to know whether Ball's criticism goaded Mari into improving his book in the fourth edition, but, unfortunately, I have been unable to find a copy for comparison.

Mari spent time in study abroad in Austria, France, Germany, and Switzerland during the years 1892, 1896, and 1898, but I do not know with whom he worked.[224] He left Warsaw in 1902 for St. Petersburg, where he was appointed professor of comparative pathology at the Military-Medical Academy (see Chapter 4).

We return now to Nikolai D. Ball (Fig. 47). Born in Podolsk, Russia, in 1872, he first studied animal husbandry and later veterinary medicine, the latter at Dorpat, graduating in 1897. He stayed on at Dorpat for two years as prosector in the pathology department, working under Waldmann, Semmer's successor in the chair of pathology. During 1897, he was awarded a gold medal in a prize competition for research papers. His topic dealt with the healing of fractures in the chicken; he did this work during his last months as an undergraduate.[36,417]

Ball expanded the above work into a larger research project on experimental osseous pathology and wrote up the results in his dissertation for the M.V.Sc. degree, awarded in 1899.[628] As related by Chernyak,[151] the world of veterinary pathology in Russia at that time consisted of four one- or two-man departments, and there was no place where Ball

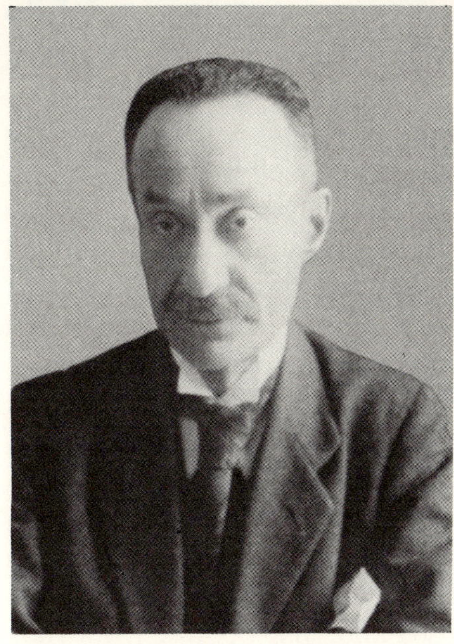

Figure 47. Nikolai D. Ball, about 1929.

could go for further study or to work in his specialty. He took a job as director of a veterinary assistant's (*feldsher*) school which he organized in Tomsk, Siberia. Eventually (in 1903) he was appointed assistant professor* at the Warsaw Veterinary Institute as successor to N. N. Mari.

One of Ball's early interests at Warsaw was teratology, and he began a collection of malformations in 1904.[297] From this

*There was no *professor* of pathology; the Warsaw Veterinary Institute was never granted the same status, posts, or salaries by the imperial Russian government as the other three veterinary schools in the empire at Dorpat, Kazan, and Kharkov.[356] Thus pathology did not enjoy the distinction of a chair, and as Millak (p. 91) shows, in 1904, Ball was paid but 1,200 rubles per year as compared to the 1,500 rubles paid to the professor of therapy and 2,800 rubles to the bacteriologist.[356] As a Russian, however, Ball was entitled to a 300-ruble increase every five years, whereas the Polish faculty members were not allowed to receive this. The annual budgets of the four schools in 1912 were: Kharkov, 75,573 rubles; Kazan, 73,850; Dorpat, 57,000; and Warsaw, 46,962 (Koropov,[264] p. 124).

collection resulted a publication on ectopic lungs in 1910[40] and another, by his student Lindtrop, on malformations of the spleen.[297]

In 1907, Ball wrote a lengthy description of the Pathological Institute at the Berlin Veterinary College, tracing veterinary pathology in that institution from its beginnings by Gurlt in the early nineteenth century up to 1904, when Ball worked there under Schütz.[38] From this paper it is clear that Ball knew of the best in German veterinary pathology and was impatient to raise the Russian discipline to that status. Ball acquired his familiarity with German, Austrian, and Swiss pathology also by working in the veterinary colleges in Vienna (Johann Csokor) and Bern (Karl Guillebeau) in 1904, the pathology department of the medical school in Leipzig (Felix Marchand*) in 1906, and with Ernst Joest in Dresden in 1908.[532] I believe that he was able to travel so much in Europe between 1904 and 1908 because from 1905 to 1907 the Warsaw Veterinary Institute was closed in reprisal for the student participation in the revolution of 1905 (Millak,[356] p. 379).

In his historical paper, Ball points out the influence of Virchow, Müller, Meckel, and others on human and hence veterinary pathology and expresses gratitude to the Berlin Veterinary College and to Professor Schütz for their kindness and helpfulness in training veterinarians from the Russian Empire."† Clearly, Schütz, who did not suffer fools gladly,[469] had made Ball feel at home during his sojourn—which tells us something about Ball's aptitude and ability.

Ball's historical paper, designed to acquaint the Russian

*Professor Marchand also contributed to the education of another veterinary pathologist, the Danish A. F. Følger, who studied with him in 1909.[175]

†Ball was at this time in Warsaw even though this paper was published in the Dorpat journal. Whether this gratitude is for help to the Dorpat faculty, the Warsaw faculty, or both is not clearly indicated.

veterinary reader with how much he is indebted to the traditions, discoveries, and advances made by the Berlin College—particularly its Pathological Institute—suggests to me that Ball considered himself to have inherited this tradition, that he had benefited from it, and was inspired by it to introduce modern pathology, its ideas, and its methods to whatever extent he could to his compatriots. Thus, when the Dorpat Veterinary Institute commenced publication of its own scientific journal in 1906, Ball collaborated by submitting abstracts of the foreign literature on pathology.[39] I believe his later career can be explained (in part) by thinking of him as motivated by an amalgam of pride in the achievements of German veterinary pathology and a boundless determination to impart these achievements—and, if possible, greater ones—to his colleagues at home.*

Thus we see that Bohl and Ball, the founders of the respective schools of veterinary pathology in Russia, were both products of and influenced by their German training—an exposure that imprinted its stamp deeply upon them and was in turn conveyed by them to their scientific descendants. (It is of interest that both of them were members of the Russian delegation to the Ninth International Veterinary Congress in The Hague in 1909 and appear in the picture of that group [see frontispiece] with I. I. Shukevich and N. N. Mari, two more of the historical figures described in this book.[182] The delegation was heavily weighted with pathologists.)

By 1913 or 1914, Ball had acquired an assistant, N. V. Landa, who published a paper in the latter year on ossification of the myocardium in the horse.[290] Although Landa is

*His interest in history was still evident two decades later, when he gave three lectures in Leningrad entitled: "History of the veterinary schools of Western Europe," "History of the development of Russian veterinary schools," and "History of pathologic anatomy of animals as a scientific discipline."[45] (His prosector, Belkin, had attended and reported on the first All-Union meeting of pathologists in Kiev in 1927.)

not mentioned in Millak's book on the Warsaw Veterinary Institute,[356] he is listed in this paper as being from the pathology department of that Institute. Landa later worked with Ball in Moscow[291] and then received the chair of pathology at the Saratov Veterinary Institute in the middle 1920s.[292]

In 1915 the German army was threatening Warsaw, and the imperial Russian government took the decision to evacuate the Veterinary Institute to prevent its falling into enemy hands.* The Institute was moved, and Ball with it, first to Moscow† and shortly thereafter (1916) to Novocherkassk[356,553] where it was directed by N. N. Mari, who left Petrograd to assume this post. Because the pathological museum had perforce been left behind in Warsaw (Millak,[356] p. 250), Ball had to build a department of pathology under war conditions (and later revolution and civil war) as best he could.

How terrible these conditions were, the chaos and often anarchy that prevailed in those times, we can hardly imagine. It helps to know that Novocherkassk changed hands four times in two years during the Civil War.[174]‡ The economy of

*This evacuation involved many institutions, particularly factories, and Westwood tells us that during the three months that it lasted, it produced a railway crisis "choking junctions, disorganizing stations, and exacerbating the car shortage."[632] Warsaw was occupied by the Germans on August 5.

†Apparently, no clinical or laboratory teaching was conducted during the brief period that the faculty was in Moscow, although a British observer reported that life went on there much as usual. Lockhart[302] writes: "Theatres and places of amusement flourished as in peace time, and, although the proletariat and peasantry were deprived of their alcohol, no such restrictions were imposed on the well-to-do classes. To replenish their private stock of wine they required a permit, but, as the cost of living rose and since Russian officials were badly paid, permits were easily obtainable. In restaurants the only difference was that one drank one's alcohol from a teapot instead of from a bottle."

‡Following the Tsar's abdication in February 1917, there was a brief period of democratic government. After the Bolshevik seizure of power in

the region was in ruins, much of the land unploughed, the harvests meager, and food short.[306] Nevertheless, some teaching of sorts went on despite all of the disruptions. For example, Władysław Walkiewicz (1896–1941), a Polish refugee student, who accompanied the faculty in its flight from Warsaw, studied under Ball at Novocherkassk and graduated as a veterinarian in 1919 (Fig. 48). He emigrated to Poland in 1920 and, after serving in the Polish Veterinary Corps, taught veterinary pathology at Warsaw in 1922–1924 and from 1927 to 1939 (Millak,[356] pp. 196 and 251). He perished in the Katyn Forest massacre, in which Stalin had four thousand Polish officers murdered.

One of the students at the Novocherkassk Veterinary Institute was Aleksandr A. Pinus (1896–1963), who likewise graduated in 1919 (Fig. 49). He joined the Red Army as a veterinary officer and received further training in pathology under N. D. Ball during the years 1922–1926. Stationed in Kiev during the late 1920s, he worked in the department of pathology of the Kiev Medical Institute under Professor Pavlo A. Kucherenko, a medical pathologist. During his Kiev sojourn, he published two scientific papers,[415] and later he wrote the obituary of his mentor, Ball, within the time span to which I am restricting this book.[418] Although he was one of the best of the Soviet veterinary pathologists, the rest of

---

Petrograd in October 1917, the Don Cossacks set up an independent local government in Novocherkassk. This collapsed in February 1918, when the Bolsheviks occupied the city and established their authority over the region for the first time. Longworth[306] relates that Bolshevik rule on the Don quickly became very unpopular. This was not only because of the forced requisitioning of grain; for example, the Reds showed their contempt for religion by stabling their horses in Novocherkassk Cathedral! An anti-Bolshevik rebel Cossack band took the city from the Reds in April and held it for several days.[306] Then the Bolsheviks retook it, but they were again driven out by a Cossack rising in May of 1918, at which time Footman[174] writes: "Novocherkassk had no public services and no police." The final occupation of the city by the Red Army occurred late in 1919.

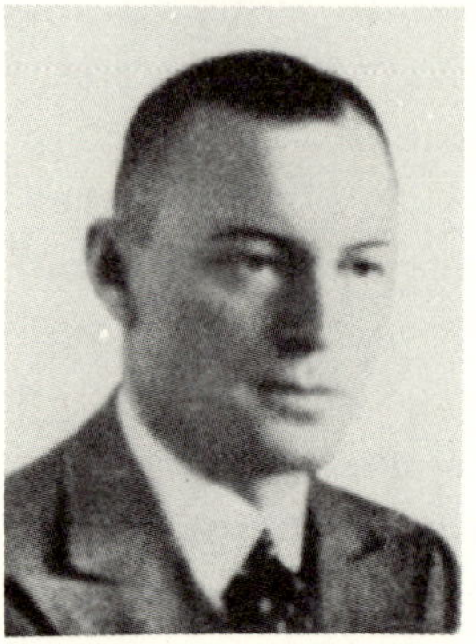

Figure 48. Władysław Walkiewicz.

Pinus' scientific work falls outside of our historical compass, and I have therefore omitted allusion to it. An exception is his very useful historical account of veterinary pathology in Russia, which he presented during the first All-Union Conference of Veterinary Pathologists in Voronezh in 1961.[418] Although unsupported by specific bibliographic citations, the allusions, clues, and hints with which it is replete have often guided me to more detailed sources of information. The greatest value of Pinus' historical paper lies in the perspective it provided—a panoramic view of veterinary pathology in Russia during the period I am discussing here.

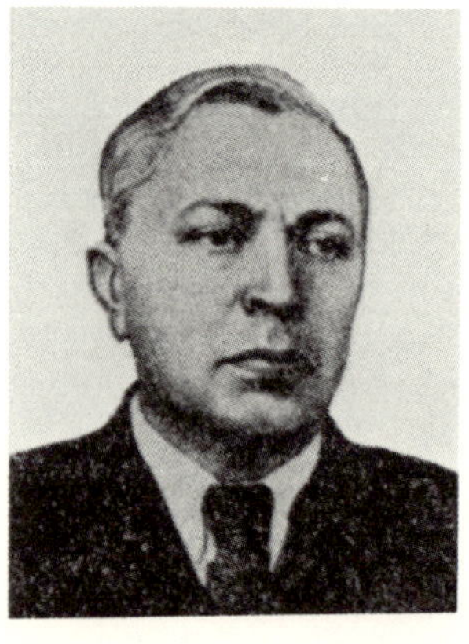

Figure 49. Aleksander A. Pinus.

Somehow, in the midst of all the chaos that reigned in Novocherkassk, Ball managed to write two papers in 1919, one on the pathology of gout in chickens[41] and one on hepatic amyloidosis in a cat[42], and even found photographic film to illustrate them! In addition, he supervised the work of a student, Lipnik, who published a study on myocardial lesions in horses.[298] The cat, incidentally, had been autopsied by Ball in February of 1916 in the Hospital of the Society for the Protection of Animals in Moscow during his brief sojourn there between Warsaw and Novocherkassk. One must marvel at his ability not to lose the autopsy record in the course of the move. One does not know whom to admire more, Skryabin, the editor of the newly founded journal of the Novocherkassk Veterinary Institute, for scrounging enough paper to print it on in times of extreme scarcity,[393] or Ball for managing to publish on this paper, which by 1978 was yellow, brittle, and shortly due to crumble into dust. Ball remained in Novocherkassk* as head of the pathology department until 1920. That year he was invited to come to Moscow to join the founding faculty of the newly established Moscow Veterinary Institute, later renamed the Moscow Veterinary Academy.

Professor Mari published his last paper[341] in Novocherkassk in 1920 and died in Moscow a year later.

*Arndt[30] states (p. 223) that the Novocherkassk Veterinary Institute was obliged under the terms of the peace treaty with Poland to return most of the "inventory" of items that had been removed from the Warsaw Veterinary Institute. I have found no reference to this return in Millak's history of the Warsaw school. He says, in fact (p. 250), that when the Institute was evacuated in 1915, the collections of the pathological institute had to be left behind, and that because of lack of care and supervision, many items were lost. The chances are that Arndt is right about the terms of the treaty, but that, as with many other treaties, the Bolsheviks did not fulfill it.

8 The Moscow Veterinary Institute

The belly is ungrateful—it always forgets we already gave it something.

—Russian proverb

By 1920, the Civil War was raging, but there was no fighting near Moscow itself, and the men who shaped events there took the decision to found the Moscow Veterinary Institute. Of the four veterinary schools that had existed within the Russian Empire until 1917, two had been lost to the emerging newly independent nations of Poland and Estonia; there was thus an urgent need to replace them with schools within the borders of the new republic.* It was decided to commence veterinary education in Omsk and in Moscow. Once the decision had been taken to establish a veterinary school in Moscow, Professor Ball was a natural choice for its faculty; the Veterinary Directorate could not afford to let a man of his caliber languish in the provinces. Thus, in the short space of three years, Ball moved once again, from Novocherkassk back to Moscow, and spent the next two years, along with the rest of the founding faculty, getting things ready to receive the entering students in 1922. (According to Shishkov,[535] Ball made the move in 1919, not 1920, but this is in conflict with other sources.)[151,418]

*Part of the Dorpat faculty was in Saratov and of the Warsaw faculty in Novocherkassk, but the former veterinary school was barely viable and the latter was very small.

That year, veterinary education began again in Moscow after a lapse of almost 80 years, with Ball as head of the Institute's pathology department. For the second—but not last—time in his life, he had to organize a laboratory and a teaching department from scratch, and that while organizing teaching and diagnostic activities at the Military Veterinary Bacteriological Institute and fulfilling both scientific and administrative duties at VIEV.

By 1919, the Bolsheviks had seized and held power in Russia for almost two years, but were still threatened by civil war and foreign intervention. The previous year they had organized the Red Army, which in lieu of motor transport contained a large complement of horse-drawn vehicles, horse artillery, and, to aid in recruiting volunteers, a prestige cavalry corps, Budenny's* 1st Mounted Army.[343a] The Red Army was at first known as the Workers' and Peasants' Red Army, and only they and no one from the bourgeoisie or nobility was allowed to serve as a combatant. This stricture could not, of course, be applied to medical or veterinary officers, and those who wished to volunteer were accepted eagerly even though they had served in the tsarist medical or veterinary corps.[21]

It was not easy to recruit for even the cavalry portion of this Red Army among the war-weary tsarist troops and civilians, and the poster artists resorted to no little artistic license in depicting the mounts that awaited potential cavalrymen (Fig. 50). As one can see from a picture of one of Professor Ball's visits to the field (Fig. 51), the horseflesh in reality looked somewhat less ideal even in 1922, by which time most of the

*Named after Semeon M. Budenny (see Appendix II).

†It was soon found necessary to also accept tsarist combatant officers, as there were not nearly enough workers and peasants capable of reading and writing, let alone exercising command or carrying out staff duties. Later, when voluntary recruiting failed, conscription was introduced for enlisted men, and coercion was used when staff or field officers of experience and ability were needed.

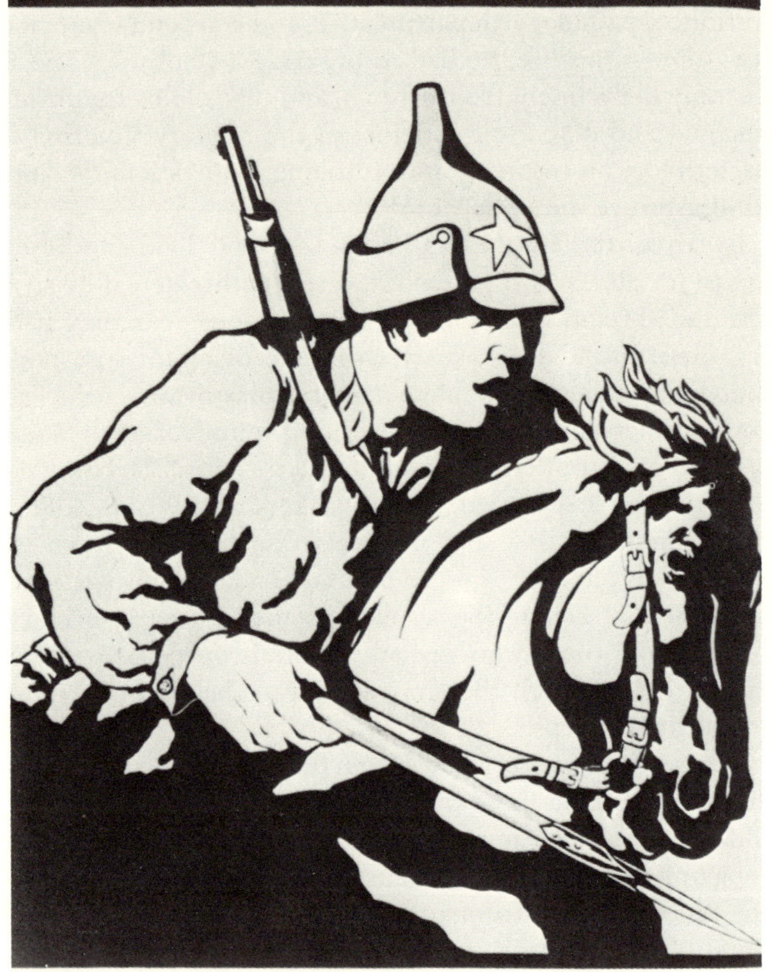

Figure 50. A recruiting poster in Ukrainian, inviting one to "Join the Red Cavalry!"

fighting was over. But during 1918–1920 it must have been difficult to find a heroic looking animal among the thousands of underfed, overworked, mangy, glandered, and otherwise afflicted troop horses that served loyally in both the Red and the White armies. When one considers their

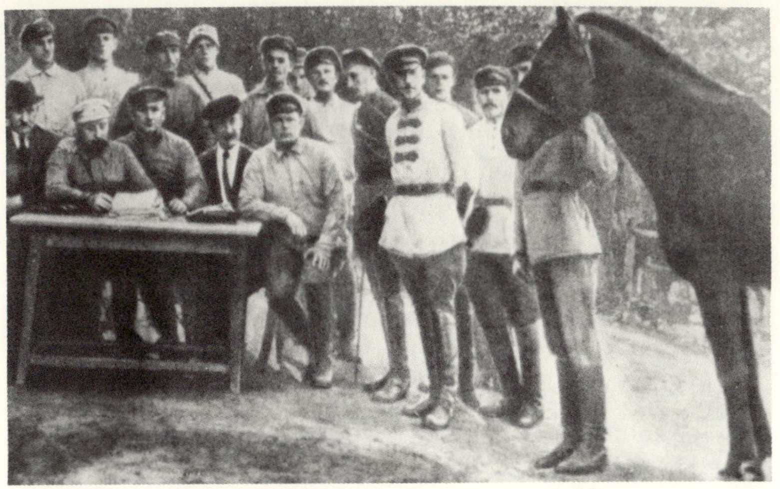

Figure 51. Professor N. D. Ball at a field inspection of horses in a cavalry formation in 1922. Seated from left to right are Professor Vyshelesskii, divisional veterinarian Grigorov, divisional commander Kotovskii, Professor Ball, and deputy chief of the Red Army Veterinary Corps Vlasov.

incredible suffering from hunger or poor fodder, forced marches, exposure to voracious Siberian mosquitoes and biting flies, heat, dust, rain and frost, lack of blankets, horseshoes,[127] and decent saddlery, one can only rejoice that horses are no longer employed in warfare.*

The head of the Red Army veterinary corps, N. M. Nikolskii, soon realized that it was necessary to organize a military bacteriological laboratory to diagnose the infectious diseases that were raging across the country, particularly glanders and other respiratory afflictions, affecting military and farm animals alike.[186] This laboratory was founded in

*The suffering of a stallion carrying an untutored rider on its back, its festering saddle sores aggravated by the flies, is nowhere more vividly portrayed than by Isaac Babel, in his story "Argamak" in the book *Red Cavalry.*[33] This deals with the year 1920; writing as late as 1937, Trotsky, the first Bolshevik Commissar of War, mentioned that the quality of the horses in the Soviet Union was still far below that of France or the United States.[599]

Moscow in 1922 and at first experienced severe problems. Zagrodzki[642] relates that it occupied several rooms on the fourth floor of a house at 51 Arbat Street, rooms that were dirty, dark, and without heat, so that the cultures froze solid inside the incubators! Later conditions improved somewhat. Undaunted, as usual, Professor Ball organized its department of pathology. From this laboratory he trained the pathologist staff for several branch military diagnostic laboratories throughout the country. Ball later (about 1924) temporarily gave up direction of this laboratory as he assumed other duties, but he never gave up his interest in military veterinary medicine and its problems. He served on the editorial board of the short-lived (1920–1921) *Voenno-Veterinarnyi Vestnik* (Military Veterinary Herald), and during the Civil War and afterward he kept in touch with practical military problems* by visiting formations in the field (Fig. 51).

In 1926, when the Central Military Veterinary Bacteriologic Institute† moved to Leningrad, he resumed direction of its pathology department. His contributions as consultant to the veterinary corps were recognized during the celebration of the tenth anniversary of the Red Army.[418] Ball's considerable talents as an organizer were quickly recognized by the new regime, desperate for officials with even

*Of these there was no dearth, and he set his brightest pupil, Chernyak, to work on pulmonary lesions caused by worms and by fungi and on the distinction of both from glanders. This problem was of critical significance to the Red Army, because, on the one hand, glanders was taking a terrible toll of horses and, on the other, animals were being killed with lesions that resembled glanders, but were not. To help one understand the prevailing conditions, Chernyak reported that in 1922, near the end of the Civil War, the cavalry horses not infrequently were fed moldy hay and oats. In one formation, from which he got 16 cases of pneumomycosis out of 62 autopsies, it had been necessary to resort to straw from thatched roofs as fodder for the horses![143]

†Just a few years later, Sir Frederick Hobday visited it and reported that it was well staffed and well equipped.[210]

minimum competence, and were used repeatedly in a series of new situations where he was asked to undertake the creation of something out of nothing. He always succeeded. Although his organizational talents were unmatched by any other veterinary pathologist in Russia, it is as a teacher that he left his deepest mark on our specialty.

Simultaneously with his teaching duties, Professor Ball also reorganized the Veterinary Laboratory of the Ministry of Internal Affairs. In an ill-considered move, opposed by all of its staff, but insisted upon by the government, it had been evacuated in October 1918 from Petrograd to a suburb of Moscow, to be the national veterinary research center. It was first named the Government Institute of Experimental Veterinary Medicine (GIEV), and later the All-Union Institute (VIEV).† Ball took it over in 1922, at which time it had been floundering for four years, never having recovered from its disastrous move, in the course of which most of its equipment had been lost, stolen, or destroyed. He headed it for two years, until 1924, and got it more or less on its feet, turning out a small amount of useful research work, but chiefly making vaccines and diagnostic reagents.[43] I think it is fair to say that during the period of time covered by this book, from 1922 to 1930, the VIEV did not amount to much except on paper. This was because of lack of material resources rather than lack of adequate direction on Ball's part. The recovery from the Civil War was slow, and trying to build an institute of national rather than local scope must have been monumentally frustrating. In the first volume of VIEV's scientific proceedings, some of this can be read between the lines of Ball's annual report.[43] One paper dating from this period, by N. V. Landa, who had earlier been Ball's

†Moscow bureaucrats are even fonder of acronyms than our own. These two are derived as follows: GIEV (*Gosudarstvennyi Institut Eksperimentalnoi Veterinarii*); VIEV (*Vsesoyuznyi Institut Eksperimentalnoi Veterinarii*).

assistant in Warsaw, indicates that veterinary pathologists were participating in meetings of the Moscow Section of the Russian Society of Pathologists as far back as 1923.[291]

The reason Ball gave up the direction of VIEV, or was replaced, is not given by the sources I have read,[114,151,532] but can perhaps be surmised from the fact that he reorganized and headed its pathology department during the subsequent two years. I am assuming, admittedly with little evidence, that his interest in pathology and, above all, in teaching, overcame his interest in administration. Ball was a conscientious man, with a high sense of duty, but there must always have been others waiting in the wings ready to take over prestigious posts. It would be nice to be able to find some detailed historical data, to know what actually took place and why, but I do not have access to the necessary sources. Even assuming that the information was published, the publication of veterinary journals in the early 1920s was so erratic and the availability of such journals as did appear so limited—none in North America and few in Western Europe as far as I can find out—that I cannot pursue this further. While considerable useful research work emanated from the pathology department of VIEV, which was headed from 1926 to 1959 by B. G. Ivanov, a pupil of Bohl's, it falls outside the era discussed in this book.

In 1924, Ball was one of the delegates from Russian academic institutions who attended the 50-year jubilee of the Kazan Veterinary Institute.[18] Also that year, in concert with an editorial board that included K. H. Bohl and K. I. Skryabin, Ball helped found the journal *Prakticheskaya Veterinariya i Konevodstvo* (Practical Veterinary Medicine and Horse Husbandry) which later became *Veterinariya,* the national veterinary journal of the country.[203] This venture was actively supported by Nikolskii, the chief of the veterinary corps, and Budenny, the Inspector of Cavalry.[128,203]

9 The Leningrad Veterinary Institute

I tell everyone very plainly that I take bribes, but what kind of bribes? Why, greyhound puppies.

—Nikolai Gogol, *The Inspector-General*

In 1926, four years after teaching had begun, the new Moscow Veterinary Institute was forced to close for a time because the proliferating bureaucracy in the capital had created a shortage of buildings. After a long lapse—40 years—veterinary instruction was being resumed in Petrograd—newly renamed Leningrad—and Ball transferred to the recently organized Leningrad Veterinary Institute* as head of its pathology department. For the fifth—and last—time, he organized a new pathology laboratory, a museum, and both an undergraduate and a graduate teaching department from the ground up. In the meantime, as already mentioned, the Military Veterinary Bacteriological Institute was also moved to Leningrad, and Ball resumed direction of its pathology department. This provided him with abundant equine material for research and for teaching.

In 1929, Ball assumed editorship of the annual scientific publication of the Leningrad Veterinary Insttitute, of which volume 1 had appeared in 1927, complete with German summaries of each article. He served as rector of the Institute for two years,[418] which means he was responsible for

*It had apparently commenced limited operations in 1920, but a listing of the teaching staff of 1921-1925 shows that many disciplines were not then represented.[288]

directing the whole operation during its formative period, as well as his own department.

From 1926 until his death, Ball also collaborated editorially on the *Jahresbericht der Veterinärmedizin,* published in Berlin, by abstracting Russian articles on pathology and enlisting his assistants Belkin* and Chernyak to do likewise. Where he found time to do all this among his other duties can only be guessed. Certainly he could not have been lacking in energy or drive.

Ball's accomplishments and contributions do not lend themselves to facile analysis. They cannot be measured by the customary yardstick of books and papers published, for he lived and worked in chaotic times, his country rent by war, revolution, and civil war, and his life must have been in constant turmoil for at least the decade between 1916 and 1926. One's imagination falters at the thought of a person imbued with such zeal in the pursuit of excellence under such adverse circumstances. Being repeatedly uprooted does not conduce to the calm necessary for observing, thinking, and writing, even if one is moving between already existing, well-staffed, and well-equipped institutes in a country without food, fuel, equipment, and paper shortages. In these respects, Ball's lot was not a happy one, but three obituaries (by his Estonian student Laas,[289] by Pinus and Romanov,[418] and by Chernyak[151]) leave no doubt that Ball was undaunted by it, and that he had a tremendous impact on all with whom he entered into a teacher-student relationship. Ball's creative drive found expression in his teaching—he was an enthusiastic and inspiring teacher, whose fervor kindled the spark of interest in his students that is the hallmark of all great teachers. He saw clearly what had to be done in his specialty

*After training under Ball,[50–52] Grigorii Yakovlevich Belkin (1896–1954) became professor of pathology in the newly founded Belorussian Veterinary Institute in Vitebsk in 1926. Most of his publications are beyond the era covered in this book.[133,548] In the early 1930s he also served as acting professor in the Vitebsk Medical Institute.[568]

to improve it and with it veterinary medicine as a whole, and he did it with élan and originality of approach—in a backward country, during ruinous times, and beset by ill health—by the sheer force of his personality, tenacity of purpose, and intellect.

Ball left pathology firmly entrenched in the veterinary corps of the army* and on a solid scientific footing in three newly founded veterinary schools and the national veterinary research establishment (VIEV). Veterinarians trained by him established branch diagnostic laboratories in military formations stationed throughout the Soviet Union. The main one did research on anthrax[392] and the one in Kiev also was used for research on anthrax vaccines and on swine erysipelas.[367] Ball's lasting contribution was in the institutions he organized and left in flourishing condition and in the men he taught who staffed them, able to go on to practice their specialty on their own, with a thorough scientific preparation and inspired with zest and enthusiasm.†

As already mentioned, Ball was on the editorial board of the *Archiv für Tierheilkunde,* and in the June 1931 issue we find a moving dedication‡ at the head of an article in German by his most gifted student, Chernyak. Apart from this, his death in 1930 passed unmentioned in the non-Russian world, insofar as I can determine from my searches of the Western literature (except Laas, mentioned above). Fur-

*Horses were to remain a vital part of military transport throughout the 1930s, as pointed out by Trotsky[599] and later by Khrushchev.[242]

†In 1929, Nöller visited the Veterinary Institute in Saratov, started by the Russian faculty that had left Dorpat a decade earlier. He found the physical facilities of the pathology department rather limited, but said the rich and varied teaching material was to be envied and remarked particularly on the energy and enthusiasm with which Professor Landa and his staff worked it up. Landa was another Ball protégé, who had worked with him in Warsaw and later in Moscow, at VIEV, in the early 1920s.[290,291,292]

‡"*Dem unvergesslichen Andenken unseres teuren Lehrers, des Professors NIKOLAI BALL, in tiefster Ehrfurcht gewidmet von den Verfassern.*" (Dedicated by the authors in deepest reverence to the unforgettable memory of our dear teacher, Professor NIKOLAI BALL.)

thermore, although the pathology and pathogenesis of glanders was worked out thoroughly by Ball and his colleagues (1924–1928), this work has, to my knowledge, never been cited in foreign textbooks, including the otherwise encyclopedic Hutyra and Marek, and remains practically unknown abroad.*

By the time of Ball's death, regrettably brief though his allotted span at Leningrad had been, he had trained enough good men to assure his succession. More than that, they were of a quality to make their presence felt in the ensuing three decades, so that by the 1960s an evolutionary trend could be discerned which led Soviet veterinary pathologists to speak of two "schools": those of Ball and of K. H. Bohl. Of course, Bohl kept adding people to his "school" in the quarter century after Ball's death, but since the "schools" were already existent in 1930, it seems logical to end my chronicle of veterinary pathology in Russia at that point. The subsequent development of veterinary pathology in the Soviet Union was made by the followers of Ball and Bohl, and its history has still to be written, although an outline has been sketched by Ivanov.[214]

In limiting the era discussed in this book to the year of Ball's death in 1930, we leave our consideration of veterinary pathology in Russia before the various pupils of Bohl and Ball had had a chance to make their mark. A brief exception should be made of Valentin Z. Chernyak (1893–1963), who deserves more detailed treatment than he can be accorded here (Fig. 52). A graduate of the Warsaw Veterinary Institute in 1917 (after its evacuation to Novocherkassk) and a protégé of Ball's, under whom he studied as an under-

*It is alluded to in B. K. Bohl's *Pathologie des Lungenrotz* in the *Zeitschrift Infektkr. Haustiere 35:* 1, 1930, but no specific citations are given. Abstracts appeared in the *Jahresbericht der Veterinärmedizin 46:* 928, 934, 1926; *47:* 823, 1927; *48:* 847, 1928; *49:* 856, 1929, and in the *Berliner Tierärztl. Wochenschrift.*

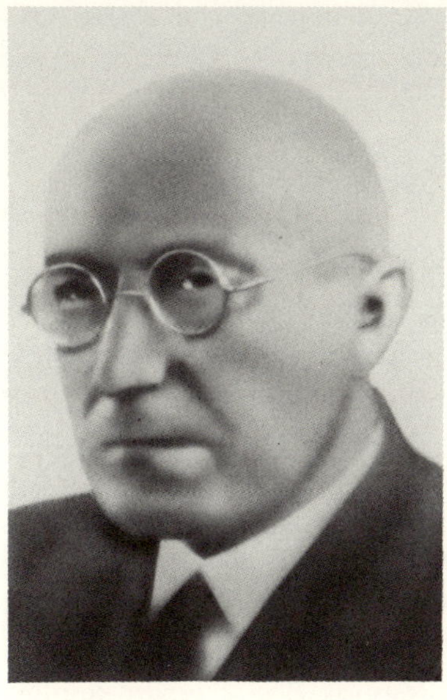

Figure 52. Valentin Z. Chernyak.

graduate, Chernyak served in the Red Army during the Civil War and then went to the Moscow Veterinary Institute in 1922. He worked there with Ball and went with him to Leningrad in 1926, continuing as his assistant.

I believe that Chernyak had become a competent pathologist by 1930, even though most of his productive work still lay ahead of him. He was to establish a reputation in the years beyond this chronicle for original contributions to the pathology of equine infectious anemia. Between 1923 and 1930 he published considerable work on glanders and mycotic infections of horses.[136–145,575] His work on the latter made him then, and for many years thereafter, the leading authority on mycotic diseases in the veterinary world.

He is also noteworthy here because, like Pinus, he was active near the end of his life as a historian, so that his views and his writings comprise part of the materials that shape this chronicle. As with Pinus' works, I have included only his historical publications for the period beyond 1930.[149–151]

10 Miscellaneous Institutions

> From the present complexity of medical science it is tempting to look back a hundred years or so as if to a golden age, when knowledge was relatively simple and new discoveries were waiting like ripe peaches to be picked.
>
> —Lester S. King, *The Growth of Medical Thought*

Most of the research and diagnostic activity in veterinary pathology took place within the larger cities described in the preceding chapters. However, a lesser amount of activity germane to the theme of this book occurred in smaller centers, some of which is briefly touched upon in this chapter.

The Omsk Veterinary Institute

The work of Professor S. A. Gryuner is treated in this chronicle for two reasons. He made several contributions to veterinary pathology, although most of his work, published and otherwise, was in ancillary fields. He is also the only Russian veterinarian I know of who spent a study leave in the United States. During that time, he lectured to an American audience about veterinary medicine in Russia, and this alone is of sufficient interest to warrant a brief sketch of Gryuner.

Sergei Aleksandrovich Gryuner (1864–1931) was born in Warsaw and received some of his preliminary education in the Mikhaelov Artillery School (Fig. 53).[549] In 1884 he studied botany in the St. Petersburg Forestry Institute. He came to the Dorpat Veterinary Institute on a state scholarship in

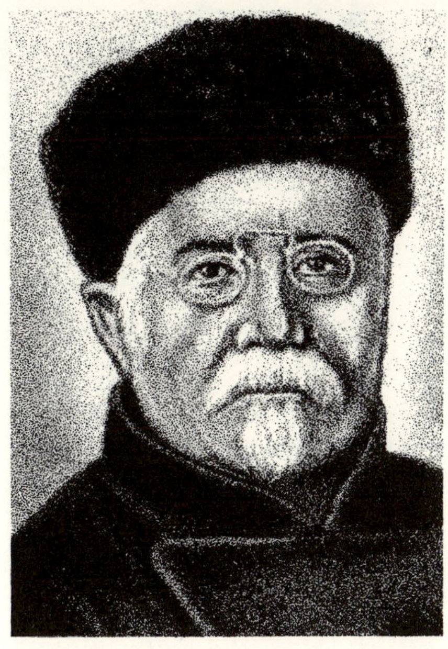

Figure 53. Sergei A. Gryuner.

1886 and graduated as a veterinarian in 1890. He was thus in one of the last classes to be taught pathology by Eugen Semmer. Gryuner then served in the army as a veterinary officer in a variety of cavalry and artillery units from 1890 to 1898. During one of these assignments, in 1896, he was enabled to do advanced study and take the examination for the M.V.Sc. degree at the Warsaw Veterinary Institute. The following year he was posted temporarily to the Dorpat Veterinary Institute, where he wrote and defended his dissertation and was awarded the degree. He was then assigned to a military post in Khabarovsk.

In 1899, Gryuner studied bacteriology with Professor G. N. Gabrichevsky in Moscow, and from 1899 to 1900 he worked as veterinarian of the Poltava *Zemstvo,** then from

**Zemstvo,* an elected district council in prerevolutionary Russia, which had a limited amount of autonomy in the running of local affairs, including the hiring of physicians and veterinarians.

1901 to 1902 of the Voronezh *Zemstvo.* During this period, he enjoyed a brief study leave at the Veterinary College of Munich. In 1905–1906 he went on an official study tour to Berlin, Copenhagen, Stockholm, and Vienna. In the latter city he learned applied bacteriology from Professor Anton Weichselbaum, head of the pathology department of the medical school and pioneer research worker in pneumococcal pneumonia and meningitis. Gryuner's biography in the *Veterinarnaya Entsiklopediya*[553] stated that he also visited Japan, Alaska, and the continental United States during the above years; however, this information was wrong with respect to the latter countries. This biography does not mention that he also made a study trip abroad in 1902, but his bibliography shows that he published a report of this trip in an obscure provincial veterinary journal.[190]

Upon his return to Russia in 1906, Gryuner worked for the Moscow *Zemstvo* in the Moscow rendering plant* and the following year in the Odessa abattoir. He published case reports of some of the pathological material he encountered in these institutions.[417] In 1907 he worked as assistant director of the Chita research station, a laboratory in Siberia that prepared antirinderpest serum and other biological agents. In 1908 he was appointed veterinary inspector in the city of Yakutsk in Siberia and concurrently lecturer in the school for *feldshers* (medical assistants). Here he organized a veterinary diagnostic laboratory and began what was to remain a lifelong interest: studying diseases of the reindeer—economically vital in this region—and their causes. In 1910, Gryuner was transferred to Petropavlovsk as district veterinary inspector for the whole of the Kamchatka province. He organized a new diagnostic laboratory in that city as well.[549]

I recount Gryuner's civilian appointments in possibly tedi-

*A factory in which condemned carcasses are rendered into tallow or otherwise reduced to inedible products.

ous detail, because they seem to me to indicate that he was given positions of increasing responsibility (as well as a two-year study leave abroad) from the time he left the military service. But an anonymous author of Gryuner's capsule biolgraphy in the *Sibirskaya Sovetskaya Entsiklopediya*[19] writes: "Because of his participation in the revolutionary movement he was often persecuted." One of his eulogists explains that Gryuner was kept in Siberia because he was suspected of revolutionary activities: "For his participation in the revolutionary movement he was exposed many times to persecution from the tsarist regime. His banishment to Siberia probably contributed to his exploration of the land where he was forced to live until the revolution."[301] If one accepts these statements at their face value, it becomes difficult to reconcile them with the fact that Gryuner was then permitted to go abroad, at state expense, for another two-year study tour to Alaska and the United States in 1911 and 1912! Gryuner spoke and read numerous languages, including English, and during his visits to the several countries mentioned, he availed himself of the facilities of various libraries and laboratories to further his knowledge. Perhaps the above statements are attempts to claim the fame of a cultured gentleman of the old regime for the new one. Alternatively, Gryuner may really have been a revolutionary, who succeeded in outwitting the tsarist regime at least as often as they succeeded in becoming informed of his activities and returning him to Siberia. Certainly his eulogy of Bauman* would support the thought that his sympathies were far to the left.[199]

On April 24, 1911, Gryuner read a paper before the Veterinary Medical Association of the Colorado Agricultural College, acquainting his American audience with veterinary education and practice in Russia. He published this paper

*See footnote on page 147.

later that year in the *American Veterinary Review.*[194] In this lecture he permitted himself some criticism of the Russian veterinary educational system, which he probably would not have dared if he were back in Russia. He pointed out that the United States had numerous veterinary colleges, with comparatively few students in each, whereas Russia had but four colleges, each with a large enrollment. He wrote, "I believe the system in the United States is the better, because a great many students in one college cannot get enough practical work as well as receive the proper instruction in crowded laboratories, and therefore gain only the theoretical knowledge."

Gryuner pointed out that in America the students were required to take only three years of study to be awarded the doctor's degree, whereas in Russia the students spent four and one half years completing their curriculum, but graduated only with the title "Veterinary Surgeon." Even if they then pursued the prescribed additional work for a graduate degree they could receive only the Master of Veterinary Science. The degree "doctor" was not given to veterinarians in Russia.

Gryuner explained that in other branches of science, one could obtain a master's degree, and then by further work and another dissertation, proceed to the doctorate. Physicians, who graduated with the diploma "physician," could proceed directly to the doctorate by taking an examination and preparing and defending a dissertation, without having to take the intervening master's degree as did botanists or chemists. He wrote: "In Russia you can be a Doctor of Mathematics, Astronomy, Greek, Literature or Medicine, but never of Veterinary Science." This was the same iniquitous system which Semmer had earlier railed against (see p. 40), but only after his retirement, and only in the relatively safe haven of an obscure Austrian veterinary journal[521] of limited circulation in Russia.

After spending some time in Alaska and publishing a case report based on this trip in the *American Veterinary Review,*[193] he spent part of the years 1911–1912 in Colorado. There he worked in the laboratory of Dr. Benjamin F. Kaupp, professor of pathology and bacteriology in the Veterinary Division of the Colorado Agricultural College in Fort Collins. The results of his joint research with Dr. Kaupp, on the complement-fixation test in the diagnosis of glanders, were published upon his return to Russia.[195]

While in the United States, Gryuner commenced a column called "Russian Review" in the *American Veterinary Review.*[192] In this (paralleling similar columns entitled "French Review" and "British Review," edited by others), Gryuner translated and abstracted the Russian veterinary literature, thus making it available for the American reader. This column was short-lived, appearing but twice in 1912 and not at all thereafter; however, Gryuner's name remained on the masthead of the Board of Contributors to the *American Veterinary Review* for another couple of years.

Gryuner also visited American meat-packing establishments and, following his return to Russia, published a lengthy article describing for his compatriots the status of meat hygiene in the abattoirs of Chicago, Kansas City, Denver, and Seattle.[196] He pointed out that trichinosis in swine was nowhere so widespread as in the United States, but that, paradoxically, it was in this very country that microscopic examination for trichinae* was not carried out! He also re-

*After several outbreaks of human trichinosis in Germany, Rudolf Virchow had advocated microscopic examination of all slaughtered swine. This was instituted there in 1866, and has been continued until today; it is also conducted in many other European countries and in Chile. The examination consists of compressing a sample of pork between two glass plates until it is very thin and projecting an enlarged view of it onto a screen, upon which the worms can readily be seen. Such inspection was initiated in the United States (for pork to be *exported* only) in 1889, but discontinued in 1906, apparently because the method was too expensive.[350] This left the

ported in the same journal his observations on deer husbandry in Alaska, comparing them with the practices in Siberia.[197] It is likely that in coming to the United States to study, which he did by way of Alaska, he followed the same route by boat as had the reindeer imported from eastern Siberia some two decades earlier (see Appendix VI). In his brief report on his visit to Alaska in the *American Veterinary Review* in 1911, he wrote: "With reindeer imported from Siberia were also introduced into Alaska certain diseases and parasites peculiar to these animals."[193]

Around the turn of the century, Gryuner's initial contributions in the field of pathology were based on packing house materials from the abattoirs in Moscow and Odessa. Somewhat later he began to publish on Arctic animals and fish and their diseases.[191] As far as I can trace his career, he held the job of district veterinary inspector of Kamchatka province until 1917. I do not know what his activities were between 1917 and 1925. In 1925 he was appointed to the chair of husbandry of cervidae* at the newly founded (1919) Siberian Veterinary Institute at Omsk.

According to Pinus,[417] Gryuner published about 70 scientific studies, of which he lists over a dozen that dealt with pathology. These contributions, several of which I have cited, qualify for inclusion in this book even without the aspects mentioned at the beginning of this section. Gryuner made

---

United States veterinary service subject to ridicule from foreigners, even visiting Russians. As we have seen, although Russia was a backward country, the ability, intellect, and education of its veterinary pathologists, such as Gryuner, were second to none.

*My designation; in Russian, the chair of deer husbandry and Siberian stag husbandry. For some reason, his appointment in the 1969 biography[553a] has been revised to read "deer husbandry and camel husbandry," but none of the accounts written during his life make any allusion to camel husbandry. However, he did write a review article on diseases of camels.

wide-ranging observations on the diseases of the wild and domesticated fauna of Siberia and created a museum in Omsk devoted to these animals. By the time of his death in 1931, he had contributed more than anyone previously to our knowledge of the diseases of cervidae.

The Siberian Veterinary Institute (now called the Omsk Veterinary Institute) started without a chair of pathology, and at first K. H. Bohl of Kazan acted as visiting professor of this discipline.[181,593] Bohl placed A. D. Balzamentov, who had done research under him in Kazan,[18] in charge of pathology at Omsk. By 1925, Balzamentov was a professor with two assistants: his wife, N. A. Balzamentova, and K. I. Vertinskii. (The latter worked in Kazan under Bohl in 1931, and later held the chair of pathology at the Moscow Veterinary Academy*). In the mid-1930s Balzamentov did research on bovine mastitis with Karl Nieberle in Leipzig;[47] apart from this I could find no biographical details of his career.

The Moscow Agricultural Academy

Gavriil I. Gurin, M.V.Sc. (1858–1933), a Kazan graduate of 1882, wrote a book *Kratkoe Rukovdstvo Obshchei Patologii Zhivotnykh* (Short Manual on General Pathology of Animals) (Moscow, 1912), which reached a second edition in 1924.[201] Gurin held the chair of veterinary science at the Moscow Agricultural Academy from 1898 to 1930 and specialized in meat hygiene. He spent 1902–1903 in postgraduate studies in Germany, Holland, and Denmark. The title of Gurin's book in the Index Catalogue to the U.S. Surgeon-General's Library led me to believe that I had over-

*See Khrushchev[242] for a fascinating acount of the discovery of Stachybothryotoxicosis in which Vertinskii participated.

looked a significant pathologist and his work. I was able to find a copy of the second edition; it is a modest volume, aimed at an audience of agriculturists rather than veterinarians.

Gurin seems to have been outside the mainstream of veterinary pathology being treated in this book. He devoted years to popularizing veterinary science,[226] and perhaps for this reason is not mentioned by contemporary Soviet writers on the history of veterinary pathology. Allusion to him here is only to spare others the effort of seeking his book because of its enticing title.

The Women's Medical Institute

In his historical sketch on veterinary pathology in prerevolutionary Russia, Pinus[417] mentions Nikolai P. Savvaitov (1861–1918), who was professor of epizootiology at the Women's Medical Institute (Fig. 54). This was a teaching

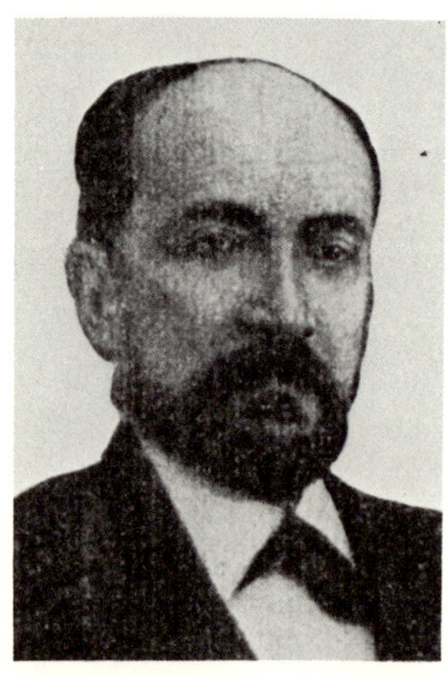

Figure 54. Nikolai P. Savvaitov.

institution for physicians, and I have not been able to find out why they had a veterinarian to teach epizootiology on the staff.[164] Savvaitov's contributions to Russian veterinary medicine were chiefly in infectious and parasitic diseases and in meat hygiene rather than pathology, so that we need dwell on him but briefly here.

Born in St. Petersburg, he graduated from the veterinary division of the Medico-Chirurgical Academy there in 1883; that is, in its last class. He early showed an interest in pathology and learned all he could from Vorontsov and Raevskii (see pp. 64 and 69). From 1883 to 1902 he worked as the St. Petersburg city veterinarian and published a number of papers in the field of meat hygiene. His dissertation "Materials for the Study of St. Petersburg from the Sanitary, Zoohygienic and Veterinary Statistical Standpoints" was also published as a large book in 1897.[461] He got the M.V.Sc. that year from the (by this time) Military-Medical Academy; apparently it still granted the advanced degree although no longer educating veterinary students or granting veterinary diplomas. The book looks like a good source for historical research; for example, considerable space is devoted by Savvaitov to a discussion of autopsy rooms in various Russian veterinary institutions, and a detailed description is given of the one in the Institute for Experimental Medicine.

Savvaitov also published a number of case reports of lesions he had encountered during meat inspection.[462-464] The illustrations from several of these were used by Mari in his textbook of pathology.[338] It is of interest that Savvaitov lists his address on these papers as "From the St. Petersburg City Autopsy Room," an indication that pathology was being practiced there rather than cursory meat inspection.

When the First All-Russian Veterinary Convention met in St. Petersburg in 1903, Savvaitov was one of the chief organizers; he also edited its published proceedings.[465] In these volumes are papers by himself and others which provide valuable historical information on veterinary pathology in Russia at the turn of thc century.

The Kiev Medical Institute

A leading Ukrainian pathologist, Professor Pavlo O. Kucherenko (1882–1936), headed the department of pathologic anatomy of the above institution from 1921 (Fig. 55).[24] An enthusiastic research worker, he was also a very effective teacher and trained numerous pathologists despite his relatively short life span.[299] Veterinary pathologists were also welcome in his laboratory, and Kucherenko is mentioned here because of the training in pathology and research support which he provided for two of them. A. A. Pinus and B. M. Gurvich were military veterinarians, stationed at the District Military-Veterinary Laboratory in Kiev during the mid-1920s. Pinus had already received some training from N. D. Ball, but I have no biographical details on Gurvich. Both were interested in the pathology of glanders, and although Kiev had a new veterinary school, this did

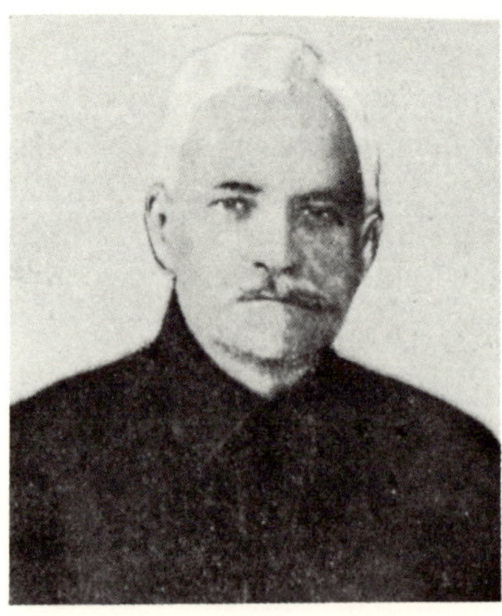

Figure 55. Pavlo O. Kucherenko.

not yet have a functioning pathology department during the period covered here. Pinus and Gurvich might therefore have found themselves in relative scientific isolation had it not been that Kucherenko hospitably provided some facilities for them in his laboratory.

Kucherenko's eulogists,[299,349] although stressing how hospitable he was to young physicians training in his institute, do not mention the above two veterinarians. Some of the work that they published on glanders[415] lists Kucherenko's laboratory as the scientific source of the work, and in other papers this is shared with the Military-Veterinary Laboratory. In 1925, Kucherenko also indicated his support of and interest in veterinary medicine by contributing a review article on the recent advances in pathology to the journal of the Kiev Veterinary Institute.[283] Thus another medical pathologist whose comparative interests have been forgotten deserves a place in this book because of those interests.

11 Research on Infectious Diseases

The names connected with the beginning of pathogenic bacteriology—Pasteur, Koch, Klebs, and their contemporaries—are known all over the scientific world. Less well known is that this discipline got its start not so much from the study of human infections as from the problems inherent in infectious diseases—some of them transmissible to man—of domesticated animals and birds. Fowl cholera, anthrax, swine erysipelas, and rabies were the diseases wherein Pasteur worked out his theory of attenuation of pathogenic agents for the production of vaccines (Fig. 56). If we add tuberculosis to this list, a disease affecting both man and lower animals, all the infections that provided the foundation for the beginning of the discipline of pathogenic bacteriology are represented. In the study of three of these, anthrax, fowl cholera, and tuberculosis, the veterinary pathologists of Russia made noteworthy contributions. Although these have already been mentioned in connection with the lives of individual men, they can best be brought into focus in a chapter dealing with the diseases themselves. To this chapter I have added four more diseases that seem to be apposite to its subject.

The Great Rinderpest Controversy

The export of cattle to England and Continental Europe was an important source of income to the Russian

Empire. The Russian herds were often ravaged by outbreaks of rinderpest, which caused losses both within the country and in the countries that imported Russian cattle. Between the years 1865 and 1866 alone, more than 400,000 cattle perished in the United Kingdom from a diseased lot said to have been imported from Reval (now Talinn), Estonia, a Baltic port. The British buyer, James Burchell, noted that some of the animals were ill before they were shipped, but the Russians forced him to buy them nevertheless.*

In addition to the intimidation of buyers, however, the Russian government was taking more constructive steps toward elucidating the cause and control of the epizootics. This was during the years 1860 to 1880, just before the discovery of the role of bacteria and long before the discovery of the role of viruses in the causation of disease. Experiments were set up, using several thousand head of livestock, in several places in the Russian Empire.

From the results obtained in these stations, Semmer, Jessen, and Tartakovskii, whom I will call "the Dorpat faction," came to the conclusion that preventive inoculation was the way to control the disease and recommended to the government that this should be undertaken. True, they reached this conclusion on the basis of inadequate evidence; a more effective and less dangerous vaccine was needed but was not to be forthcoming until several years later. Ravich and "the St. Petersburg faction," however, reached the opposite conclusion—that vaccination was dangerous, killing more animals than would die if a herd were left unvaccinated. They further claimed that vaccinated animals often would still succumb to the disease when challenged later with tissue extracts from

*He testified to the British Royal Commission on Cattle Plague about some visibly diseased cattle: "I had purchased them because they insisted upon my taking them. They stopped my passport and thought to frighten me very much. It is an awkward thing to be in a country like that, and to have your passport stopped, and you doing no harm."[7]

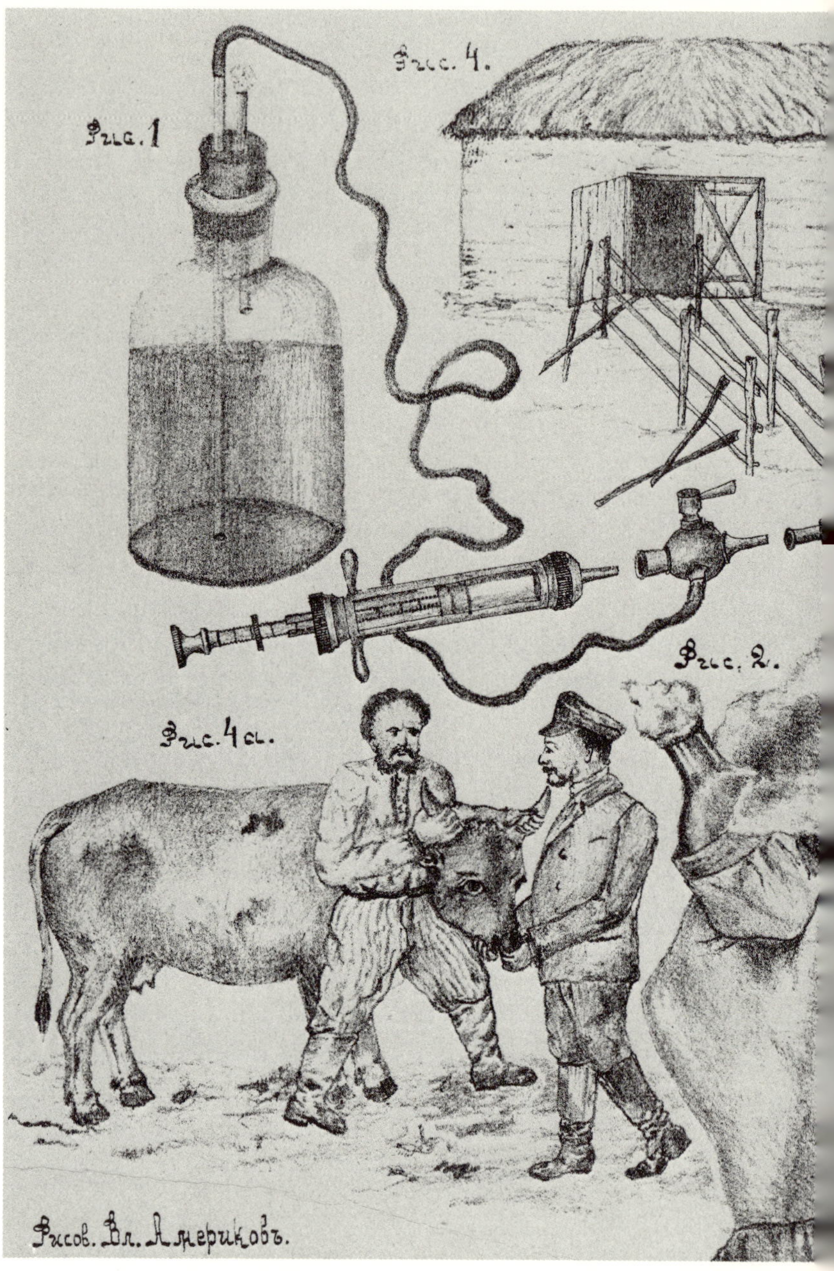

Figure 56. Anthrax inoculation of sheep in the late nineteenth century.
Apparatus for mass inoculations. 2, The mass of cotton on which the needle
wiped is held to the vaccine bottle with paper. 3, Container for vaccine if onl
few animals are to be inoculated. 4, Enclosure for restraint of cattle to

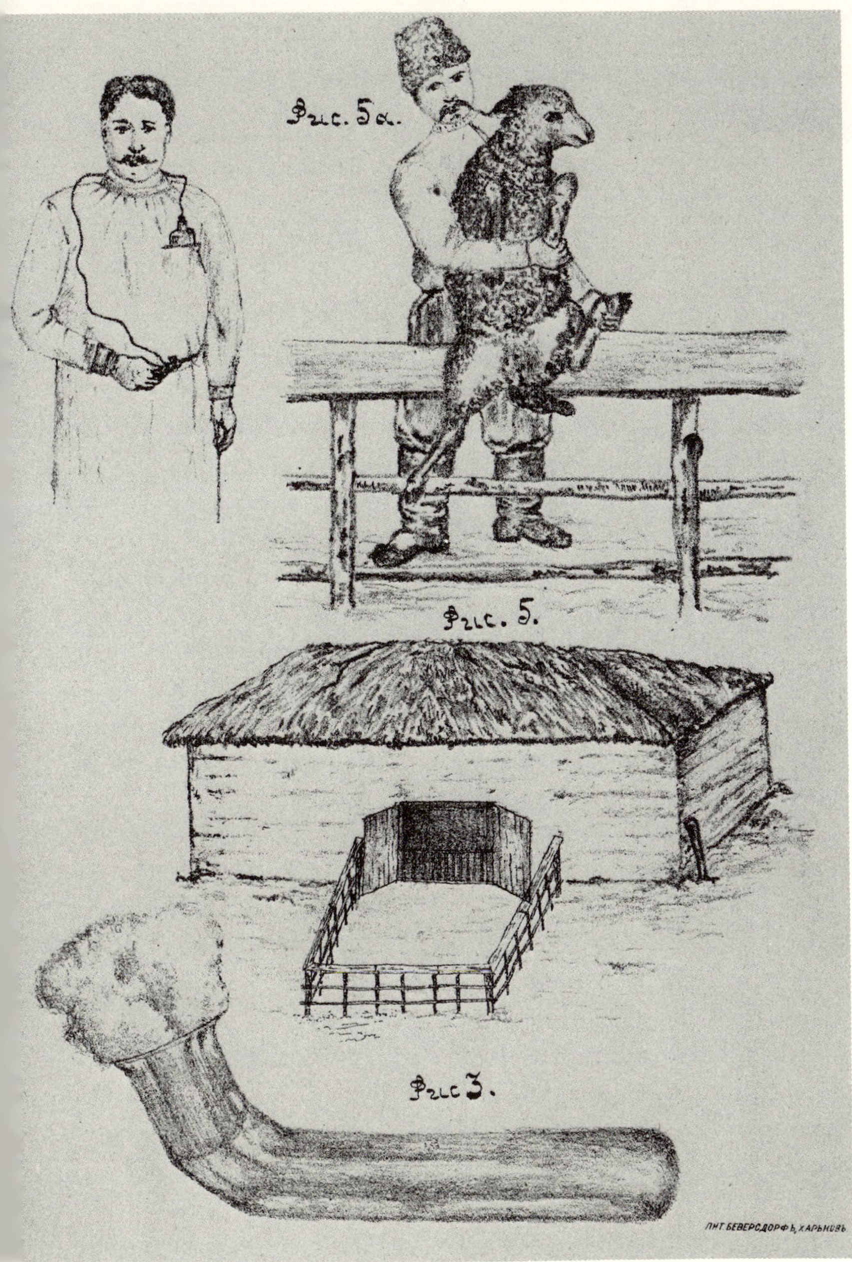

noculated. 4a, Two men restraining an animal for inoculation (the Russian egend explains that an excitable animal should be tied by the horns to a post). , Enclosure for restraint of sheep to be inoculated. 5a, The sheep is restrained n a sitting position on the top board of the enclosure.

diseased animals. Their conclusion that vaccination was not a useful control measure was also premature, failing to take two factors into account—the varying resistance of steppe versus northern breeds of cattle, already known, and the varying antigenicity and virulence of different viral strains, which would not be known until years later. On the basis of *their* work, however, they recommended that the only reliable method of control of the disease was eradication by slaughter.

This was not merely an academic disagreement; in view of the fear of rinderpest in Europe and the disrepute of the Russian cattle, which were—erroneously—thought to be responsible for all of the outbreaks in the West, most of the Western countries had in effect already closed their borders to Russian cattle by enforcing prolonged quarantine periods. The consequences to the Russian cattle trade were drastic, and the government was ready to take any steps—even the very expensive ones of setting up research stations—that might lead to control of the disease and resumption of foreign cattle exports. Thus arose what I think may fairly be termed "The Great Rinderpest Controversy."

The two factions in this controversy, Dorpat versus St. Petersburg, are so designated by me; while hinted at, they have never been clearly identified as antagonists in any Russian historical writing that I have found. Nevertheless, their existence and their antagonism emerge clearly enough; indeed, their bickering was even carried on before an audience of foreigners in Zurich at the Third International Veterinary Congress.[648] Although the records of the congress have been published, it would require access to the primary source material, i.e., records of the Russian government from 1860 to 1890 to do justice historically to this controversy. Nevertheless, its outline can be sketched in well enough from the secondary sources which I have read.

Unfortunately, the St. Petersburg faction was able to convince the government that the research stations had served their purpose in demonstrating the uselessness of rinderpest vaccination and should therefore be closed down. Later, "swimming against the tide," a new research station was opened by Semmer in the Ukraine under the auspices of the Institute for Experimental Medicine in St. Petersurg and supported by private funds. The group within the government, however, the so-called "Veterinary Committee," succeeded in stirring up so much local opposition that Semmer was forced to abandon his field work.[518] Thus, an effective method of immunization, with an improved vaccine, which Semmer's lead in this field would probably have resulted in discovering, was denied to him and had to await discovery abroad.

It is often the lot of those who espouse extreme positions that history shows them to have been just as wrong as their opponents; the truth, when it is finally discovered, is seen to lie between the extremes. Thus Ravich and Semmer were almost equally right, but also equally wrong—Ravich perhaps a little more wrong than Semmer. The faction that had the ear of the officials wielding political power in St. Petersburg triumphed in the short run; but Russia was the loser, and with it veterinary science worldwide. Its representatives at the International Veterinary Congress in Zurich were waiting to get the results of what they termed the largest series of experiments in the world;[648] they were given instead a biased presentation of the results together with the wrong conclusions drawn from them.

Since eventually (by the early twentieth century), vaccination and not slaughter was proved to be the way to control rinderpest in countries where it was enzootic, it is incredible to read the opposite view being defended in Russia as late as 1959! In a paper on Leningrad's history, Professor V. Z. Chernyak, a pupil of N. D. Ball and a veterinary pathologist of considerable erudition, was apparently obsessed by either civic chauvinism (Leningrad versus Tartu-Dorpat) or

Slavophilism.[150] Whichever it was betrayed him into retrospectively extolling Ravich's virtues in this controversy, at the expense of Semmer's, and glossing over Semmer's work as hardly worthy of mention. That an otherwise objective writer could be guilty of a lapse of such magnitude is deplorable indeed. Despite Chernyak's opinion, the verdict of history has awarded the decision to Semmer. Although he was unduly optimistic in thinking that the vaccine which he had developed would be of great practical value in controlling rinderpest, he was right both in contending that slaughter would not and also in the reasons he gave for why it would not. And he was also right in principle that vaccination would serve to control the disease. A truly effective vaccine had to await the accrual of additional basic knowledge after the turn of the century.

The first published investigations to adequately describe the pathology of rinderpest appear to have been carried out in Russia; the authors were Brauell, 1862, Ravich, 1864, and Semmer, 1875. Of the three, I believe Ravich gave the most comprehensive description of the lesions. Ravich's work (Figs. 57 and 58), gained almost instant recognition in the West because the following year an epizootic of rinderpest broke out in Great Britain that was to claim the lives of 400,000 cattle before it subsided. The British government appointed a Royal Commission to "Inquire Into the Nature and Origin &c. of the Cattle Plague"; it retained several leading British medical scientists to study (among other things) the pathology of the disease.[7,8]

In the report of the Royal Commission, the British scientists cited the work of Brauell and Ravich in laudatory terms, saying that they had confirmed their findings. The British Ministry of Agriculture's history book,[359] published a century later, likewise praised the Russian work, although one cannot tell readily that it is this work to which they are referring. (The useful knowledge they are alluding to can only be

Neue Untersuchungen

über die

pathologische Anatomie

der

Rinderpest

von

Joseph Ravitsch.

Magister der Thierheilkunde, ausserordentlichem Professor am Veterinairinstitute der K. Medico-chirurgischen Akademie zu St. Petersburg.

Mit 2 Tafeln Abbildungen.

Berlin, 1864.

Verlag von August Hirschwald,

Unter den Linden, 68.

Figure 57. Title page of Ravich's book on pathology of rinderpest.

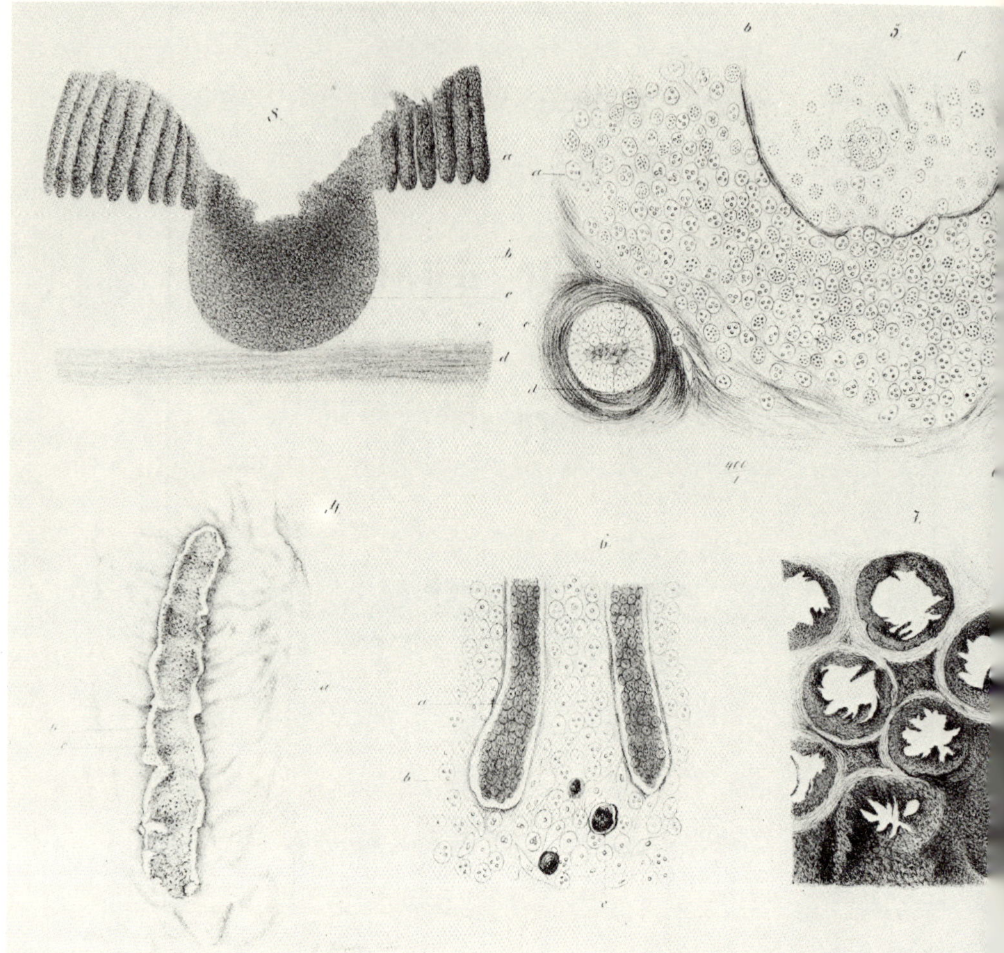

Figure 58. Plate from Ravich's book with drawings of rinderpest lesions. At lower left is a gross lesion—erosions at the periphery of a Peyer's patch. Histologic changes in the tongue are depicted in 5, changes in the alimentary canal in 6, 7, and 8.

Brauell's and Ravich's contributions—at that time there was little else that could be considered useful.) Deprecating the investigation of the British Royal Commission in the nineteenth century, the 1964 book states (p. 132): "Although these added little to the useful knowledge of the disease, they provided a fine series of colored plates illustrating the lesions." This is a far harsher judgment* than the British work of 1865–1866 merits; but it highlights the fact that there was little left for anyone to add to Ravich's thorough description of the pathology of rinderpest after he published it in 1864. As I point out later, this is among Russian veterinary work that is now forgotten and unknown in the West.

The Russian work, however, evoked contemporary interest on the Continent as well as in England. Professor Gerlach, Director of the Royal Veterinary College in Hanover, who had testified at the hearings of the British Royal Commission, took cognizance of Brauell's and Ravich's work in his book on rinderpest published in 1867. Gerlach pointed out that Röll and his colleagues at the Vienna Veterinary College considered the lesions to be of a croupous exudative character, which he said was a reasonable interpretation in view of their gross appearance.[179] Gerlach also said he could understand how such an interpretation would arise particularly in Vienna, under the influence of Rokitansky's teaching and ideas. In pointing out that Brauell and Ravich opposed Röll's interpretation, Gerlach referred to Brauell's work as "sorgfältigen and gründlichen mikroskopischen Untersuchungen" (painstaking and thorough microscopic examinations). Gerlach refers to the work from Russia on the pathology of rinderpest in several other places in his book, with a meticulousness unfortunately not shared by authors in the twentieth century.

In his textbook on infectious diseases published in 1881, Röll likewise cited the work of Brauell and Ravich on the

*I believe these authors are wrong in their judgment. Since their view could not have been motivated by chauvinism, we are left with ignorance as the only explanation. One can forgive wrong judgment about a classical piece of work; however, it is deplorable to disparage a scholarly treatise in this way. The criticism was leveled by anonymous authors perhaps best described in Churchill's terms as "modest men with much to be modest about," who abused their cloak of anonymity by sniping from behind it.

pathology of rinderpest.[445] Although he was a leading Austrian professor with a reputation to uphold, Röll was big enough to indicate that these workers had refuted his own previous report (of 1850) that the plaques in this disease were of a croupous nature. Röll's seems to be the last allusion to Brauell's and Ravich's work in any important Western book on infectious diseases of animals.

The work on rinderpest in Russia was not all in the scientific domain, that is, pathology or immunology. Some of it was of an immediate, practical character, not requiring the application of hard-won basic scientific knowledge. I leave a description of this to George Kennan, correspondent for the *Century Magazine* (and great-uncle of George Kennan, our later ambassador to the U.S.S.R.). In 1891 he wrote the following vivid passage (Fig. 59):[239]

> Instead of following the Yenisei River back to Krasnoyarsk, which would have been going far out of our way, we decided to leave it a short distance below Minusinsk and proceed directly to Tomsk by a short cut across the steppes, keeping the great Siberian road on our right all the way. Nothing of interest happened to us until late in the evening, when, just as we were turning up from the river into a small peasant village, the name of which I have now forgotten, both we and our horses were startled by the sudden appearance of a wild-looking man in a long, tattered sheepskin coat, who, from the shelter of a projecting cliff, sprang into the road ahead of us, shouting a hoarse but unintelligible warning, and brandishing in the air an armful of blazing birch-bark and straw.
>
> "What's the matter?" I said to our driver, as our horses recoiled in affright.
>
> "It's the plague-guard," he replied. "He says we must be smoked."
>
> The cattle-plague was then prevailing extensively in the valley of the upper Yenisei, and it appeared that round this village the peasants had established a sanitary cordon with the hope of protecting their own live stock from contagion. They had heard of the virtues of fumigation, and were subjecting to

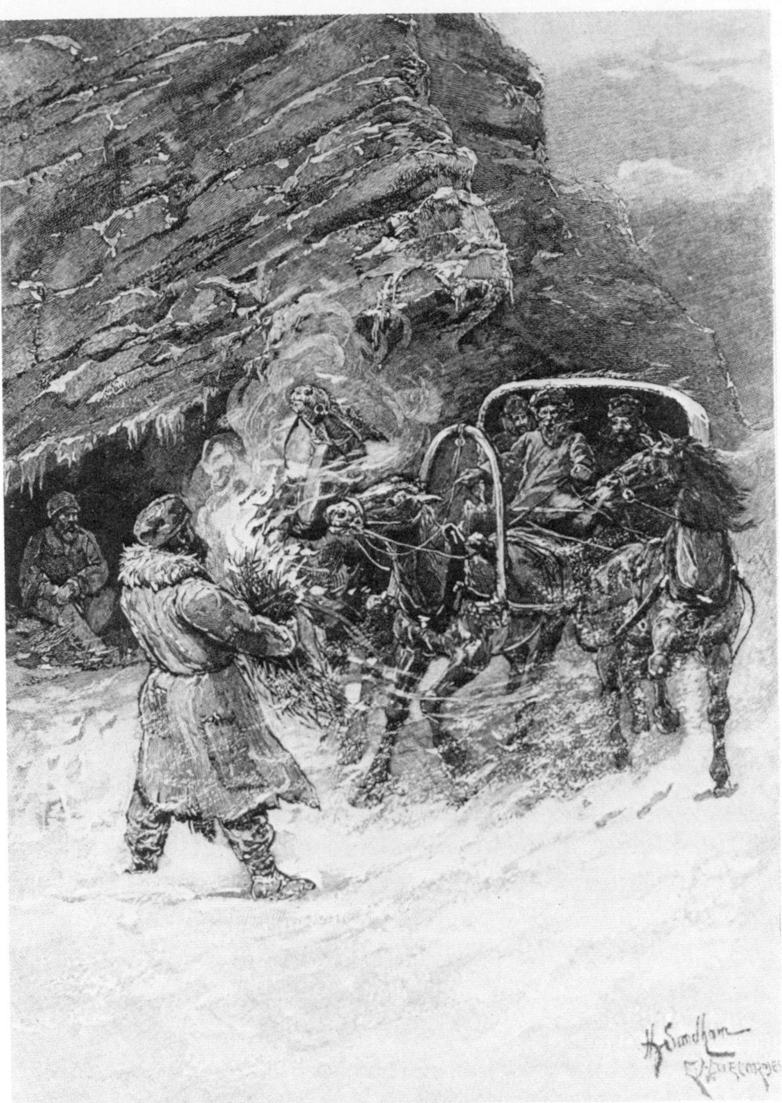

Figure 59. "Fumigation" of horses drawing George Kennan's sleigh in Siberia in 1891.

that process every vehicle that crossed the village limits. The "plague-guard" burned straw, birch-bark, and other inflammable and smoke-producing substances around and under our *pavoska* until we were half strangled and our horses were frantic with fear, and then he told us gravely that we were "purified" and might proceed.

Fowl Cholera

In contemporary textbooks of veterinary bacteriology, or of infectious diseases of domestic animals, fowl cholera is classified among the pasteurelloses. One might be forgiven, therefore, for thinking of it as just another pasteurellosis, that is, one of several such infections that affect various species of animals. Such, however, is not the case. This particular infectious disease has a claim to historical fame, being the one in which Pasteur first succeeded (in 1880) in attenuating a living agent to make a prophylactic vaccine.

That same year, in a short note in *Virchow's Archiv,* Eugen Semmer wrote: "Recently a dispute has broken out between Perroncito in Turin, Toussaint in Toulouse, and Pasteur in Paris, regarding which of them had first discovered the transmissibility of fowl cholera and the significance of the bacteria encountered in this disease."[500] According to Semmer, all of these authors had observed the disease in the year 1878. "However," he goes on, "the dispute is a futile one, inasmuch as the disease had already been investigated by me in Dorpat in 1877, its transmissibility demonstrated, and the significance of bacteria in it emphasized, as can be seen in my article *Die Hühnerpest,* published in the *Deutsche Zeitschrift für Thiermedicin und vergleichende Pathologie* in February 1878."[492]

It was easy enough to find that a literary conflict was indeed being waged by some of the individuals named; in fact, most of it can be read in a single volume (57) of the *Recueil de Médecine Vétérinaire* for 1880, although some of it had appeared elsewhere the year before. Untangling who had really done what and when was somewhat less easy and not made more so by a standard reference work, Bulloch's *History of Bacteriology.*[130] Bulloch (p. 241) states that fowl cholera "had been recognized as bacterial by the Italian worker Perroncito (1879), and the organism described by him had been cultivated by H. Toussaint (1879), a professor of the Lyons Veterinary School."

One begins to wonder about Bulloch's scholarship upon reading elsewhere in his book that Toussaint was a professor at the *Toulouse* Veterinary School, but he can be forgiven for not knowing that Gaul is divided into different parts. Reference to Perroncito's paper cited above,[398] however, elicits that the latter wrote (page 46, line 9): "Nie habe ich im Blute Bacterien oder Vibrionen gefunden." (I have never found bacteria or vibrios in the blood.) And again (page 49, para. 6, line 1): "Obwohl sehr häufig im Blutplasma der Seuche erlegenen Hühner freie Körnchen gefunden werden, wie ich sie beschrieben und abgebildet habe, so wage ich doch nicht zu behaupten, ob es Mikrokokken in Hallier's Sinne seien." (Although free granules were very often found in the blood plasma of chickens dead of the disease, as I have described and illustrated them, still I do not dare to contend that they are micrococci in Hallier's sense.) To make of this that fowl cholera had been "recognized as bacterial," as Bulloch puts it, when Perroncito was clearly too timorous to ascribe a pathogenetic role to the organisms he saw, *and said so,* strikes me as unwarranted tampering with history.

What credit *can* we give to Perroncito on the basis of his publications? First, he gave an excellent description of the epizootiology and pathologic anatomy of the disease, one that was not improved upon for many years thereafter. Second, he succeeded in transmitting the disease to unaffected chickens by inoculating them with blood or tissues from diseased ones; however, that had been done by some French workers over 20 years previously. Third, he recognized what were undoubtedly the causative Pasteurella bacteria in the blood of affected chickens, even though his scientific caution kept him from ascribing a pathogenic or etiologic role to them.

Perroncito published his paper in 1879, but the period of his observations on fowl cholera spans the years 1877 (beginning in October) and 1878. As he pointed out in his polemics with the French critics, he had given a preliminary paper on the subject, which contained an illustration of the organisms observed, to the Royal Agricultural Academy of Turin in February 1878.

To return now to Semmer, how much of what he had accomplished was being claimed in 1880 by others, whether Italians or Frenchmen? Certain it is that his work on fowl cholera, published in a distinguished German journal on March 12, 1878, was not cited by either Perroncito or his French competitors. This journal must have been available to both groups of workers. Nor was it cited by Bulloch,[130] who likewise found no room for Semmer in the 50-page biographical section of his book, which contains 327 sketches of bacteriologists, some important and others whose place in history is less secure.

In the autumn of 1877, an outbreak of fowl cholera occurred in Dorpat and was studied by Semmer. His description of the lesions is not nearly as detailed as that provided by Perroncito, who was studying the outbreak near Turin that same autumn (in 1877 and not in 1878 as claimed by Semmer). Semmer transmitted the disease by feeding pieces of intestine from affected birds, but as already mentioned in summarizing Perroncito's work, that had already been done by others. Semmer, however, found micrococci and short rodlike bacteria both in the intestinal contents and in the blood of affected birds, *and stated unequivocally his view that they played an etiologic role* in the disease. In this attribution he has undoubted priority, both over Perroncito, who made similar observations but was too cautious to draw a conclusion regarding their significance, and Toussaint, who isolated the organisms in pure culture the following year, 1879.

Events moved swiftly thereafter. By 1880, Pasteur, working with bacteria isolated from chickens with fowl cholera, had succeeded both in proving his theory that living organisms could be attenuated to make vaccines and in providing a practical control method for a devastating avian disease. There would seem to have been enough credit to go around for everyone. I do not know why neither Perroncito, Toussaint, nor Pasteur deigned to mention Semmer's observations. But the strident tone of the French and the Italians' polemics with each other makes it hard to shake off the feeling that the omission was deliberate. (Figure 60 shows Semmer and Perroncito together at the International Veterinary Congress in Paris 10 years later).*

Should the organism of fowl cholera—the type name for the whole genus Pasteurella—be renamed *Semmerella choleragallinarum?* The proper name for this organism has given taxonomic bacteriologists trouble for decades, and they are unlikely to welcome the intrusion of this question into an already messy situation. But now that Yersinia and Francisella have been separated from the formerly larger genus Pasteurella, it seems timely to suggest that an organism be named Semmerella in honor of a great veterinary scientist, whose contributions have been ignored in Italy, France, and the United Kingdom.

*It would be interesting to know what, if anything, Semmer said to Perroncito about fowl cholera on the occasion of their meeting! Unfortunately, I have no information on this; Semmer's trip report on his return to Dorpat makes no mention of anything personal.[514]

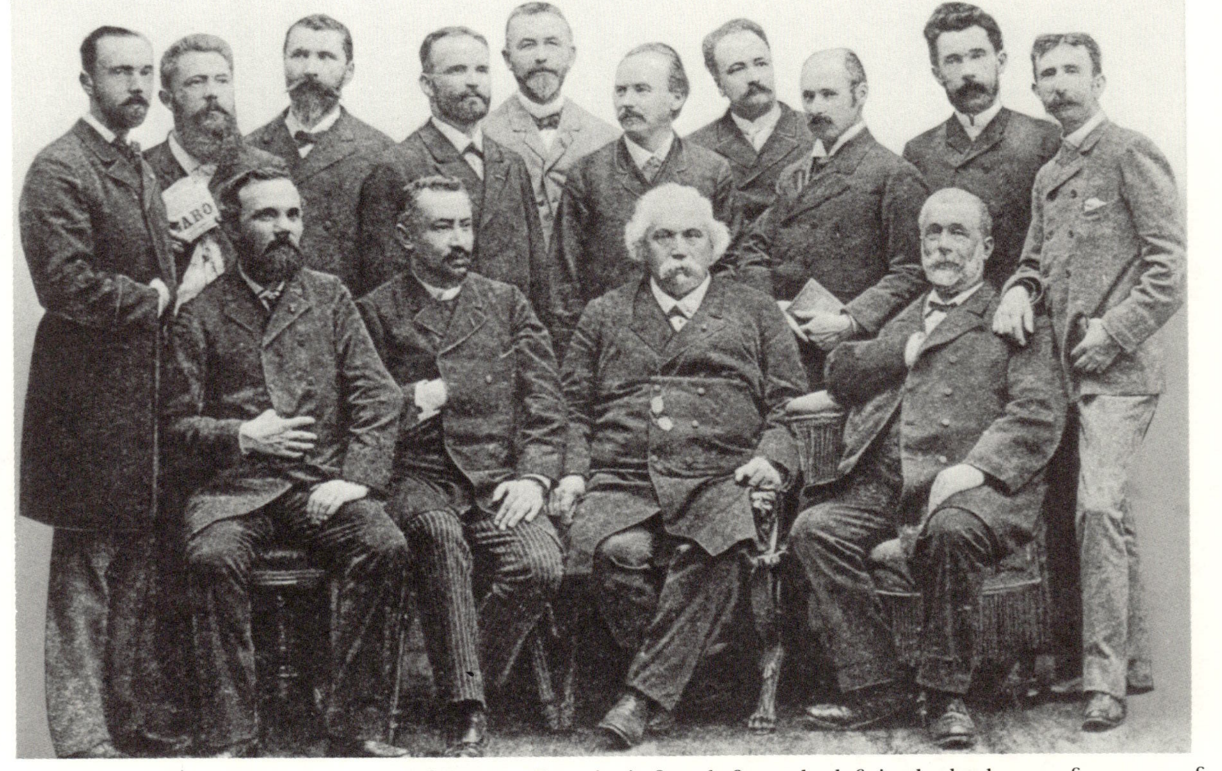

Figure 60. Professor E. Semmer, of Dorpat, Estonia, is fourth from the left in the back row of a group of delegates to the Fifth International Veterinary Congress in Paris, September 1889. The other delegates (including several destined to acquire international repute) from left to right are, standing: B. Bang, Copenhagen; A. Koch, Vienna; Potterat, Bern; Semmer; Remy, Belgium; Degive, Brussels; Robinson, United [illegible] Utrecht; Fraers, Belgium. Sitting: Perroncito, Turin; Nocard, Alfort;

Glanders

The data on the pathology and pathogenesis of glanders in the horse have never been compiled in any one textbook. There are treatises of the pulmonary lesions in the eight-volume *Joest's Handbuch,* but the disease is split up on a regional basis, with the volume on the skin still to appear several years after that on the lungs has been in print! The only comprehensive presentation which adequately takes into account the voluminous Russian literature is the monograph by Tsvetkov and Chernyak.[601] It likewise considers the German literature, as well as some French contributions. An attempt must therefore be made to compile background material on our knowledge of the pathology of the disease from Nieberle's contribution to glanders in the first edition of *Joest's Handbuch,* the last edition of it, the pathology book of Nieberle and Cohrs, the book by Tsvetkov and Chernyak, plus whatever important papers are cited by these books.

In compiling the literature on pathology, one realizes at the outset that much of it is Russian and most of that is based on work done in the decade 1920 to 1930. The major question that then comes to mind is: Why did the Russians put so much time and effort into studying the pathogenesis of glanders, when perhaps all that was needed was to test all of the horses in the country, slaughter the reactors, and then go on to something else?

From the report of Zagrodzki,[642] I am not at all sure that it would have been possible to carry out such a national testing effort. He tells about the primitive conditions prevailing in the various laboratories that had to manufacture mallein—for example, in the Central Military Veterinary Bacteriologic Station there was no heat in the buildings or incubators, no light except when the staff could find candles, and no running water. Once the cultures *froze* inside the incubator! He tells even more about the purposeless meetings of veterinary officials, where nothing was ever decided, and the hopeless dissemination of the disease by the stupid shipment of animals from one part of the country to the other. (There was famine in southeast Russia, so the plan was to ship the horses out of there—an epizootic area—to the north to keep them from being eaten. In the north, most of the horses were free of glanders, until the southern ones arrived!) What an irony that in the country in which mallein had been discovered, the facilities for producing it should have become so woefully inadequate that it was not to be had in anything like the needed quantities.

Responsible for this irony was the appointment in 1918 of a veterinary assistant (*feldsher*), K. G. Martin, to head the civil veterinary administration in Moscow. Martin had little to recommend him except his membership in the Bolshevik party, which dated back to 1903. This gesture of defiance by the Bolshevik rulers at the university-educated class, which they detested and mistrusted, cost them dearly in maladroit disease control until, in 1921, stark reality prevailed over dogma and Martin was replaced.*

Paul Scheffer, who reported from Moscow for a leading Berlin newspaper, wrote of the disorganization affecting all but one of the ministries in the Kremlin in 1921.[466] He found

*His replacement, V. S. Bobrovskii, although a veterinarian rather than a *feldsher,* was not much better, if judged by how well epizootic diseases were controlled during his administration. An 1897 graduate of the Kharkov Veterinary Institute, he had spent much of his time as a student and also after graduation as a professional revolutionary. His appeal to Lenin was thus obvious, in a year when Lenin had not yet learned some bitter lessons—that to keep his regime afloat he needed competence rather than political loyalty. Some of the mistrust that the rulers in the Kremlin felt toward academic holdovers from the old regime was heard by the pathologist Hamperl when he was in Russia in 1929. The then current belief about a professor, even one outwardly docile and toeing the party line, was that he is "like a radish—a thin layer of Red on the outside, but White to the core on the inside!"[205]

only Trotsky's ministry (war) to be orderly and operating with a modern concept of organization. His account conjures up images of bedlam in countless ministerial offices—small wonder that what emerged from the government was mostly futile talk and very little action.

As related at the beginning of Chapter 8, Trotsky had become aware during the Civil War that it was better to appoint former tsarist officers whose loyalty to the Bolsheviks was dubious, but who could organize and act, than to lose battles with loyal agitators who could not. In the civilian sphere, this lesson was slow in being learned, and, in fact, 60 years later it is still unpalatable to the rulers in the Kremlin. Lenin grasped it near the end of his life, and in his address to the All-Russian Soviet of June 1922, he recommended fewer revolutionary words and more deeds, as well as the return of common sense in lieu of wild ideas (Scheffer,[466] p. 83). Despite his exhortations, one seeks in vain for any effect from his words as mirrored by veterinary events during that year.

The veterinary problem of glanders was aggravated in the 1920s by its public health aspects. McGilvray writes that during the Civil War the incidence of human glanders was appallingly high because of the lack of control measures for the equine disease. This is true; what he does not mention is that it was also appallingly high because of the lack of food, causing hungry vagrant children and also members of the Workers' and Peasants' Red Army to seek and consume the flesh of glandered horses that had been condemned as infected and shot. The carcasses were supposed to be buried, not eaten.

McGilvray's* statement[311] is also echoed by Jennings.[219]

*My interest in glanders dates from the early 1940s, when my teacher Dr. C. D. McGilvray regaled his veterinary students with tales of how he had eradicated glanders in Canada. His method, which was to shoot first and ask questions afterward, caused us to call him "Shotgun Charlie" behind his back.

Otherwise, the literature of the past 50 years is peculiarly silent on the topic of human glanders in Russia, at least from an epidemiologic standpoint. All one can find are scattered case reports. There is not even a hint of the dreadful epidemics in Russia in 1920–1924 in modern textbooks of epidemiology or bacteriology.

Statements additional to McGilvray's are Zagrodzki's,[642–644] published in Polish (and, more briefly, also in French and German) in 1921, which indicate that cases of human glanders were so numerous that special hospitals for their confinement had to be established in Kiev and in the Crimea during the 1920s. There were 400 deaths in Kiev alone in 1921, over 100 in the month of June.[642]

Another statement is by Sir Frederick Hobday in 1922.[209] In a British morning paper of June 6, he mentions a Reuter's dispatch from Helsinki citing a report in the Soviet *Red Gazette* that some children infected with glanders had been shot for "humanitarian and sanitary reasons." (Those who believe that man's inhumanity to man in Soviet Russia was inaugurated by Stalin should remember that this occurred during Lenin's rule. Further documentation of Lenin's cruelties are amply supplied by Solzhenitsyn.[564]) I have been unable to find which British morning paper he meant; a newspaper called *Krasnaya Gazeta* was published in Leningrad during the 1920s, but only a few scattered issues exist in American libraries.

There is also a report by Dr. Henry Podgaez in the *Veterinary Journal* in July 1922, dealing with human glanders in Kharkov.[421] He relates that a group of soldiers of the Red Army became infected after eating the meat of condemned horses. Once their disease had been bacteriologically confirmed, they were taken from the hospital to a military prison, ostensibly as deserters, and shot.

The fact that one of the reports is reputed to have been published in the Soviet public press suggests that similar ones may also have appeared in the medical press before the subject became taboo. I have scanned the pages of the major Russian medical journals for the years 1921 and 1922 to the extent they are held in American libraries. These, however, were years of severe paper shortages and scant deliveries of journals to subscribers abroad. None of the available issues have dealt with human glanders.

Finally, Mikhail Bulgakov, in his historical novel *The White Guard,* writes of newspaper accounts of "how the Moscow shopkeepers were selling horsemeat* infected with glanders.[129]

The disease in horses was a serious threat both to the Soviet army and to Soviet agriculture, but the human infection must have made the Bolsheviks frantic to control the disease in horses—it turned a situation that was drastic into one that was desperate. Because they were unable to produce or buy enough mallein, I surmise that the authorities hoped that more refined methods of pathological diagnosis might show that some of the cases were actually nonglanderous. In fact, this approach served not only to delineate the pathology of glanders, but also to support some outstanding work on pseudo-glanderous lesions: from it developed a knowledge of parasitic and mycotic lesions that might never have resulted from a less intensive effort.*

Three major groups worked on the pathogenesis of glanders during the early to mid-1920s. The first, at the All-Union Institute of Experimental Veterinary Medicine in

*Isaac Babel writes of visiting the Petrograd abattoir in 1918 and finding it closed for lack of cattle. A short distance away he finds a horse abattoir in which starving and sick horses are being slaughtered for human food at more than 10 times the prewar rate.[34]

*Considerable information of this kind had already been published by Eberbeck, the pathologist on the staff of the German Army Veterinary Corps Infectious Disease Laboratory on the eastern front, during the years 1916 to 1920.[165–170] How much of this work reached Russia I do not know.

Moscow, did mostly bacteriological work. The second, under Professor N. D. Ball at the Central Military Veterinary Bacteriological station (at first in Moscow and later in Leningrad), concerned itself chiefly with the correlation of the various diagnostic tests and lesions found at autopsy. From these, it appears that the complement-fixation test, when positive, had the highest (91.6 percent) incidence of correlation with the presence of postmortem lesions.[52] Professor Ball's group (Belkin, Chernyak, Landa) also worked on the pathology and pathogenesis of glanders, but I have not been able to obtain their publications, and there are not enough details in the available abstracts to permit an assessment of their work. The third group was that of Professor K. H. Bohl in Kazan, and its members are given on page 143.

As reported by Vereshchagin,[613] the methods used to control glanders, both before World War I, when only clinically ill animals were condemned, and after it, when all horses reacting positively to mallein were killed, failed to achieve their goal. He states that the cardinal problem lay in the nature of the inflammatory process, which was a granulomatous one.

The concept of the nature of this inflammation, as described by Professor Bohl, was not shared by other pathologists, including Bohl's teacher Schütz.* However (writes Vereshchagin), when Schütz became acquainted with chronic Russian glanders during World War I, he then confirmed Bohl's hypothesis.

A direct conclusion from Bohl's concept was that no matter how malignant glanders may appear, it can also pursue a milder, more benign course in horses and some of them can consequently be completely cured. As a result, the killing of

*I do not know what the nature of this controversy was. Schütz denied for a long time that glanders lesions could calcify—perhaps this is the point on which Bohl differed with him.

all infected horses, even if the only evidence that they had glanders was merely that they reacted positively to mallein, was not an appropriate way to reach the goal.

Vereshchagin says that, based on Bohl's work, the Red Army was able to eliminate glanders completely between 1921 and 1925. Despite his lengthy discourse, he does not make clear how a better understanding of the pathogenesis of the disease led to its eradication.

Someone—Bohl and his team in Kazan, Ball and his in Leningrad, or Eberbeck in Germany—made the important discovery that despite the fact that ultimately most of the lesions in glanders involved the lungs, *the mode of initial infection was not pulmonary.* On the contrary, it was by ingestion of the infected nasal discharges with fodder or water soiled by them, and the primary lesions occurred in the pharynx and alimentary canal. Subsequent spread of infection to the lungs from those sites was hematogenous. This knowledge enabled the proper control measures to be introduced, and the useless ones, designed to control inhalation of the bacteria, to be abandoned. I have not been able to sort out whether Bohl, Ball, or Eberbeck actually made the important pathogenetic discovery.

In abstracting some of the Russian work (by Bohl and his group) on glanders in 1927 and 1929, Eberbeck said that not all that they claimed as new discovery really was.[169,170] Since Eberbeck had himself done extensive research on the pathology of glanders, one may be forgiven for wondering whether he was possibly a biased critic.

Tsvetkov and Chernyak[601] (p. 54) give credit to Eberbeck, saying that his systematic autopsy and histologic work on more than 300 horses was undoubtedly of great merit. They add, "However, the Soviet investigators reached similar conclusions completely independently" in the early 1920s. Is this statement true? To answer this question it would be necessary to know whether Ball, Bohl, and their colleagues had read the reports of Eberbeck's work before commencing their own or whether they were unaware of it. Unfortunately, I have been unable to obtain most of the published Russian articles on glanders, especially those by N. D. Ball and his group. I am acquainted with the Russian work only from brief abstracts in the German *Jahresbericht Veterinärmedizin,* which do not contain detailed information. Hence I cannot comment on its extent, its quality, or its originality. The judgment by an impartial critic of how much the Russian veterinary pathologists really contributed to our knowledge of the pathogenesis of glanders still remains to be made.

All of the work I have discussed above was done either during World War I, by Eberbeck, or shortly thereafter by the Russians. Therefore it is of interest that Kokurichev, who wrote a large atlas of veterinary pathology in 1973, still referred to Eberbeck's research.[252] Apparently it is still respected in the Soviet Union, but knowing this does not answer the question raised in the previous paragraph.

Viral Encephalomyelitides

Investigation of infectious diseases of the nervous system has a long tradition in Russia, dating back to the third quarter of the nineteenth century. We have already seen that both Eugen Semmer in Dorpat and Constantin Blumberg in Kazan were wont to examine the central nervous system in the course of their autopsies, a practice that was to remain neglected by veterinary pathologists in many countries for decades thereafter.* The neurologic diseases that were stud-

*In fact, in 1906, senior veterinarians of the U.S. Bureau of Animal Industry were writing papers such as "Epizootic cerebro-spinal meningitis of horses" *without doing any autopsy at all.*[191]

ied in Russia were canine distemper and rabies, followed, near the end of the period we are considering here, by equine encephalomyelitis.

To aver that veterinary neuropathology first emerged as a discipline in Russia would be exaggeration; nevertheless, the dim outlines of the shape it was later to be given in Vienna and Prague by H. Dexler can be seen emerging in nineteenth-century Russia. From the efforts of the veterinarians and physicians in Russia who were examining the brain and spinal cord histologically between 1875 and 1900, there resulted, by the turn of the century, a number of publications which, though small, was unmatched in most other countries. What little attracted attention in the West was soon forgotten; eventually, almost all of it was, even in Russia!

Following the initial report of the lesions in the spinal cord in canine distemper by Gowers and Sankey in England, two papers in Russian expanded this knowledge. The first was by K. Matsulevich in 1884[342] and the next by A. Kraevskii in 1887.[272] It was not then the custom to identify the institute from which a scientific paper emanated, so that in discussing the above two workers, I once wrote, erroneously as it turned out, "Other than that they were Russian veterinarians, I have been unable to find out who Kraevskii or Matsulevich were, and whether they made any subsequent contributions to neuropathology."[460] In the case of Matsulevich, I have still found no biographical information. Kraevskii's biography, however, which I found too late to avoid the above faux pas, turned out to be in the Biographical Dictionary of Polish Veterinarians![355]

Alfred A. Krajewski (as it is written in Polish) was born near Vilna in 1855. He attended the Dorpat Veterinary Institute, graduating in 1875. In 1880 he received the degree M.V.Sc. from Dorpat, with the dissertation *Über die Wirkung der gebräuchlichsten Antiseptica auf einige Kontagien.* Krajewski served in a number of different posts in the Russian Empire as a provincial veterinarian and later as a veterinary inspector. None of these posts ostensibly involved scientific work; however, he published a number of studies which must have required either a bacteriological laboratory, a histological one, or both.[270–272] Where he got the laboratory facilities to carry out these studies is obscure to me and is unfortunately not mentioned in the above biographical source. Krajewski went to Poland after the Revolution in 1917 and died in Warsaw in 1920.

The most important of the early publications on the neuropathology of canine distemper was made by Karl H. Bohl, who did this as his dissertation research for the M.V.Sc. degree under N. M. Lyubimov in Kazan.[77] In this report, Bohl described in considerable detail the lesions in the spinal cord of nine dogs. He used the recently developed stains of Nissl and Weigert to very good purpose, being the first veterinarian to do so. I have discussed this work elsewhere[460] and will add here only that he followed it up with other neuropathological contributions shortly after the turn of the century.[81,97,98]

Bohl retained an interest in neuropathology through many years. In the early 1930s, a strange, new neurologic disorder appeared among horses in the Soviet Union. Although other veterinary scientists thought it was a forage poisoning, Bohl studied its neuropathology and contended on the basis of the lesions that it was of viral etiology. He stated, however, that it was not Borna encephalitis, which affected horses in Germany. Within a year or two, his etiologic predictions turned out to be correct, as virologists were able to isolate a new, filterable infectious agent from the brains.[593] No doubt Bohl was acquainted with Borna encephalitis from having worked with Joest in Dresden before World War I. His knowledge of equine neuropathology enabled him to focus the efforts at finding the etiology of the new disease in the proper direction.

To discuss rabies, we must return now to the last quarter of the nineteenth century and to the Military-Medical Academy in St. Petersburg. Interest in the pathology of rabies was first shown by Professor M. M. Rudnev, with the false start related earlier. The work soon got onto the right track, and Rudnev's assistant Kolesnikov, beginning in 1875, published three papers that described the inflammatory changes in the spinal cord and brain of the dog.[254,257,258] He augmented this work slightly in his dissertation for the M.D. degree in 1885.[259] Neither he nor workers in other countries during the nineteenth century stumbled onto the inclusion bodies that were later found by A. Negri; but the location and attributes of the other lesions were well mapped and thoroughly described. Like the papers by the Russian authors just mentioned on canine distemper, Kolesnikov's work was soon forgotten in the West. Although one of Kolesnikov's papers was in *Virchows Archiv,*[258] which makes missing it hardly excusable, J. Innes and I managed to write a book, *Comparative Neuropathology,* in 1962, in which we deplored the fact that the lesions of rabies in animals had not been sought out sufficiently and studied!

Another early worker on the histopathology of rabies was S. A. Ivanov, a veterinarian in the Military-Medical Academy in St. Petersburg.[215] He likewise studied the histopathology of the lesions in dogs, under the direction of Professor A. Raevskii, Rudnev's successor as teacher of pathology in the veterinary division of the Academy. Applying somewhat different stains than Kolesnikov, chiefly osmic acid, Ivanov found fatty deposits around the walls of cerebral vessels in rabid dogs. These changes were apparently secondary to the cerebral inflammation. Ivanov used this material in a dissertation for the M.V.Sc. degree and published it in a veterinary journal as well.[215] Unlike Kolesnikov, he chose a Russian rather than a German journal, making it easier to overlook his work in the West.

Veterinary Pathology in Russia

In this section, I have placed the emphasis on who the five early workers in neuropathology were, rather than dwelling on details of their work. These early Russian contributions to our present knowledge of the neuropathology of rabies and of canine distemper (1) were among the very first on the respective diseases, and (2) provided important information, much of which has stood the test of time. But to attempt to analyze it in detail and relate it to the development of neuropathological knowledge of these diseases would take us too far afield. My aim here is merely to reveal that this early activity existed at all, something that has been forgotten since Dexler wrote about it in 1900.[158]

Trichinosis

A classic example of the bumbling Russian medical officialdom is given by Krylow and Favr, from the pathology department of the University of Kharkov, in 1876.[282] Their paper on trichinosis was published—in an apparent choice of discretion over valor—in a German journal, safely beyond the reach of the Russian censors.* It reads like the plot for a comic opera by Gilbert and Sullivan, wanting only to be set to music to be ready for the stage. (The costumes would already have been provided by the uniforms which all of the main actors wore in the course of their official duties.)

Krylow and Favr mentioned that Professor M. M. Rudnev, while performing autopsies at the Military-Medical Academy in St. Petersburg, was the first to discover human cases of trichinosis in Russia in 1865,[448,449] which he proceeded to transmit experimentally to animals by feeding them bits of

*I have cited several similar examples elsewhere in this book. The lesson seems to be: He who wishes to study Russian scientific history must be prepared to learn German.

affected human muscles. Rudnev therefore recommended the introduction of meat inspection in Russia, at least for pork. All that resulted from this recommendation, however, was a flurry of polemical articles in both the political and medical press, including the claim that another man should get priority for discovering human trichinosis in Russia. Regarding the latter point, which Krylow and Favr repudiated, they write, "Thus we see that the history of trichinosis in Russia is not without its mythology!"

Rudnev, as a student of Virchow, who had demonstrated the life cycle of trichinosis through feeding experiments just four years before Rudnev came to his laboratory, was of course, alert both to the human and the experimental aspects of the disease. And likewise as a student of Virchow, who had recommended and implemented the introduction of meat inspection into Prussia, Rudnev naturally made the same recommendation for his country. But Russia was not ready, and all that resulted was a prohibition on the importation of sausage from Italy and hams from Westphalia, under the pretense that the disease did not exist in Russia unless it were imported. After that, write Krylow and Favr, trichinosis in Russia was forgotten for a long time.

I have cited enough of their work here to indicate that the path of those studying comparative pathology and/or epizootiology and epidemiology in Russia was seldom a smooth one. Following a small epidemic of trichinosis in Moscow, the subject was reopened and subsequently dealt with more intelligently; this went as far as actually admitting officially that trichinae existed in native (Russian) rats and swine! But rational control measures were still a long way off, and the authors, apparently both Ukrainians, end their paper on a note of pessimistic resignation, indicating that they did not expect anything sensible or useful to happen in the Russian Empire in the foreseeable future.

12 Russian Contributions to Veterinary Pathology

> This I know—if all men should take their troubles to market to barter with their neighbors, not one when he had seen the troubles of other men but would be glad to carry his own home again.
>
> —Herodotus, *History* VII

The Role of Pathology in Russian Veterinary Medicine

As explained in the Preface, this book is an outgrowth of a wider historical treatise on veterinary pathology that is still being written. Dealing with a segment of the projected whole, this book identifies—for the first time for the English-speaking reader—the people who worked in Russian veterinary pathology during its formative years, 1860 to 1930. Some of these men are worthy of more detailed historical and biographical treatment than they have received here. This can be provided only by someone more conversant with their language, history, and country than I, and someone who has access to sources of information within that country.

Organizationally, pathology was taken much more seriously in Russian veterinary education than in the American, British, or Canadian counterparts, especially in the nineteenth century. Much that is claimed by Soviet propagandists, beginning about 1947, to be Russian priority in science is really American, British, German, or French. Between 1917 and 1947 the Russians recognized this, but that year Stalin's propagandists began making sweeping claims for priority in all branches of science. According to Parry, the purpose of the drastic switch in the party line was to reassure the Russian people in their own country and "to spread and strengthen antagonism towards the West, particularly towards America."[390] However, some claims can legitimately be made; one of these is that by the late 1880s, three of the four veterinary schools in the Russian Empire had a full-time professor of pathology and the one in Warsaw had an assistant professor. This was undoubtedly because these schools were following the organizational example of the German ones, just as pedagogically they were using the same textbooks. The Russians heeded Virchow's admonition "dass die Pathologie eine selbstständige Wissenschaft sein muss." (that pathology must be an independent branch of science).[615]

By contrast, at the turn of the century, not one Canadian or American veterinary school had a full-time chair of pathology, and this state of affairs was reflected by the paucity of original contributions coming from our schools. At this time in some parts of the English-speaking world, veterinary medicine was still being taught in two-year schools (rather than four-year ones as in Russia) and pathology was hardly recognized as an individual discipline, let alone having any representatives. Furthermore, by 1885 the Russian curriculum required that each veterinary student complete and write up at least one postmortem examination,[171] something that was still not required in most veterinary schools in North America 50 years later!

The situation of pathology could hardly have been better in American or British veterinary medicine than it was in human medicine, and there it was bad indeed! To illustrate this point, Esmond Long writes of the nineteenth century, in his *History of Pathology:*[305] "Great Britain, in spite of its important individual contributions to the science, was even more indifferent to the merits of pathology for independent development. For many years the only chairs for the teaching of the subject were in Edinburgh and the University College of London, and *strenuous efforts were being made to do away with the Edinburgh position as an unwarranted academic burden and expense*" (italics added). Still referring to the nineteenth century, Long writes: "American pathology failed to establish itself in this period, and Americans in quest of training in morbid anatomy continued for years to visit the great deadhouses of Europe." Long is referring to human pathology, but the situation was even worse in veterinary medicine, as shown by the list in my Introduction, which contains no English-speaking school at all. Judged in this context, Russian veterinary pathology, both in organization and in the education and professional knowledge of its professors, was literally decades ahead of the discipline in Britain, the United States, and Canada.

The question now arises whether the early recognition of pathology as a valuable discipline and the according of academic status to it, which certainly look good on paper, actually enabled the Russian veterinary pathologists to record real accomplishments. In posing this question, but particularly in attempting to answer it, my aim, paraphrased from Seton-Watson[526] (p. ix), is to try to see the developments and the people in terms of what was possible in their time, rather than to try to impose on them the standards accepted in our own.

The achievements of the veterinary pathologists in Russia can be assessed from two aspects, international and national. The first entails their contribution to the general body of knowledge of veterinary pathology as a discipline. The second involves their contribution to the teaching of veterinary students and to the diagnosis and control of animal diseases in their own country. There was never more than a handful of pathologists—four when this chronicle begins and little more than twice that number when it ends—to cope with the animal disease problems of this vast empire.

What were some of the problems that required solution between 1860 and 1930? Which of these were solved during this period, and to what extent did Russians contribute to their solution? These are the major questions that can help us to make the needed assessments. They can also help us to understand how Russian veterinary pathology evolved and how its evolution fits into the general picture of the evolution of this specialty worldwide. Such a historical inquiry has not been undertaken by the Russians themselves. The three papers that survey the subject, those of Ivanov,[214] Kokurichev,[251] and Pinus,[417] do not really come to grips with it, nor does Chernyak's paper on comparative pathology.[149]

Thus reduced to a few basic questions, these points appear disarmingly simple to pursue. This appearance of simplicity might in fact be true, had anyone provided a general historical picture of the development of veterinary pathology worldwide during the period in question. Such a survey could serve as a background against which specific questions pertaining to individual countries could be posed. However, such a documentation, much as one would wish it, does not in fact exist. In its absence, while I have touched on a few salient points that shed light on the problem, an inquiry of this kind and scope, pursued on a scale that would provide the answers, is beyond my capacity. Pursuing history as an avocation, I must leave it to others to explore the paths I have surveyed, and—at least in outline—mapped. The outline appears to me as follows.

Contributions of International Significance

At the beginning of the period surveyed here (1860), delineation of diseases, and hence the possibilities of distinguishing them from one another, was imprecise. For example, rinderpest and contagious pleuropneumonia were often confused with one another, as was the latter with shipping fever and all three with malignant catarrhal fever. Thus, the advances in veterinary pathology consisted in part of careful and precise study of the lesions in each disease and the description of how similar ones could be distinguished. The use of the microscope in pathologic anatomy, which came widely into vogue at the beginning of the period we are considering, made such distinctions meaningful for the first time.

Many advances in the nineteenth century were discoveries of the causes of disease. The new science of bacteriology came into its own between 1875 and 1880—shortly after the period covered here began—and, as Long (p. 142) puts it, "solved some of the major problems which had puzzled medicine for twenty centuries."[305] Viruses were discovered as a cause of disease in 1898, when Loeffler and Frosch implicated the first one in foot and mouth disease.

As I have mentioned, those who held chairs of pathology in Russian veterinary schools in the nineteenth century often did research and taught bacteriology as well. Thus, in assessing their achievements, we must look also at their activities in determining the causes of infectious diseases. In this respect, the contributions of Brauell and Semmer are considerable, and those of Blumberg, while less important, are still noteworthy. As Long has said:[305] "Etiology has always been the weakest portion of pathology." Certainly Brauell and Semmer did much to improve this situation with respect to anthrax, fowl cholera, and rinderpest.

We must not think that whatever Semmer and his contemporaries accomplished in research was merely their job. Not so! Today we consider it axiomatic that teaching and research belong together, although evidence that they do is not really convincing. In nineteenth-century Russia, however, the duty of the teacher was *to teach;* research was done in separate places, outside of schools and universities such as the Imperial Academy of Sciences. The idea that a teacher could do both, was in Russia in the literal sense of the word *revolutionary,* and people who did both—even if the research benefited the country—were swimming against the stream. Indulging their curiosity as scientists, they got little moral or pecuniary support and were in fact apt to be looked upon with suspicion. Viewed in this historical context, the bacteriological investigations of Brauell, Semmer, and Blumberg deserve more credit than if they had been made outside of Russia.

The causes of noninfectious diseases were discovered later than those of infectious ones. The importance of nutrients—vitamins and trace elements—in the scheme of physiology and pathology was understood after about 1900 and of genetic diseases about the same time. The distinction of neoplasms from granulomas dates from about 1860, the understanding of metastasis from 1870, the distinction of epithelial from connective tissue tumors from 1865 (Long,[305] p. 125).

In many of these advances in understanding of disease, the development of histology played an important and obvious role. The anatomist Professor F. N. Zavarykin made histology one of the strong disciplines at the Medico-Chirurgical Academy in St. Petersburg, and two of the veterinarians on its faculty, Ravich and Raevskii, published histological studies on muscle and on the hoof.[429,437,438] The intellectual atmosphere was good because the faculty in general was superior. Because the Academy came at various times either under the Minister of Internal Affairs or the Minister of War, it was not restricted as much in its freedom as were all of the civilian educational institutions, which came under the Minister of Education. As Chernyak[150] pointed out, "Joint work carried out in closest contact with one of the largest and most powerful medical groups in the country was necessarily reflected most positively in the scholarly and scientific work of the Veterinary Department."

Undoubtedly the outstanding example of this scholarly achievement is Novinsky's work on the transmissible venereal tumor of the dog (Fig. 61). The very idea of a feat of experimental oncology similar to Novinskii's being carried out at an American, British, or Canadian veterinary school in 1877 strikes one as ludicrous. Where in the English-speaking veterinary world could one find a laboratory of experimental pathology in 1877? The four-year educational course for Russian veterinarians, which included (at St. Petersburg) the requirement of German literature in the curriculum,[217] gave them access to the latest publications carrying research results. It produced veterinarians of a quality that was not to appear on the American scene for another 50 years. Because of this educational advantage, the contributions to veterinary pathology of Russian scientists were correspondingly greater

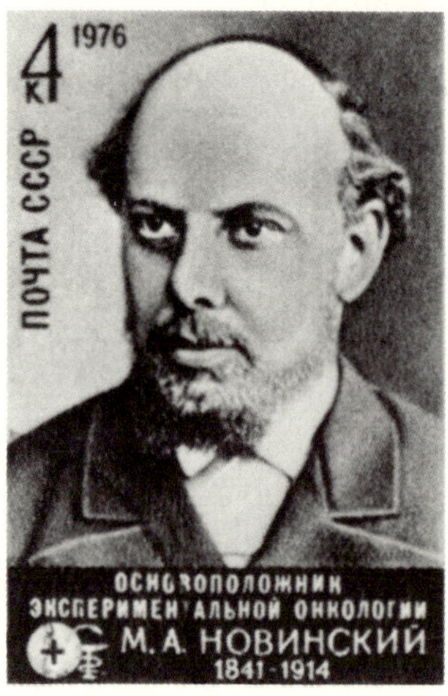

Figure 61. Four-kopeck postage stamp issued to commemorate the centenary of M. A. Novinskii's pioneer transmission of a tumor experimentally in the dog.

in the first half of the period we are considering, 1860–1895, than in the second half, to 1930.

Additional contributions were the discovery of mallein,[206] working out of the pathogenesis of glanders, and the pathology of anthrax, rinderpest, canine distemper, rabies, and equine encephalomyelitis. These contributions were of importance to veterinary pathology far beyond the borders of-Russia, but many of them are unknown in the West.

A Window to the West—But with One-Way Glass

Many articles and books emanating from Russia were overlooked in the West. Others received momentary notice but were soon forgotten and have remained so. For example, Raevski's, Ravich's, and Brauell's work in Russia on the histology of the hooves and claws received no recognition abroad. Ellenberger's comprehensive three-volume book on veterinary histology (*Handbuch der mikroskopischen Anatomie der Haustiere*), 1910–1912, cites none of it, although replete with hundreds of references. Subsequent Western authors did no better.

None of the interesting work done by Petrov on the histopathology of trematodiasis[404,405,407,408] is cited in Western books on pathology or parasitology. Neither is Melnikov-Razvedenkov's work on the pathology of echinococcosis. The Russian work on the pathogenesis of glanders has likewise been ignored in the West. A leading British authority, F. C. Minett, for example, writing in the book *Infectious Diseases of Animals* (1959), makes no mention of it.[290] Since he likewise failed to cite the pertinent German work on this topic, this lapse is probably attributable to slipshod scholarship rather than to anti-Russian or anti-Soviet bias. Neither Ravich nor Semmer are in the chapter "Biographical Notices" in Bulloch's *History of Bacteriology,* although he cites their work in his text and many less important people are sketched in his "Biographical Notices."[130]

The fact that some of the pioneer work on the etiology and epizootiology of anthrax was done in Russia by Brauell, Ravich, Semmer, and Kolesnikov likewise did not always obtain recognition in the West. Nieberle's comprehensive review of the comparative pathology of anthrax[368] does not mention any of these four authors, even though three of them had published in German. Thus, anyone depending on his review article would not even become aware that Brauell, Ravich, and Semmer had ever existed!

Unfortunately, the contributions of Brauell, Ravich, and Semmer to the pathology of rinderpest have likewise been forgotten, undeservedly, for they are classic pieces of work, Ravich's particularly so, and beautifully illustrated as well. The definitive modern paper on the pathology of rinderpest[343] says not a word about the pioneering Russian contributions, nor are these cited in the monograph by Hutyra and Marek,[213] even though their book is illustrated by a dozen colored plates borrowed from the British Royal Commission report[8] in which Ravich's work is repeatedly cited. The latest encyclopedia of viral diseases of animals likewise omits reference to the Russian contributions, but, as I have pointed out elsewhere,[459] the chapter on rinderpest is so poorly written that this is but one of many lapses. Thus, the major works dealing with pathology of rinderpest in English, French, and German, far from being a source of information on the original contributions from Russia, constitute an impenetrable barrier to obtaining it.

Much early Russian work on amyloidosis was also forgotten. Bohl reported on it in horses,[80,83,87,94] long before its widespread occurrence in Russia became known. He also reported on the rare nasal amyloidosis in horses,[107] as did Chernyak.[140] Ball reported on hepatic amyloidosis in cats,[42] and Shukevich on hepatic amyloidosis in horses,[537,538] and in camels.[543] Arndt is one of the few Western authors to have cited this work.[29]

Why was so much Russian work ignored in the West and remains so until this day? I do not know and can only speculate. The language barrier suggests itself as the obvious reason, but all of the important work was published, either initially or eventually, in German. Anti-Russian (later coupled with anti-Soviet) prejudice seems a more plausible reason, albeit supporting evidence is hard to come by. Lack of thorough scholarship on the part of Western veterinary pathologists writing papers and books is undoubtedly another reason.

Peter the Great had founded St. Petersburg as "a window to the West" through which he hoped that his subjects would view the rest of Europe and adopt its ways. Some of his subjects did so, some did not want to look out, but neither were there many veterinary scientists in the West who wanted to look in through this window.

Impediments to Scientific Progress in Russia

From an international standpoint, the achievements of the veterinary pathologists in Russia may seem at first glance not to loom very large when gauged against those of their German contemporaries. This judgment alters, however, if the Russian achievements are viewed from a special perspective—within their own framework—that determines what was actually possible in Russia at any given time. By this I mean a framework bounded by the educational level of the country and by the amount of freedom available to the intelligentsia—mistrusted by both Tsars and Bolsheviks—within the social structure.

Russia was, in the literal sense of the word, a regimented society under the tsars,* as is apparent from the illustrations

*In the nineteenth century, travelers from abroad commented on the colorful uniforms that abounded in every town. These were worn not only by the soldiery, civil servants of every rank, as well as university students, were obliged to wear them. A few, such as I. P. Pavlov, avoided wearing his

of uniforms in Figures 13 and 40 and the imperial coat of arms worn on these uniforms (Fig. 62). It became even more regimented under the Bolsheviks. Such conditions do not conduce to optimum research accomplishments. The following paragraphs sketch in an outline of the social, geographic, and climatic impediments to achievement in Russia. Only after reflecting on these can one fairly decide whether the veterinary pathologists there accomplished more or less than could be expected.

Beginning with Tsarist times, we can reflect on the milieu in which Brauell, Blumberg, and Semmer worked. The bulk of the population was kept illiterate by deliberate policy of the Tsar, which must have made it extremely difficult to recruit even an occasional technician to work in a laboratory. The few scientists who worked in nineteenth-century Russia were, in the words of Olga Mechnikov, "struggling against the inertia and reactionary forces which were shackling the normal development of culture and science in Russia."[351] These forces hung like a pall over a country in which only an occasional ray of light penetrated from the West. The universities were especially suspect as harboring radical elements and hence subject to particular repression, as I was reminded forcibly not long ago, when I opened an old book by Unterberger, published in Dorpat, and found the censor's imprimatur.[604] And this on a subject as politically innocuous as horse breeding! In nineteenth-century Russia, *nothing* could be published without prior approval,* and this

---

uniform and managed to stay out of official disfavor, but professors of lesser fame could not do so. I have illustrated Professor Bohl in Figure 40 wearing his uniform in front of the uniformed students, so that a class in veterinary pathology gives the appearance of one on military tactics. An individual student in uniform is shown in Figure 13.

*It is not so different in 1978, but Russian scientists have had over a century to learn how to outwit the censor. Andersohn,[6] a Baltic veterinarian, published a harmless article on the history of anthrax in an Austrian journal, with the frank explanation "Als aber mein Artikel dem Ermessen hiesiger Censur gemäss, zum Abdruck in den Zeitschriften der Ostsee-

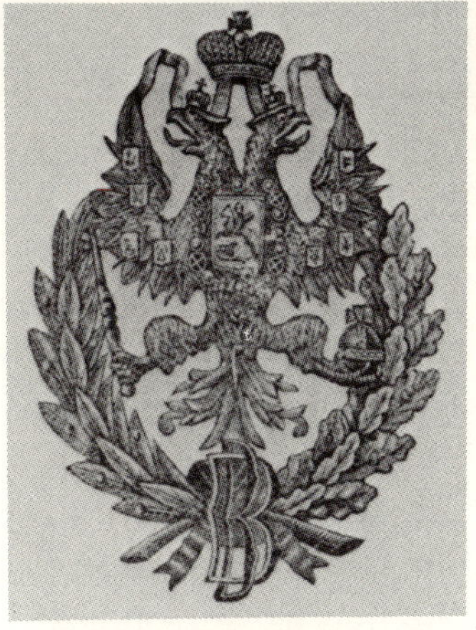

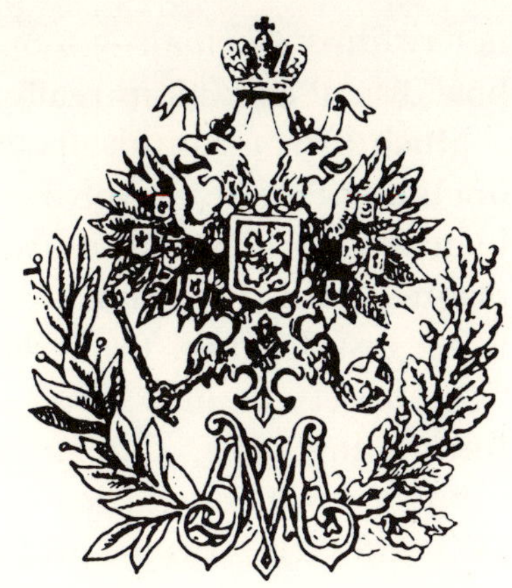

Figure 62. Metal badges for the uniform jackets of veterinarians, each embodying the Russian imperial coat of arms. The one at left is for holders of the diploma of veterinarian. Superimposed at the base of the wreath are the intertwined letters **ВВ**, of the words **Ветеринарный Врач** (Veterinarnyi Vrach, or veterinary physician). At the right is the badge for holders of the degree Master of Veterinary Science, the initial letters of which are likewise on the wreath.

had a very stultifying effect. Thus we understand how Blumberg could begin an article with a sentence lauding the Russian government for its support of veterinary education and then—counting on the censor not reading further* or

---

provizen unzulässig erkannt worden ist, wende ich mich damit an ein dazu geeignetes veterinärärztliches Blatt." (However, as my article, in the view of the local censor, was determined to be inadmissible for publication in the press of the Baltic provinces, I am submitting it to a suitable veterinary publication.)

*Carmichael[131] put it nicely in describing the situation in Russia a few years previous to this: "The increasing harshness of the autocracy, propped up by a comprehensive censorship mitigated only by the incompetence of the officials." In 1862 the oppressive preventive censorship was replaced by what Seton-Watson[526] (p. 358) calls a "more tolerable punitive censorship." In 1865, however, we find that Semmer's M.V.Sc. dissertation on the pharyngeal muscles of animals still carried a censor's approval! Perhaps this was because at that time, as Monas[361] tells us, "there were more censors than books," and, like all bureaucrats everywhere, they wanted to keep their jobs!

not reading German—go on to relate in the next sentence how dismal conditions really are in Kazan![60]

Much of Russian history between 1860 and 1930 was an unending tragedy, involving a cast of millions, playing on a huge stage. This tragedy was comprised of overwhelming plagues—human, equine, and bovine—famines, harsh climate, vast distances traversed by few and poor roads,† (Fig. 63), shattered rail transportation—never good even when functioning—war, and revolution, which convulsed the country repeatedly during the period covered (see Appendix IV). After the 1917 Revolution, mere survival became a problem, for the veterinary pathologists as for almost everyone else. As Zagrodzki[642] pointed out in his survey of the Bolshevik veterinary service, the major preoccupations of the members of the intelligentsia were to avoid starving to death, freezing to death, or being shot by the Cheka (the terrorist secret police organized by Lenin in 1917). He added—and since he is a Pole, I cite Viktorov,[615] a Russian, in confirmation—that veterinary workers often were not paid for months on end, either in cash or in food! The famine is amply documented in a book on Herbert Hoover's famine relief during 1921–1923.[630]

The self-demobilization of the Russian armies after the Revolution resulted in the sale of many army horses by soldiers to local peasants in the provinces adjoining the former front. Glanders, strangles, and mange were rampant. The hostile White and Red armies crossed and recrossed large territories repeatedly as their fortunes changed, and in 1920 the Polish army added to the devastation. These advancing and retreating armies requisitioned cattle, pigs, and poultry as well as horses and disseminated epizootic diseases

†As late as 1934, Bohlen[112] was able to write not of the country, but of its *capital city* (!): "Charlie, Grisha and I careened around the muddy streets of Moscow all one day in search of clothes hangers."

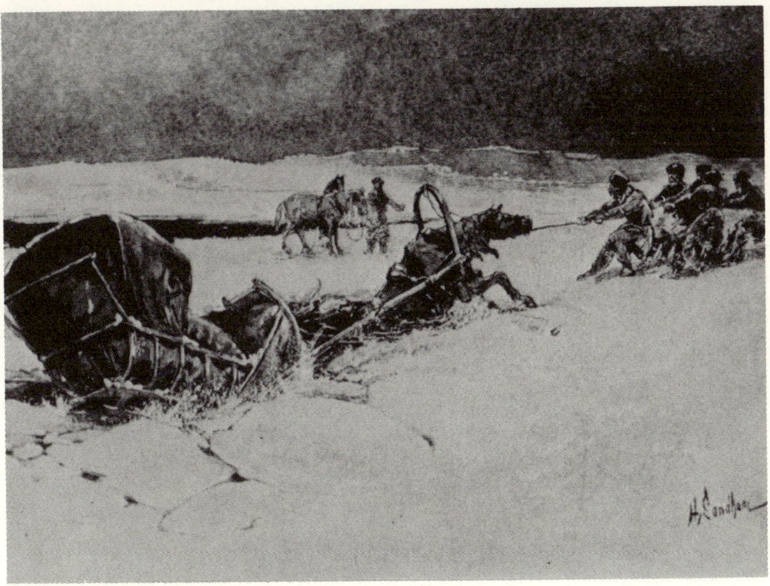

Figure 63. Getting George Kennan's sleigh back to shore. Many rivers could be crossed with safety only during the months when they were frozen solid.

widely.[420] The horse population fell from 22,000,000 in 1914 to 8,000,000 in 1922 and cattle from 18,000,000 to 6,000,000.

During the Civil War (1918–1922) and the years immediately thereafter, when famine struck the country repeatedly, Ball and Bohl were the only two veterinary pathologists with any extensive experience who were still functioning—Shukevich and Mari had died, Gryuner was at Omsk, where facilities were almost nonexistent,* Krakht-Paleev in Kharkov was trying to get teaching started in facilities that had been laid waste, and Waldmann was in Estonia. Both Ball and Bohl put their trainees to work in an

*The Omsk Veterinary Institute occupied a former seminary for priests (Arndt,[30] p. 223).

all-out program to elucidate the pathology of glanders; in a single issue of the *Jahresbericht der Veterinärmedizin* (*46:* 925–934, 1926), for example, we have papers by Ball, by three of Ball's students (Belkin, Chernyak, and Pinus), and by three of Bohl's (his son, I. Smivrov, and B. G. Ivanov).

When we think of the indispensability of the horse for agriculture in this era and of the famine that afflicted the country in 1921 and later, it is easy to see why glanders had to be controlled. The public health aspects, relative to the largest outbreaks of human glanders in the history of medicine, have already been alluded to and were no less compelling. Unlike Canada and the United States, for example, which could afford to shoot all suspect horses as well as unequivocally positive mallein reactors, the Russians could not. Their poverty thus led them to a drive to understand the pathogenesis of the disease, whereas no one in North America thought its pathology was worth studying.

Although infectious diseases were mainly responsible for the losses of horseflesh in the Red Army and on the farms during the Civil War and thereafter, neglect of horses by Red soldiers, many of whom had been recruited into the cavalry ignorant of horse husbandry, was also damaging. In his book *Red Cavalry,* one of these soldiers, Isaac Babel,[33] gives a vivid rendition of how he ruined a horse's back during the Polish campaign in 1920. When the stories that comprise this book first appeared, S. M. Budenny, who had commanded the Soviet troops (see Appendix II), complained that Babel had libeled his forces. Writing as late as 1924, however, Budenny, then Inspector of Cavalry, was himself appalled at the conditions he found upon inspecting several Soviet military districts.[127] Neglect of proper trimming of feet, improper shoeing, and the use of nails either too long or too short were all widespread. He deplored the shortage of adequate blacksmith shops and shoes and realized the need for setting up farrier's schools. The fundamental problems to be solved, however, were illiteracy and ignorance of horse husbandry among the troops and inability to obtain supplies and organize their distribution among the senior Bolshevik officers.

In trying to form an image of what life was like for veterinary pathologists between 1860 and 1930, a Western reader must exercise considerable imagination. With the help of the illustrations in this book, imagine a vast, cold, arid country of eight and a half million square miles, inhabited (in 1885) by 100,000,000 people, and containing 35,000,000 cattle, 20,000,000 horses, 65,000,000 sheep, 10,000,000 swine, plus numerous camels and chickens.[513] Some of these cattle (and other species) are dying daily, sometimes in large numbers, leaving the people chronically short of food and transportation, and—because the country is largely agrarian—also short of money. The horses, too, are dying, on some days in large numbers, interfering with the country's communication, which, because of the paucity of roads and rails, depends on horses, sleds, wagons, or horse-drawn streetcars (Figs. 64 and 65).* Seldom does anyone know why the cattle and horses are dying, or—until weeks after the event—even where disease outbreaks are occurring. When foals and calves die in large numbers, replacements are slow to be made, because breeding hygiene is poor, fertility is low, and infectious abortion is prevalent.

Arrayed against all of this animal disease wastage is a profession of 1,676 veterinarians and 250 *feldshers* (veterinarian's assistants) in 1885.[513] By 1902 the number of veterina-

*The dependence on horse trams in the cities lasted considerably longer than in North America or Western Europe. Bater writes:[46] "Indeed, during a period when underground transport systems were being developed in New York, London and Paris, the major programme in St. Petersburg involved replacing the horse tram with the electric tramcar, a programme not started until 1907." All of the main lines in the inner city had been electrified by 1914, but 261 horse trams still remained on many peripheral lines.

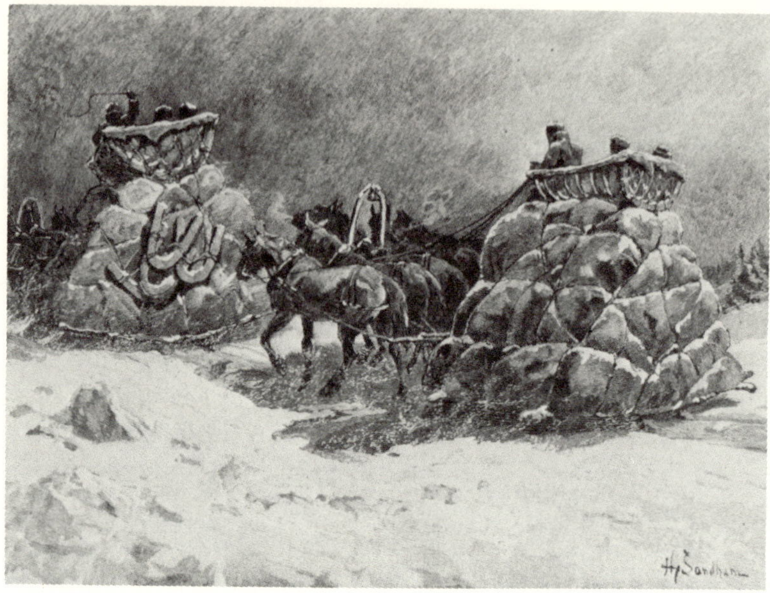

Figure 64. Larger freight sledges were drawn by teams of three or more horses.

rians has risen to 3,000[265] but there are more people and more animals in the country, so that the proportion of veterinarians to the number of animals has not improved. These veterinarians attempt to funnel information, carcasses, and requests for diagnostic assistance to a group of four to six (later eight to twelve) overworked pathologists, who are responsible also for the teaching of their subject as well as ancillary subjects, such as bacteriology and meat hygiene, in the country's four veterinary schools. Even teaching alone would not have been easy once the students began participating in revolutionary activities. And participate they did, during 1905–1907 at all four schools—Dorpat, Kazan, Kharkov, and Warsaw.[639]

Higher education is under the national government, and it is in the government's interest to support these half dozen pathologists munificently, with money, equipment, experi-

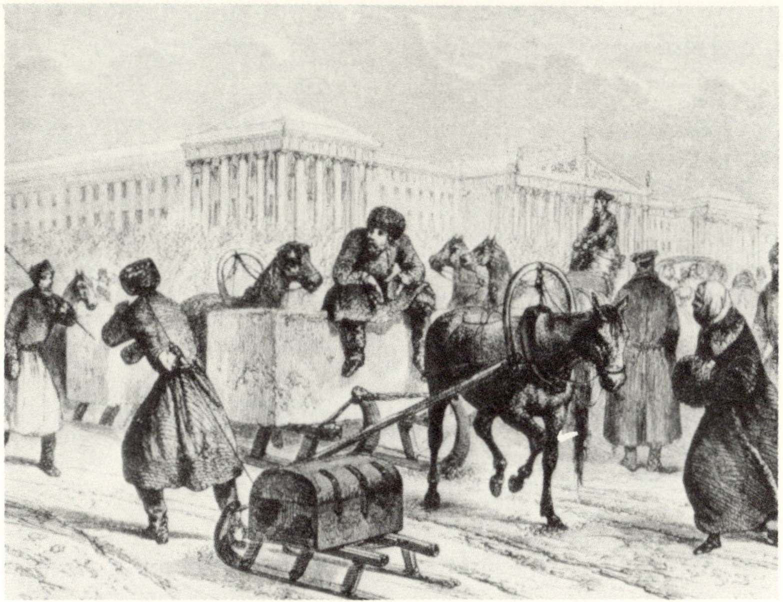

Figure 65. Blocks of ice were transported to storage houses for summer use by horse-drawn sleighs, items of luggage by human-drawn ones.

mental animals, and above all with assistants. Such enlightened self-interest would lead—as in Western countries—to control of some of the animal diseases and reduction in the incidence of others. But, the handful of pathologists do not get this support because the government is manned by mediocre men* of narrow vision and limited intellect, who mistrust all professors—even veterinary pathologists! Instead, the money is spent on such luxuries as Russian Orthodox chapels in the European spas frequented by the Russian royalty, of which the one in Wiesbaden, Ger-

*Some of them would have had to rise far to *attain* mediocrity. But perhaps one should not generalize about Russian bureaucrats. Fodor writes of the Intourist "service bureaus" today; "Amiability and competence alternate with staggering inefficiency and boorishness" (*Fodor's Europe,* p. 895, 1974). In the nineteenth century, too, both kinds of officials were in the service of the empire, but there were not many of the former.

many, still standing in 1977, gilded roof and all, shows that the priests wielded considerable influence at court even if the scientists did not.

For most of the period 1860–1930, financial support of the pathology laboratories—as for the veterinary schools as a whole—was niggardly; however, this is also true of the British and North American schools, many of which had to exist as private ventures. During the last five years of this period, 1925–1930, the laboratories were somewhat better equipped and, according to one German observer,[371] they were comparable to the best in the West. The dean of the Kharkov Veterinary Institute, however, was still complaining that equipment and budgets were far behind those in Germany.[427]

Many historians of Russia, such as Kennan (see Appendix V), have stressed the inefficiency of its unwieldy, bungling bureaucracy, centrally directed but unable to function efficiently at any distance from St. Petersburg, venal, but unable to get out of its own tracks even when bribed. The Soviet authors Ginzburg and Ivanov especially emphasize that nothing very effective was done to control animal plagues until the Bolsheviks came to power.[180] Nevertheless, someone in the tsarist Ministry of Public Instruction saw to it that there were four veterinary schools in operation, and, even if the minister in 1909 fired the pathologist (and director) of one of them, he saw that they continued in operation. Thus, in writing about Russia's backwardness in the nineteenth century, we must avoid what Seton-Watson calls "comparisons between two propaganda pictures, between a caricature of European imperial rule, with all negative aspects stressed or magnified and all positive achievements ignored, and an idealized version of Soviet rule, in which the promised blessings of the future communist utopia are treated as contemporary facts. This fantastic distortion has long passed for truth in a large part of the world."[525]

Contributions to the National Welfare

From the national standpoint, the pathologists were the important leaders in Russian veterinary education and above all in Russian veterinary journalism. Fulfilling editorial functions comparable to those of Gurlt, Schütz, Kitt, and Cohrs in Germany, pathologists founded and edited the most important and influential veterinary journals in Russia. The veterinary pathologists in Russia also wrote both textbooks and research monographs. To some extent books are landmarks of the stage of development of a scientific discipline. They are not the ultimate landmarks, especially of original research work, because most such work is not published first in books. But they do provide an indication of whether a branch of knowledge has emerged from its infancy or is still embryonic.

Almost all of the major figures treated in this chronicle wrote books—Brauell, Blumberg, Ravich, Raevskii, Semmer, Ostapenko, Krakht-Paleev, and Bohl. Their titles have been cited in the discussions of each person and need not be repeated here. Such extensive literary activity on the part of almost all of the veterinary pathologists in Russia is indeed noteworthy and can be construed in several ways.

The books published in German, or translated into it from Russian, betoken a wish to communicate knowledge to the veterinary world outside of Russia. Both these and the books published only in Russian are an indication of intense interest in their discipline among a dedicated group of men and, further, of a desire to propagate a knowledge of that discipline to their colleagues in Russia. Last but not least is the desire to communicate such a knowledge to veterinarians in the Russian Empire in the Russian or Ukrainian language, either to reach people who read only their mother tongue or to indicate that these languages had come of age as media of scientific communication.

Laugh as we will at the backwardness of the Russian Empire and its largely illiterate subjects—and certainly there is much to laugh at—the nineteenth century brought forth no British or American counterparts of any of the books produced by Russian veterinarians. And in the first three decades of the twentieth century, that is, to the end of the 60-year period covered herein, A. T. Kinsley's *Veterinary Pathology,* published in 1910, and W. J. Crocker's *Veterinary Post-Mortem Technic,* in 1918, were the sole such books emanating from the English-language countries.

The intensive production of so many books by so few people seems to have been part of a wider historical process. Igor Vinogradoff[618] tells us that during the reign of Nicholas II, Russia had an industrial growth rate of 6 to 8 percent, "by far the highest in Europe," and enjoyed a philosophic, literary, musical, and dramatic revival; its visual arts were beginning to astound the West by their freshness and originality. "The 'Great October Revolution' . . . reversed her economic growth and retarded her recovery, distorted her social and political destiny and destroyed a great flowering of civilization and art." This retardation was perhaps less obvious in veterinary pathology than in other branches of science and certainly less than in the arts.

Veterinary pathologists represented their country at several international veterinary congresses, in the days when these served their original purpose of facilitating the control of epizootics in Europe.* Without their help and that of the veterinarians they educated, the agriculture of the country would undoubtedly have come even closer to the brink of collapse from the effects of equine and bovine diseases than it did on several occasions.

*The congresses and the veterinary pathologists representing Russia were: Vienna, 1865 (Ravich), Zurich, 1867 (Ravich), Brussels, 1884 (Semmer), Paris, 1889 (Semmer), Bern, 1895 (Semmer), Budapest, 1905 (Tartakovskii), The Hague, 1909 (Ball, Bohl, Mari, Shukevich).

In addition to their work in veterinary pathology, two of the veterinarians mentioned in this book, Belkin and Bohl, contributed to the beginning of newly founded medical institutions. A third, Krakht-Paleev, who also held a medical degree, lectured in the medical faculty of Kharkov University in addition to his veterinary duties.

Almost all of the pathologists mentioned in this book had an interest in veterinary history. At least they wrote about it; probably more for the edification of their colleagues than in order to report the results of any historical research. This is not the place to enlarge on such ancillary activity, hence I will merely cite the pertinent papers. These were by Ball,[38,45] Blumberg,[58] Bohl,[110] Brauell,[116] Mari,[325] Ostapenko,[381] Raevskii,[427] and Semmer.[509]

"To Prevent Virtuous Actions from Being Forgotten . . ."

How did veterinary pathology evolve in Russia? We can discern two main streams of evolution.

In the first, Russian veterinarians learned the German language, read German veterinary books and journals, went to Germany* for postgraduate work with the authors of such publications, and returned home to teach. They organized the veterinary schools on German lines and equipped them as much as possible like the ones they had seen in Germany. They used German instruments and German autopsy, histologic, and bacteriologic techniques to study diseases in Russia. They taught the details of these techniques to their stu-

*The term "Germany" is used generically here, to indicate the three countries within the German-language sphere: Austria, Germany, and Switzerland. Even among the few people illustrated in Appendix VII, we find Germans teaching in Austria and Switzerland (Klebs), Swiss teaching in Germany (Ziegler), and people from all three countries changing their location without regard to national boundaries.

dents and published the results of their observations or experiments in German journals and books.

For advances to be made today in pathology, sharp powers of observation, ingenuity of experimental approach, and keen intellect are required; seldom must one wait for techniques to be discovered. It is perhaps laboring the obvious to point out that in the nineteenth century, advances in pathology could only follow—they could not lead—the development of microtomes, fixing, embedding, and staining techniques and quality microscopes. The work in Russia kept pace with these technological advances, the highlights of which are given in the section "Some Historical Events."

As advances in knowledge were made in Germany (and elsewhere in Europe), they were reflected by the German-educated Russians in their teaching and applied in their research work. Thus veterinary pathology in Russia evolved along parallel lines with German veterinary pathology, keeping pace with it or almost so, and remaining far in advance of American or British veterinary pathology. At international veterinary congresses, the Russian veterinary pathologists met their American, British, French, Austrian, Dutch, German, Italian, Scandinavian, and Swiss colleagues and through personal contact kept up with what was going on in this specialty in Western countries.

In the second stream of evolution, which was concurrent with the first one, veterinary pathologists in Russia were in the vanguard of those making original contributions, and in certain aspects of animal pathology they worked independently of progress being made elsewhere. Russians led in experimental oncology, in the discovery of mallein, in the pathology of rinderpest, and in research on an effective immunization against it. The evolution of veterinary pathology on independent lines also includes the delineation of the neural lesions in canine distemper, rabies, and equine encephalomyelitis, basic contributions to the bacteriology of anthrax and of fowl cholera, and the demonstration that the presence of a bacterial organism can be used to establish the diagnosis of a disease (Brauell). In its evolution along these lines, veterinary pathology in Russia was up to or ahead of the best elsewhere, perhaps because several of the people involved in it were not Russians (Brauell, Jessen, Blumberg, Semmer).

Taking the two streams of evolution together, the final question is, did the veterinary pathologists working in Russia between 1860 and 1930 accomplish anything worthy of mention, let alone of a whole book?

I find it difficult to make an impartial judgment because I am torn between rejection of Soviet propaganda with its contempt for truth and distortions of history, and admiration for the indomitable spirit of many of the men whom I have mentioned here—the whole clouded by the notorious Russian secretiveness which defeats all but the professional historian in obtaining data and attaining a sharp focus on events. I judge that in the circumstances I have described, prevailing against incredible adversity, our half dozen or so scattered Estonian, Latvian, Polish, Ukrainian, and Russian colleagues (and Brauell and Jessen, Germans in the service of Russia) acquitted themselves creditably, one could even say remarkably, in practicing veterinary pathology in Russia. They availed themselves of German training, books, journals, and microscopes (as we did also in the United States). With the help of these, they made original and lasting contributions to our knowledge of the cause and pathology of anthrax, canine distemper, rabies, tuberculous mastitis, fowl cholera, equine viral anemia, equine encephalitis, glanders, rinderpest, and the mycoses, as well as being the first to experimentally transmit a tumor. They advocated and conducted carefully done autopsies.* They also wrote a dozen

*Had Blumberg's book on autopsy technique been translated into English in 1895, it would have greatly advanced veterinary pathology in all of the English-speaking world from that year until 1919, when Crocker pub-

books. While these accomplishments by no means loom as large as certain Soviet propagandists would have us believe, they are nevertheless substantial, and many are unknown in the West.

In writing this book, I have attempted, as Taylor[588] suggested all historians do, "to shape into a version a tangle of events that was not designed as a pattern." He also said that "history is not just a catalogue of events put in the right order like a railway timetable. History is a version of events. . . . The historian tries to impose on events some kind of rational pattern: how they happened and even why they happened." I have aspired to meet this challenge, but I have seldom been able to determine why events happened and not always how. I hope I have revealed the outline of the major events themselves with sufficient clarity to indicate *which* ones happened! I hope also that my version of events has untangled them enough to reveal those questions which remain to be answered, so that others may be encouraged to seek answers.

My reward has been in heeding Tacitus' admonition to prevent virtuous actions from being forgotten and Pliny's to rescue from oblivion those who deserve to be remembered.

> Eine Chronik schreibt nur derjenige, dem die Gegenwart wichtig ist. (A chronicle is written only by him to whom the present is important.)
>
> Goethe,
> *Maximen und Reflexionen aus Kunst und Altertum,* 1826.

---

lished the first book on this subject in English. Because it was not translated, Blumberg's book remained a potential rather than an actual contribution to international veterinary pathology.

Appendix I. The Anti-Virchow Nonsense

Koropov, the author of the major book on the history of Russian veterinary medicine, forfeits our confidence straightaway with distortions of one kind or another—particularly about Rudolph Virchow.[265] Not only does he put words in Ravich's mouth (Chapter 4) which the latter never uttered, but as a historian Koropov manages to "forget" that Virchow was the first foreign scientist to be elected an honorary member of the Moscow Society of Veterinarians. This occurred on his seventieth birthday, September 27, 1891. It is documented in a 10 page obituary in the journal *Veterinarnoe Obozrenie* embellished with a full-page portrait, which shows how Russian veterinarians really felt about Virchow.[13]

Although Koropov's book was published a year after Stalin's death in 1953, it must have been in press during that year and was undoubtedly written before Stalin died. Very likely, Koropov was obliged to echo the then current Communist party line, which switched in 1950 from previous recognition (Fig. 66)* to condemnation of Virchow.[176] By 1961 (eight years after

*This recognition was high in tsarist times[53] and remained essentially undimmed during the early Soviet years. Thus, at the first All-Union Congress of Pathologists, held in Kiev in 1927 to coincide with the twenty-fifth anniversary of Virchow's death, not only did Professor N. N. Anichkov of Leningrad give a memorial address, but to further honor Virchow's memory, *he gave it in German!*[563]

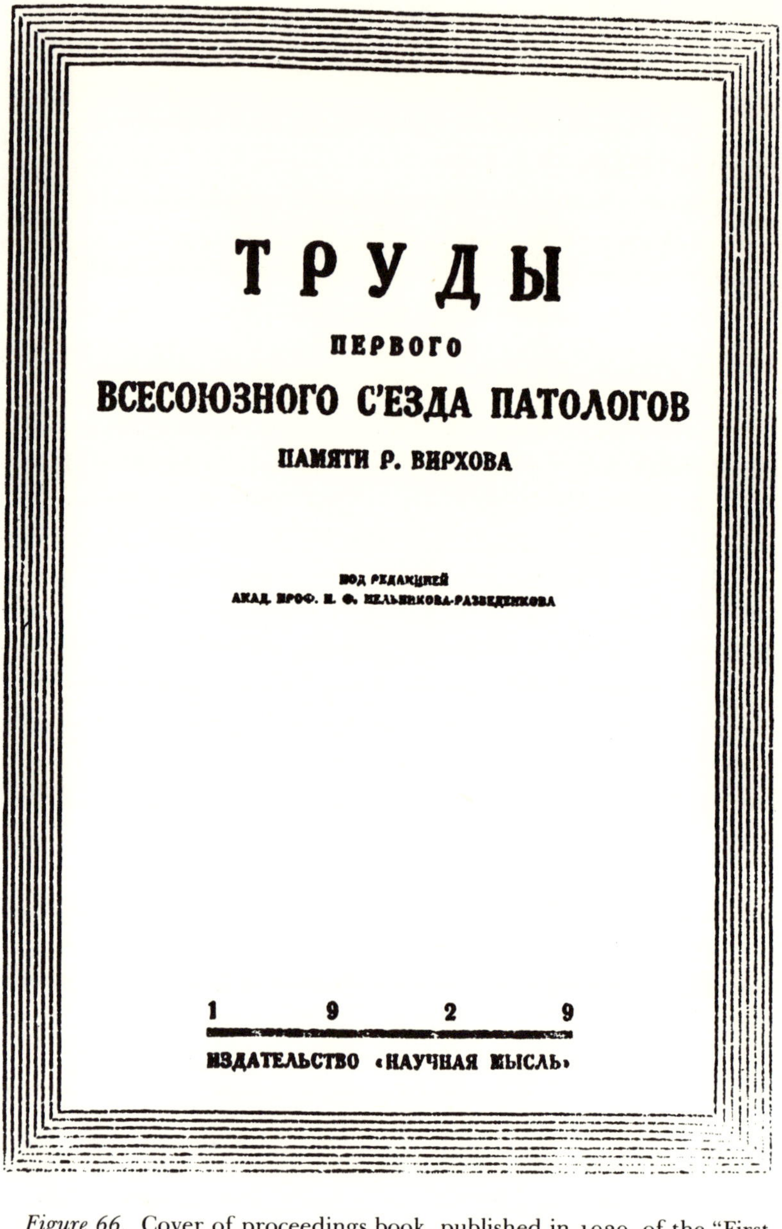

ТРУДЫ

ПЕРВОГО

ВСЕСОЮЗНОГО С'ЕЗДА ПАТОЛОГОВ

ПАМЯТИ Р. ВИРХОВА

ПОД РЕДАКЦИЕЙ
АКАД. ПРОФ. Н. Ф. МЕЛЬНИКОВА-РАЗВЕДЕНКОВА

1 9 2 9

ИЗДАТЕЛЬСТВО «НАУЧНАЯ МЫСЛЬ»

Figure 66. Cover of proceedings book, published in 1929, of the "First All-Union Conference of Pathologists, in Memory of R. Virchow," held in Kiev in 1927. The editor is N. F. Melnikov-Razvedenkov.

Stalin's death), the party line had veered back again sufficiently that the leading Soviet medical pathologist, Davydovsky, addressing a conference of veterinary pathologists, not only mentioned Virchow in the same breath as Pavlov, but even had the audacity to say: "There have been mistakes connected, for example, with cell theory criticism. . . . There have been mistakes in the interpretation of the role of the nervous system . . . which transformed Pavlov's excellent theory into an oligarchic despotic 'nervism,' which in fact blocked the road to thought."[156]

Davydovsky, who, as president of the Soviet All-Union Society of Pathologists and chief editor of its journal, had also been obliged to toe the party line during the last Stalin years, was no doubt relieved by 1961 once more to be able to tell the truth. The party line in biology during the preceding years had been formulated by T. D. Lysenko in genetics and by a crank known as O. Lepeshinskaya* in cytology.[294] Lerner tells us that her "delirious biology" included "half-baked notions on spontaneous generation."[295] Whereas Graham[187] describes her (and Lysenko) as third-rate scientists, Lerner objects to this designation as an undeserved compliment and points out that these people were in reality not scientists at all. I agree with Lerner. They were charlatans, exploiting their scientific education and Stalin's paranoia, with his backing, at the expense of genuine scientists and of the welfare of their country.

The condemnation of Virchow was part of Stalin's neo-Slavism and anti-Westernism that ushered in the cold war. This era was characterized also by a purge in the world of music (Prokofiev, Khachaturian, Shostakovich—all later rehabilitated and even lionized) even more stupid than the ones in biology and medicine.[634] Although Davydovsky abandoned

*Not to be confused with the Olga Lepeshinskaya who earned her renown as a ballerina!

his enforced anti-Virchowism after Stalin's death, Koropov had not yet done so by 1954, either for the reason given above or perhaps because he was a Stalinist at heart. By 1973, however, the Soviet textbook[614] officially approved for teaching veterinary pathology had not only "rehabilitated" Virchow, but even had a portrait of him in its chapter on history! Whether this was a fleeting moment of truth or a final reconciliation with the realities of history, only subsequent editions and the passage of time will reveal.

Appendix II.

S. M. Budenny

Marshall Semeon M. Budenny (1883–1973) (Fig. 67), a former tsarist noncommissioned officer, fought with the Russian Army in World War I and cast his lot with the Red Army in early 1918. After a series of rapid promotions, he organized and led his First Mounted Army in the Civil War with brilliant tactics, or as well as could be expected of a sergeant-major, depending on whether one reads his admirers or his detractors. Like the other Soviet commanders, he could not prevail against the Poles in the Battle of Warsaw in August of 1920. Whatever his talents, they were not equal to the challenge of the German invasion of 1941, and Budennyi soon had to be removed from command in the field.

He survived this debacle and lived to congratulate the journal *Veterinariya,* which he had helped to found, on the occasion of its fortieth anniversary in 1964[128] and the Moscow Veterinary Academy on its fiftieth anniversary in 1969. He also celebrated his own ninetieth birthday in 1973!

A man of humble origins, as a senior cavalry commander, Budenny was in one respect much better than many other cavalry generals. He had a far firmer grasp of the importance of veterinary medicine in military horse husbandry than many of his better educated contemporaries abroad, and this is reflected in the wide range of responsibilities which he assigned to the veterinary officers of the Red Army.[244]

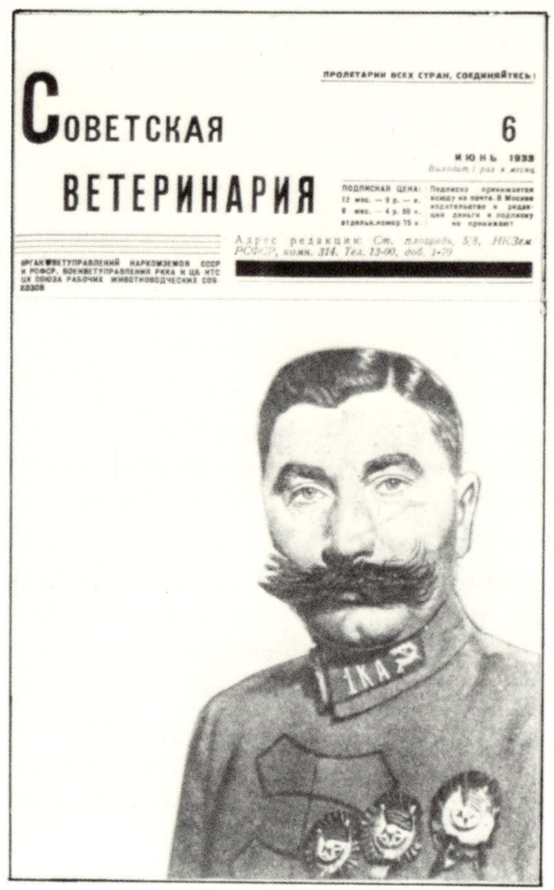

ПРОЛЕТАРИИ ВСЕХ СТРАН, СОЕДИНЯЙТЕСЬ!

СОВЕТСКАЯ

ВЕТЕРИНАРИЯ

6

ИЮНЬ 1933

Выходит 1 раз в месяц

ПОДПИСНАЯ ЦЕНА:

Адрес редакции: Ст. площадь, 5/8, НКЗем РСФСР, комн. 314. Тел. 13-00, доб. 1-70

ОРГАН ВЕТУПРАВЛЕНИЙ НАРКОМЗЕМОВ СССР И РСФСР, ВОЕНВЕТУПРАВЛЕНИЯ РККА И ЦБ ИТС ЦК СОЮЗА РАБОЧИХ ЖИВОТНОВОДЧЕСКИХ СОВХОЗОВ

Figure 67. Semeon M. Budenny, during the 1920s, as commander of the First Mounted Army. This portrait appeared on the cover of the journal *Sovetskaya Veterinariya* in June 1933.

Budenny is mentioned in this chronicle because of his staunch support of the Army Veterinary Corps and of its consultant, Professor N. D. Ball, while he was commander of the First Mounted Army and later inspector of cavalry for the whole Red Army (see Chapter 12).

Appendix III.

Ukrainian Culture

You cannot drive straight on a twisting lane.
—Russian proverb

The Ukrainian language, explains deBray in his book on the Slavonic languages,[124] "was not allowed to evolve smoothly under the Czars, who regarded its development as an effort to tear away Ukraine from Russia. In 1863, Ukrainian was forbidden as a language of instruction in the schools; and in 1876 printing and publishing in proper Ukrainian was forbidden altogether within the Russian Empire. The ukase promulgating this was a secret one, so that the Russian public learnt of it only some years later.... In 1905, the ban on the use of Ukrainian was lifted with the establishment of the new constitution."

The Ukrainian language, which had evolved up to the Bolshevik seizure of power in 1917, was adequate for literary expression but not for scientific or technical use. Several conferences were held to decide on what form the newly evolved language was to take.[124] During the period of the new economic policy (NEP), a policy of ukrainization was allowed to begin. During it, on August 1, 1923, a Language Act proclaimed the priority of Ukrainian over Russian in the Ukraine. Seton-Watson[525] points out that "this cultural progress to some extent compensated for the lack of political freedom. The progress was the work of Ukrainian Bolsheviks, chief among whom was Mykola Skrypnik, who held the Commissariat of Education from 1927 to 1933." A decade after NEP had begun, however, Ukrainian scientific words were still not widely known, so that Krakht-Paleev felt obliged to publish a glossary of Ukrainian-Russian terms in his book on veterinary pathology in 1932 (see Fig. 32). Shortly thereafter, in 1936, Professor P. O. Kucherenko of Kiev, a medical pathologist, published his book *Patolohichna Anatomiya*, on human pathology, also in the Ukrainian language. He was able to avail himself of a Ukrainian terminology newly created for medical science by a Medical Terminology Commission of which he was a member.[419]

In 1928, Stalin abandoned the NEP, and thereafter stopped the policy of ukrainization. Its momentum kept it going for a while after that, but in 1930, 1931, and 1933 the Ukrainian Communist leadership was purged, ostensibly for treasonable plotting against the Soviet state. The actual reason was the leadership's nationalistic leanings, which Stalin feared and hated as much as had the tsars. Numerous leaders of the government of the Ukrainian Republic, and later their replacements, were thus shot or deported on trumped-up charges, either with or without sham trials. Some, like Skrypnik, committed suicide in anticipation of their fate. Often enough, those who had acted as accusers of the murdered leaders were themselves subsequently killed. In addition to the politicians, the philologists who had helped to modernize the Ukrainian language were also killed or deported to slave labor camps, where they died.[267]

During this period, use of the Ukrainian language in science again went into a decline,* although a few exceptions were tolerated for a time, such as the books by Krakht-Paleev

*This decline itself pursued a zigzag course. Thus, I am informed that for a time during the early 1930s (in conformity with a shifting trend that soon reverted to Russian), Russians who taught in Ukrainian universities were obliged to lecture in Ukrainian, even though they did not speak the language! Most of them complied by reading a few introductory sentences in Ukrainian and then reverting to Russian.[391]

and Kucherenko. By the 1950s, however, almost everything published by members of the Kharkov and Kiev Veterinary Institutes had, for 15 years or more, been in the Russian language; only a small number of publications had appeared in Ukrainian. An exception was made, probably to stir up patriotic feelings, during World War II. Bazhenov[48] writes that during the "Great Fatherland War" the Ukrainian veterinary journal was resurrected for a few years (see Table 4). He does not mention that it was killed again as soon as the war was over, or a little before!

Except for volumes 15 to 17 (1929–1935), published in the Ukrainian language as *Zbirnyk Prats,* the *Sbornik Rabot* (Collected Works) of the Kharkov Veterinary Institute have been in Russian from their inception in 1890 until today. The veterinary periodicals that have been published in the Ukrainian language, none of them other than short-lived, are listed in Table 4.

Suppression of the Ukrainian language in veterinary science is occasionally carried further than merely publishing work from Kharkov and Kiev in Russian. In some publications, citations of articles that appeared in Ukrainian years ago are altered to cover this up; that is, the titles are cited in Russian. Such tampering with historical materials is not restricted to veterinary medicine; it derives from general "historical" practice in the Soviet Union. Suppression is rife in all aspects of Soviet history. Thus, in the acknowledgments in the preface of his book, *The Gulag Archipelago, 1918–1956,* Solzhenitsyn writes:[564] "I would like to single out in particular those who worked to help me obtain supporting bibliographic material from books to be found in contemporary libraries or *from books long since removed from libraries and destroyed;* great persistence was often required to find even one copy which had been preserved" (italics added).*

*Although the Russians are the most practiced in rewriting history, this practice is not their exclusive domain. Thus, the English journal *New*

An example of this tampering with history is the story of Professor M. I. Samodelkin of the Kharkov Veterinary Institute. His trail begins before World War I, when he published an article as a member of the bacteriology laboratory of this Institute. He then was sent abroad for postgraduate training and published a report of his experiences in various German and Swiss veterinary schools.[454] In one of these, at Bern, he conducted a research project on the pathology of chronic arthritis of the mandibular articulations under Professor Guillebeau. He published this work in German and later in Russian.[455,456] He is next mentioned in the collected works of the Kazan Veterinary Institute. This publication carried his greetings as rector of the Kharkov Veterinary Institute on the occasion of the Kazan Institute's fiftieth anniversary in 1924.

In 1929, the Kharkov Veterinary Institute resumed publication of its "Collected Works," which had been interrupted by the war and revolution for over a decade. As mentioned above, the publication was the first in history to be in the Ukrainian language. The first issue was devoted to relating events of the previous ten years, by means of reports of the activities of each clinic and institute. Professor Samodelkin appeared in this publication as head of the Large Animal Clinic and holder of the chair of surgical pathology, ophthalmology, and obstetrics.

For the sake of authenticity, as well as to preserve the flavor of the original publication, I have reproduced by photocopy (in Fig. 68), the beginning of the report of this clinic, and have given its English translation below. From the

---

Statesman tells us that the publishers of *Who's Who* remove from their book anyone unfortunate enough to serve a jail sentence. "He is expunged from Britain's biographical Baedeker as though he had never been."[27] Since 1968, historians who tell the truth have been persecuted also in Czechoslovakia, and "their books removed from the libraries and destroyed."[28]

Table 4. Veterinary publications in the Ukrainian language

Publication and city	Dates published	Fate
Ukrainsky Vet. Visnyk (Kharkov)	No. 1, 1921	Only one issue published
Zapysky Kiyvskoho Vet.-Zootekh. Instytutu (Kiev)	Volumes 1-4 1924-1926	Ceased publication
Veterynar i Zootekhnik (Kiev)	No. 1-2, 1929	Ceased publication
Naukovi Zapysky Kiyvskoho Vet. Inst. (Kiev)	Volumes 1-3 1938-1940	Ceased publication
Veterynarne Dilo (Kharkov)	1926-1930 (successor to *Vet. Delo,* Nos. 1-25, 1922-1925, in Russian)*	Name changed to *Radyanska Veterynariya*
Radyanska Veterynariya (Kharkov)	1930-1932	Ceased publication
Naukovi Pratsi Ukrayinskoho Inst. Eksp. Vet. (Kiev-Kharkov)	Vols. 1-10 1930-1941	Continued as *Nauchnye Trudy,* in Russian, from Vol. 11, 1944.
Veterinarna Sprava (Kiev)	1936-1940	Absorbed by journal *Sotsialistychne Tvarinnytstvo*
Veterinarna Sprava (Kharkov)	1941-1944	Absorbed by Russian journal *Veterinariya*

*The name was changed from Russian to Ukrainian in 1926. Except for the mastheads and a couple of pages of news in each issue, almost all of the articles remained in the Russian language.

Bibliographic information from *Periodicheskaya Pechat SSR 1919-1949* (Moscow, 1955), from Kravchenko[261] and from Bazhenov.[48] Most of these publications are not mentioned in the six-volume *Veterinarnaya Entsiklopediya,* published between 1968 and 1976.

Хірургічна клініка великих тварин з кабінетом хірургічної патології, офтальмології та акушерства.

За звітний період часу завідуючим хірургічною клінікою та кабінетом був професор М. І. Самоделкін, викладаючи курси хірургічної патології, офтальмології та акушерства. Асистентами були: до 1/Х-26 р. М. І. Бугрімов, а з того часу В. К. Кедров. Ординаторами клініки були: А. В. Орлов, В. К. Кедров, до переведення його на посаду асистента та С. М. Корнієнко. За період часу з 18 року до осени 22 року говорити не тільки про науково-дослідчу працю клініки, але навіть про прийом хворих тварин, в нормальних умовах, не доводиться.

Більшу частину 1918, 1919 й першу третину 1920 року клініка або займалася перходячим військовими частинами, або не функціонувала через закриття інституту.

1-го травня 20 року клініки займає залоговий ветеринарний шпиталь Червоної Армії. Працю в хірургічному відділенні шпиталю несе персонал хірургічної клініки й бере участь в роботі незначне число мілітаризованих студентів-прискореників. У хірургічному відділенні провадиться велика праця.

Figure 68. Excerpt from *Zbirnik Prats Kharkivskoho Veterinarnoho Institutu* 15(1): 60, 1929.

same source I have reproduced (in Figure 69) the opening lines of the report of the chair headed by Professor Maltsev, dealing with operative surgery, topographic anatomy, farriery, and diseases of the hoof, and have given likewise its English translation.

Large Animal Surgical Clinic and Chair of Surgical Pathology, Ophthalmology, and Obstetrics

During the period being reported on, the head of the surgical clinic and of the chair was Professor M. I. Samodelkin, presenting the courses in surgical pathology, ophthalmology, and obstetrics. The assistants were two: until October 1, 1926, M. I. Buhrimov and after that date, V. K. Kedrov. The house surgeons of the clinics were: A. V. Orlov, V. K. Kedrov until his appointment as assistant, and S. M. Kornienko. During the

Кабінет оперативної хірургії з топографічною анатомією та ковки з копитними хворобами.

Кабінет Оперативної хірургії та ковки з копитними хворобами має спеціяльне самостійне приміщення, що складається з двох кімнат, з яких у меншій міститься шість шахв з колекціями хірургічного приладдя та анатомічних препаратів, що уявляють з себе необхідні допоміжні засоби при викладанні курсу Оперативної Хірургії з топографічною анатомією. В двох великих шахвах розміщені колекції зразкових підків, що вживаються для кування як нормальних копитів, так і патологічних, копитні цвяхи різних форм та инші знаряддя, що вживаються при підковуванні коней і при виробці підків; нормальні й патологічні копити та анатомічні препарати з кінця кінцівки коняки та рогатої худоби.

Зазначені практичні заняття провадились під керовництвом і при безпосередній участі професора М. О. Мальцева та асистента С. П. Постнікова.

Figure 69. Excerpt from *Zbirnik Prats Kharkivskoho Veterinarnoho Institutu 15*(1): 67, 1929.

period of time from 1918 to the autumn of 1922, not only can we not talk about scientific research work in the clinic but even about the admission of sick animals, since normal conditions did not prevail.

For most of 1918, 1919, and the first third of 1920, the clinic was requisitioned by the passing military forces or was nonfunctional due to the closing of the Institute.*

On the first of May, 1920, the clinic was used as a garrison veterinary hospital by the Red Army. The work of the surgical division of the hospital was performed by the personnel of the surgical clinic and also by a number of drafted students who had taken an accelerated course. A large amount of work was done in the surgical department.

*This refers to the Kharkov Veterinary Institute as a whole. The "passing military forces" were at various times German, White Russian, Ukrainian Patriots, and Red, which during the years mentioned alternated in their control of the city of Kharkov.

Chair of Operative Surgery, Topographic Anatomy, Farriery, and Diseases of the Hoof

The Chair of Operative Surgery, Topographic Anatomy, Farriery, and Diseases of the Hoof has a special independent facility, consisting of two rooms. In the smaller one are six cupboards with collections of surgical instruments, and anatomical preparations necessary as a means of support for lecturing in the courses in operative surgery and topographic anatomy. In two large cupboards are kept collections of sample horseshoes for shoeing of normal and pathological hoofs, horseshoe nails of different sorts, tools used in making horseshoes and in shoeing horses, normal and pathological hoof, and anatomical preparations of horse and cattle extremities.

The practical excercises were conducted under the direction and with the immediate participation of Professor M. O. Maltsev and the assistant, S. P. Postnikov.

To summarize the information shown in Figures 68 and 69: in 1929 there were two surgical chairs in Kharkov, one (which included obstetrics) headed by Samodelkin, assisted by Kedrov, Kornienko, and Orlov; the other headed by Maltsev, assisted by Postnikov. I have repeated this information to keep it in sharp focus in the reader's mind, before it becomes obscured by what follows.

In 1952 and 1954, historical articles were published (in Russian) by the parasitologist Nosik[332] (then dean of the Kharkov Veterinary Institute) and the surgeon Magda,[314] in connection with the Institute's centenary. Neither article mentions the department operated in the 1920s by Samodelkin, and one seeks in vain in these articles for any mention of Professor Samodelkin himself. Is his name missing because of an honest error of omission, say, on the part of a parasitologist unconcerned with surgery? Perhaps, but can one invoke this explanation for the same lapse on the part of a surgeon, particularly one who was teaching at the KVI in

1929 and therefore must have known Samodelkin personally?

To help answer this question (and still preserve the authenticity as well as the flavor of the original publications), I have again resorted to photocopying of extracts from the two reports of the 1950s (Fig. 70, translated below). This time the language is Russian, and the former names of the clinics have been sufficiently garbled that there is no trace of the two which were in existence in 1929. We are dealing here with no errors of omission, but ones of skillful commission. Nosik has obliterated all trace of Samodelkin's clinic, has listed Kedrov and Kornienko as Maltsev's pupils, and, because the 1929 surgical (and obstetrical) clinic has vanished, there is now no need to name its director. Continuing in this same vein of

Уже при советской власти на базе кафедры хирургии, возглавляемой старейшим воспитанником института проф. М. А. Мальцевым, выросло три самостоятельных кафедры, которые возглавили его ученики: кафедра общей и частной хирургии с ортопедией и офтальмологией, которой до ухода в отставку (1949 г.) руководил сам М. А. Мальцев, а ныне возглавил проф. В. А. Герман; кафедра акушерства с гинекологией и искусственным осеменением, которую вначале возглавлял доцент В. К. Кедров, а несколько позже доцент С. Н. Корниенко; и кафедра оперативной хирургии, которую возглавляет проф., доктор И. И. Магда.

Проф. М. А. Мальцев вместе со своими учениками широко развернул многогранную работу в области подготовки кадров. Наряду с улучше-

Укрепившаяся материальная база Института позволила совершенно по-новому организовать учебный процесс клинических кафедр и строить научную работу. Впервые при Институте учреждается научно-исследовательская кафедра клинической ветеринарии в 1923 г. с терапевтической и хирургической секциями. Руководителем этой кафедры был проф. Мальцев. С организацией этого нового научно-исследовательского отдела вводится аспирантура для подготовки научных работников клинических дисциплин. Из числа лиц, закончивших аспирантуру, в последующем стали профессорами и заведующими кафедрами: заслуженный деятель науки проф. И. И. Лукашов, проф. В. А. Герман, доктор ветеринарных наук В. К. Кедров, доц. С. Н. Корниенко, проф. И. И. Магда. Многие бывшие аспиранты этой кафедры в настоящее время работают в различных учебных и научно-исследовательских учреждениях Советского Союза.

Figure 70. Excerpts from *Sbornik Trudov Kharovskago Veterinarnogo Institutu 15*: 19, 1952 (above) and *22*: 45, 1954 (below).

socialist realism, Magda, writing two years later, implied the same line of succession from Maltsev to Kedrov and Kornienko, although he did not state it so explicitly.

> Already in the time of Soviet power, from the chair of surgery, headed by the Institute's oldest alumnus, Professor M. A. Maltsev, three independent chairs evolved, which were headed by his own pupils: The chair of general and special surgery, orthopedics, and ophthalmology, which was taken over after the retirement (in 1949) of M. A. Maltsev by Professor V. A. Herman; the chair of obstetrics, gynecology, and artificial insemination, which at first was headed by Lecturer V. K. Kedrov and somewhat later by the late Lecturer S. N. Kornienko; and the chair of operative surgery, headed by Professor Dr. I. I. Magda.

> The strengthened material base of the Institute permitted perfecting new organization of teaching by the clinical chairs and the building up of scientific work. For the first time in the Institute, a scientific research chair of clinical veterinary medicine was founded in 1923 with therapeutic and surgical sections. Head of this chair was Professor Maltsev. With the organization of this new scientific research division came the introduction of graduate students to prepare scientific work in the clinical disciplines. A number of people completed this graduate work and later became professors and heads of the chairs: Honored Scientist Professor I. I. Lukashov, Professor V. A. Herman, Dr. Vet. Sci. V. K. Kedrov, Lecturer S. N. Kornienko, Professor I. I. Magda. Many former graduates of this chair are at present working at various educational and scientific establishments in the Soviet Union.

Magda contributed his share to the general obfuscation, however, by describing a chair of clinical veterinary medicine, supposedly founded in 1923, with therapeutic and surgical sections. As far as I can determine, *this is pure fabrication.* The evidence is that the chair did not exist in 1923, because there is no mention of it in the comprehensive report of the activities of the Kharkov Veterinary Institute, published in Ukrainian in 1929. This latter report covered the period 1918–1928, and its purpose was stated by the editors to be a description of the organizational and pedagogical progress made during this decade; the scientific papers were promised for a later issue. Professor Maltsev was a member of the three-man editorial group that signed the editorial. It is reasonable to assume that either in his capacity as editor or as author of the chapter dealing with his own teaching activities, he would have described an important pedagogical innovation such as the above had it actually existed in 1929.

But we are not yet through with Magda's fabrications in the guise of history. Elsewhere in his 1954 report, in a statement I have not reproduced here, he says that the department of obstetrics and gynecology was started in 1935, evolving from the department of operative surgery, of which the head was Professor Maltsev. One need only compare this statement to the 1929 report which is illustrated (Fig. 68) to determine from which department obstetrics really branched off and who the head of this was—Samodelkin. If one then refers to the 1929 report of Maltsev's department (Fig. 69), it is obvious that it did not include obstetrics. Up to 1929 in the Soviet Union, history was still being written; it had not yet begun to be rewritten.*

By this time, by means of the misleading 1952 and 1954 information, Professor Samodelkin has been effectively effaced from the history of the Kharkov Veterinary Institute and has become a nonperson.† Once you have rewritten his-

*I will not burden the reader with yet another version of Kharkov surgical history written in 1950 by Lukashov,[308] which agrees neither with the 1929 report nor with those of 1952 and 1954. Apparently Nosik and Magda forgot to read it, confirming the adage that only a man who tells the truth can afford to have a bad memory.

†Of course, it is hard to eradicate *all* traces. Thus an article in another Soviet veterinary journal tells of a postgraduate course in Kharkov in 1929

tory to obliterate the clinic that *did* exist, no one is going to ask who the head of it was.

Samodelkin has not only become a nonperson as professor of surgery, he has also become one as rector of the Kharkov Veterinary Institute. As mentioned earlier in this appendix, the historical volume celebrating the fiftieth anniversary of the Kazan Veterinary Institute in 1924, published in 1926, carried Professor Samodelkin's greetings from the Kharkov Veterinary Institute in his capacity as rector. The historical articles on the Kharkov school make no mention of him in this capacity either, obviously for reasons of consistency.

Why has this erasing been done? I am convinced that the obfuscating stories written by Lukashov in 1950 and by Nosik and Magda in 1952 and 1954 are deliberate smoke screens thrown up to disguise some unpleasant truth about the fate of Professor Samodelkin, the nature of which I have not discovered. But the report that a group of prominent bacteriologists in the Soviet Union were tried secretly in 1930 for having "organized a horse epidemic"[154] gives one some food for thought.

---

at which Professor Samodelkin lectured on surgery and Professor Maltsev on operative surgery.[32] There is only one copy of this journal in the United States and none at all in most Western countries, so very little eradication needs to be done. Only one American library has the May 1930 issue of the journal with an article by I. Magda listing Professor Samodelkin as head of his department![314a] A mere two decades later, Magda had "forgotten" who his chief had been.

Appendix IV. The Omsk Veterinary Institute

How bad conditions were at times can perhaps be surmised from the following quotation from the year 1922:

> To the Editor of the Veterinary Journal. Gentlemen,—The Siberian Veterinary Zootechnical Institute was established at Omsk in 1918 in order to study local Siberian conditions of zootechny, to organize a struggle against animal disease, and to supply Siberia with veterinary surgeons. In spite of bad conditions of life after a great war against Germany, and the impossibility of communicating with foreign countries, the Institute widely developed its activity, thanks to the initiative and personal energy of the scientific personnel of the old Veterinary Institute at Kazan. Unfortunately, now-a-days the institute cannot do without foreign help. It needs school-books, various laboratory equipment and veterinary scientific books. Thinking it the only way to emerge from the present deplorable conditions, a group of professors have the honour to appeal to you, in the name of culture and science, for moral and material support, as much as is possible, in order to secure the existence of the Institute and its collaborators. Our misfortunes are very great, owing to the recent war and the bad harvest of last year. In the hope of receiving from our colleagues food supplies, etc., which can be sent to Siberia; A. Konerevsky, Formerly Rector of the Institute.[263]

Appendix V. The Russian Bureaucracy, as Seen in 1891 by George Kennan

Satirists in various countries, particularly France and Germany, have vied with one another in lampooning the foibles of their bureaucrats. Any country where the central government delegated little power to the provinces and tried to run everything from the capital city lent itself particularly well to such derision. I have mentioned in several places in this book that in Russia, decisions could be taken only in St. Petersburg, and that various aspects of veterinary education, meat hygiene, and animal disease control were badly mismanaged.

Lest anyone think that attempts to control epizootics from offices in St. Petersburg, by officials who knew nothing of conditions in the field, was an aberration restricted to the veterinary branch of the government, I submit the following.

The conversation, reprinted from the *Century Magazine,* is between George Kennan, correspondent for this American journal, and Colonel Zagarin, an official of the gendarmerie in a Siberian province.[238]

[If the Government would permit them to travel in summer] the exiles would reach their destination in a state of comparative health and vigor, instead of being broken down on the road by the hardships and exposures of a thousand-mile winter march.

"Why in the name of all that is reasonable has not this change been made?" I said to Colonel Zagarin when he finished explaining to me the nature of his report. "If it would be cheaper, as well as more humane, to forward the exiles only in summer and in wagons, why doesn't the Government do it? Who can have any interest in opposing a reform that is economical as well as philanthropical?"

"You had better inquire when you get to St. Petersburg," replied Colonel Zagarin, shrugging his shoulders. "All that we can do here is to suggest."

The reason why changes that are manifestly desirable, that are in the direction of economy, and that, apparently, would injure no one, are not made in Russia is one of the most puzzling and exasperating things that are forced upon a traveler's attention. In every branch of the administration one is constantly stumbling upon abuses or defects that have long been recognized, that have been commented upon for years, that are apparently prejudicial to the interests of everybody, and that, nevertheless, continue to exist. If you ask an explanation of an official in Siberia, he refers you to St. Petersburg. If you inquire of the chief of the prison department in St. Petersburg, he tells you that he has drawn up a "project" to cope with the evil, but that this "project" has not yet been approved by the Minister of the Interior. If you go to the Ministry of the Interior, you learn that the "project" requires a preliminary appropriation of money,—even although its ultimate effect may be to save money,—and that it cannot be carried into execution without the assent and coöperation of the Minister of Finance. If you follow the "project" to the Ministry of Finance, you are told that it has been sent back through the Minister of the Interior to the chief of the prison department for "modification." If you still persist in your determination to find out why this thing is not done, you may chase the modified "project" through the prison department, the Ministry of the Interior, and the Ministry of Finance to the Council of the Empire. There you discover that, inasmuch as certain cross-and-ribbon-decorated senators and generals, who barely know Siberia by name, have expressed a doubt as to the existence of the evil with which the "project" is intended to deal, a special "commission" (with salaries amounting to twenty thousand *rubles* a year and mileage) has been appointed to investigate the subject and make a report. If you pursue the commission to Siberia and back, and search diligently in the proceedings of the Council of the Empire for its report, you ascertain that the document has been sent to the Ministry of the Interior to serve as a basis for a new "project," and then, as ten or fifteen years have elapsed and all the original projectors are dead, everything begins over again. At no stage of this circumrotatory process can you lay your hand on a particular official and say, "Here! You are responsible for this—what do you mean by it?" At no stage, probably, can you find an official who is opposed to the reform or who has any personal interest in defeating it; and yet the general effect of the circumrotatory process is more certainly fatal to your reformatory project than any amount of intelligent and active opposition. The various bureaus of the provincial governor-general's office, the chief prison department, the Ministry of the Interior, the Ministry of Finance, the Ministry of Justice, the Council of Ministers, and the Council of the Empire constitute a huge administrative maelstrom of ignorance and indifference, in which a "project" revolves slowly, month after month and year after year, until it is finally sucked down out of sight, or perhaps thrown by a fortuitous eddy of personal or official interest into the great gulfstream current of real life.[1]

[1]This natural history of a Russian "project" is not imaginary nor conjectural. A plan for the transportation of exiles in wagons between Tomsk and Irkutsk has been gyrating in circles in the Sargasso Sea of Russian bureaucracy for almost thirty years. The projected reform of the exile system has been the rounds of the various circumlocution offices at least half a dozen times since 1871, and has four times reached the "commission" stage and been reported to the Council of the Empire. (The commissions were under the presidency respectively of Sollohub, Frisch, Zubof, and Grot. See *Eastern Review,* No. 17, July 22, St. Petersburg, 1882.) Mr. Kokoftsef, assistant chief of the Russian prison department, announced, in a speech that he made to the International Prison Congress at Stockholm in 1878, that his Government recognized the evils of the exile system and was about to abolish it. (See "Report of the International Prison Congress of Stockholm," by E. C. Wines, United States Com-

missioner, Government Printing Office, Washington, 1879.) That was thirteen years ago, and my latest Russian newspapers contain the information that the "project" for the reform of the exile system has been found "unsatisfactory" by the Council of the Empire, and has been sent back through the Ministry of the Interior to the chief of the prison department for "modification." In other words, this "project" in the course of thirteen years has progressed four stages backward on the return gyration.

Appendix VI. The Siberian Emigration

Professor S. A. Gryuner in 1911 wrote in the *American Veterinary Review:* "In 1892, the United States Government at different points in Alaska began the policy of establishing reindeer stations with the purpose of introducing the reindeer industry to the native population." This may well have been what Gryuner believed, but if so, it is because he was given American propaganda to misinform him when he came to visit Alaska from his station in Siberia. In the interests of providing the correct historical information, the following version is offered.

The U.S. government actually got involved in Alaskan reindeer only very reluctantly. In 1890, Sheldon Jackson, General Agent for Education in Alaska, noted that the Eskimos were suffering from a diminished yield from whaling and walrus hunting. He proposed to the U.S. government that reindeer be purchased in Siberia, brought to Alaska on revenue cutters, and given to the Eskimos. He urged that instead of being pauperized and fed by the government, the Eskimos should be given the opportunity to support themselves. Jackson pointed out the value of reindeer in the economy of eastern Siberia and northern Scandinavia, where the natives were not only supporting themselves by reindeer husbandry but actually paying taxes to the government.

The Interior Department approved Jackson's project, but

a miserly Congress refused to pass the appropriation, a paltry $15,000. Jackson thereupon appealed to public charity through letters in the newspapers of the larger cities and succeeded in raising over $2,000. With this he was able to go by ship to Siberia and purchase 16 reindeer. The following year, when Congress again defeated a $15,000 appropriation, he raised private funds enough to buy 171 more animals and also to erect a school where the Eskimos could be taught reindeer husbandry.

This effort aroused enough public interest that the Congress was induced by 1893 finally to appropriate $6,000. Meanwhile, as Greuning[189] humorously writes, the reindeer, "unmindful of congressional procrastination, had begun to procreate. Seventy-nine fawns were born on American soil that spring, and 127 more Siberian reindeer were naturalized." Jackson eventually got Congress to part with another $7,500 in 1894, and was able to transport a total of about 1,300 reindeer from Siberia to Alaska.

Gryuner reported that there were "about 25,000" descendants from these animals when he visited Alaska in 1911; and Greuning reported that by 1917 these had multiplied to an estimated 95,000. He says that for many years they contributed substantially to the economy of western Alaska and to the welfare of the Eskimos.

Appendix VII. Scientists Who Contributed to the Education of Russian Veterinary or Comparative Pathologists

A number of medical and veterinary scientists contributed to the education of the veterinary pathologists who are the chief figures in this book. Three of these, Kucherenko, Melnikov-Razvedenkov, and Rudnev have been discussed in the text. The others are depicted here, since to have intruded their pictures or biographies into the main text would have disrupted its continuity. Each has in common with the others either an interest in veterinary pathology or, if his vocation was not in this realm, an interest in contributing to the postgraduate education of veterinary pathologists.

I judge that the effect of this contribution on veterinary pathology in Russia was considerable. Yet it is hard to convey an idea of the pervasiveness of this effect when one is trying to keep in mind over 30 names. I have therefore resorted to a graphic presentation of this array of genius and talent.

With three exceptions, a capsule biography (or text reference to one) is given of each of the people portrayed. The exceptions, Virchow, Mechnikov, and Koch, are too well known to warrant biographical information here. For some of the others, citations also provide access to more detailed information. The names appearing in parenthesis after each legend are those of the Russian veterinary or comparative pathologists who studied or worked with that person.

We are considering here chiefly the mentors of those Russians who stayed in veterinary pathology and made it their vocation. A few others are mentioned in this book, albeit more briefly: Vorontsov, Samodelkin, and Petropavlovskii, who ended up in clinical pursuits, and Petrov in meat hygiene. Each of them made at least one (and some several) useful contribution to veterinary pathology despite a brief sojourn in this specialty.

The portraits of K. Nieberle and P. O. Kucherenko are shown even though B. G. Ivanov and A. A. Pinus, who respectively worked in their laboratories, are barely mentioned in this narrative. Most of Ivanov's work falls outside the scope of this book, as does Pinus', because it was done after 1930. Both of them wrote articles on the history of veterinary pathology in Russia, and I have therefore included their teachers' portraits here.

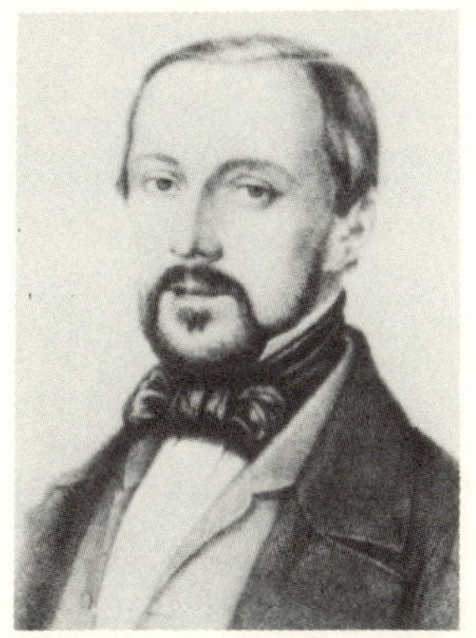

RUDOLPH VIRCHOW (1821–1902), taught pathology at the University of Berlin. (Blumberg, Ravich, Rudnev, Kolesnikov, Bohl)

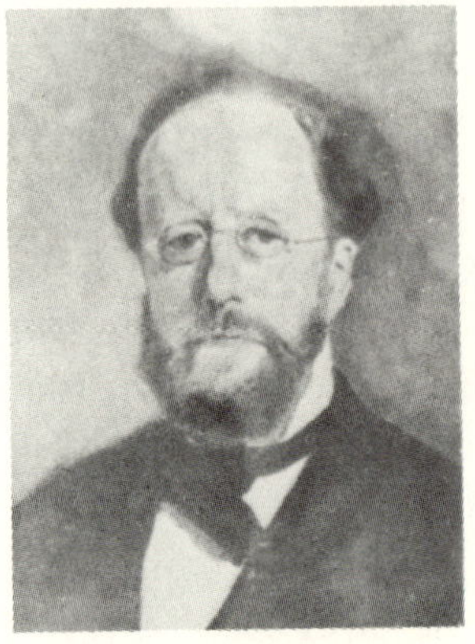

EDWIN KLEBS (1834–1913), a student of Virchow's, German pathologist and bacteriologist, taught pathology in Prague, Bern,[447] Würzburg, Zurich and Chicago. An original thinker, he made several pioneering bacteriological discoveries. The genus *Klebsiella* is named in his honor. (Semmer)

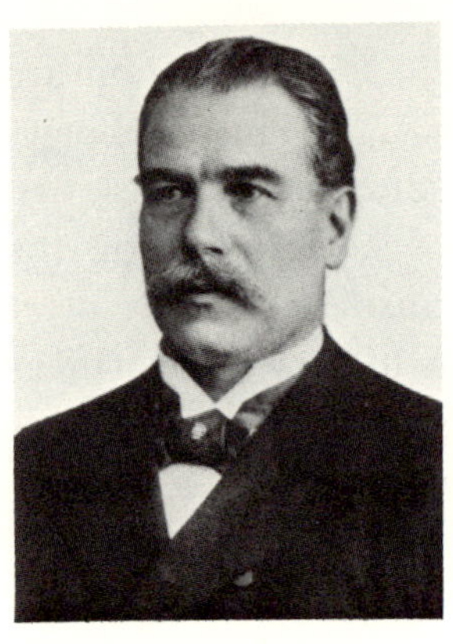

ANTON WEICHSELBAUM (1845–1920) taught pathology in Vienna from 1893. One of the first pathologists to realize the importance of bacteriology, he discovered the meningococcus of acute cerebrospinal fever in 1887. (Gryuner)

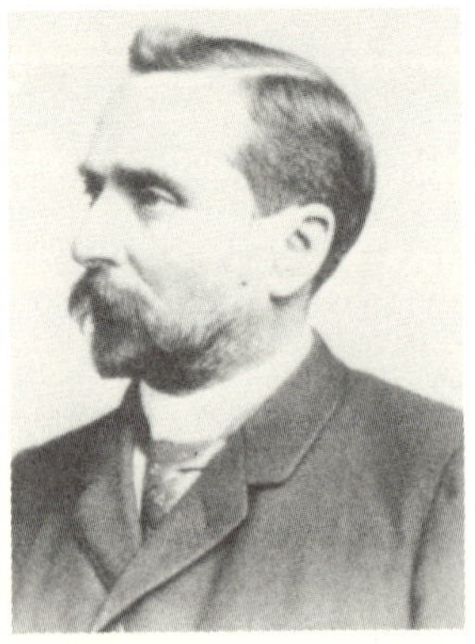

ERNST ZIEGLER (1849–1905), Swiss-born pathologist and student of Klebs, taught pathology in Freiburg im Breisgau. Physicians from all over the world congregated in his laboratory to do research and to benefit from his outstanding teaching.[357] (Melnikow-Razvedenkov)

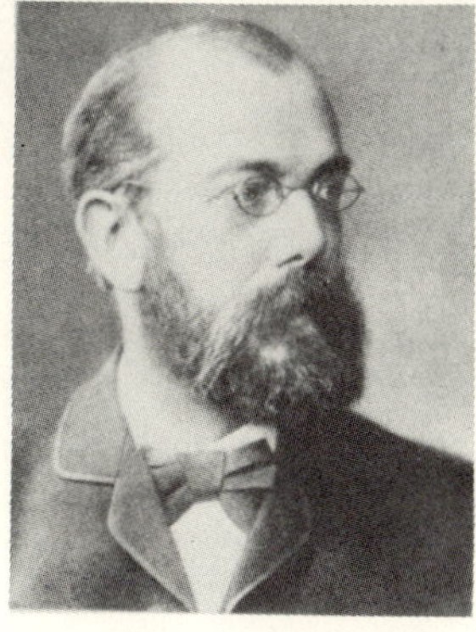

ROBERT KOCH (1843–1910), German bacteriologist. (Blumberg)

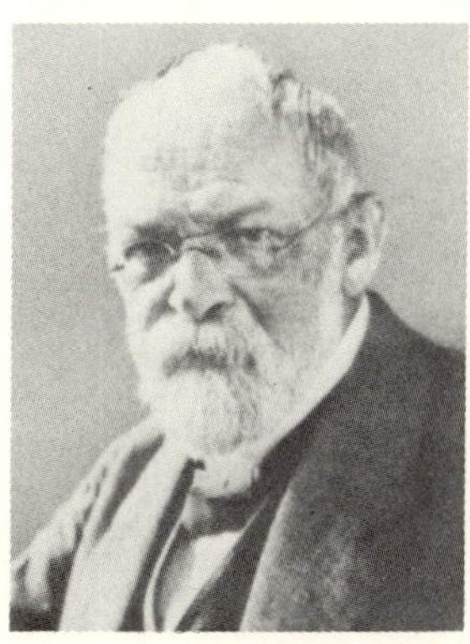

FELIX MARCHAND (1846–1928) taught pathology at the University of Leipzig.[212] (Ball)

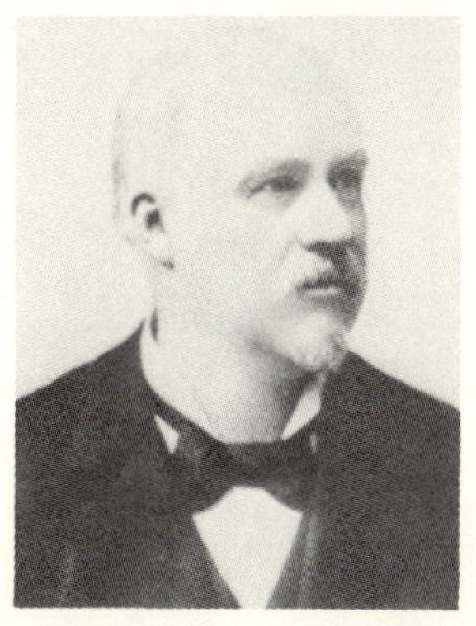

KARL GUILLEBEAU (1845–1918), Swiss physician and veterinarian, taught pathology at the veterinary school in Bern from 1876. Trained under Bollinger in Munich, he strove to bring the outstanding accomplishments of German human pathology during the nineteenth century to the field of veterinary pathology. Well known abroad, he was offered a chair at the Institute for Experimental Medicine in St. Petersburg at the time of its founding.[447] (Ball, Samodelkin)

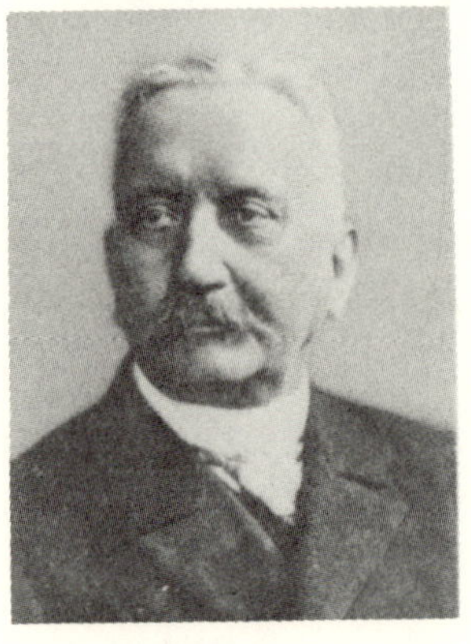

Wilhelm Schütz (1839–1920) taught pathology in the Berlin Veterinary College from 1870 to 1920. He introduced Virchow's autopsy techniques to veterinary medicine and discovered (with Loeffler) the bacilli of glanders and of swine erysipelas. He was the most important veterinary pathologist of the nineteenth century.[469] (Ball, Bohl, Krakht-Paleev)

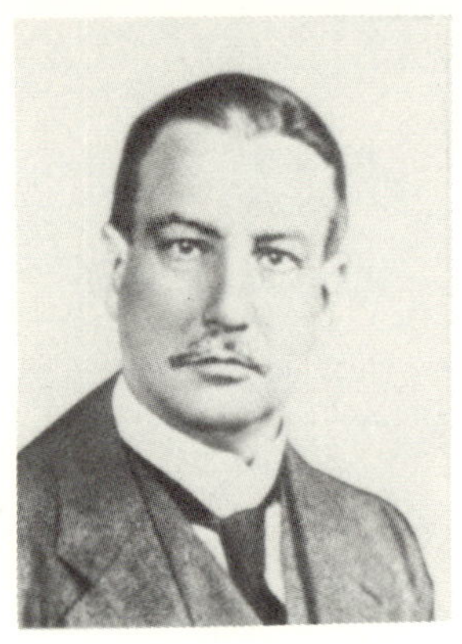

Ernst Joest (1873–1926) taught pathology at the Veterinary School in Dresden (which later moved to Leipzig) from 1904 until his death. He discovered Borna encephalitis of horses and many other disease entities. His lasting claim to fame, however, is the multivolume veterinary pathology which he edited.[369] In its third edition it is still known all over the world half a century after his death simply as "Joest." (Bohl, Krakht-Paleev)

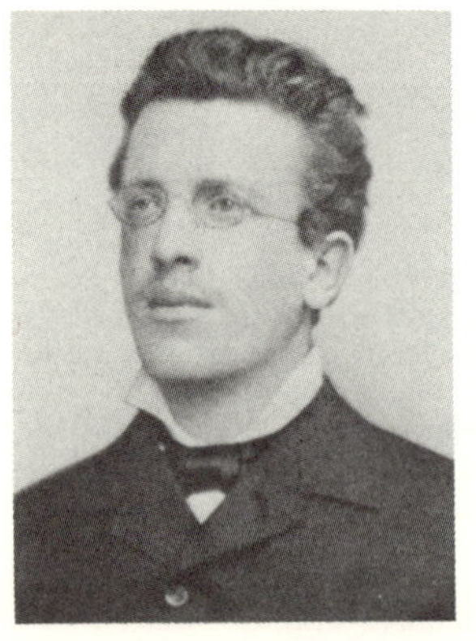

Theodor Kitt (1858–1941), a native of Munich, taught pathology and bacteriology in this city's veterinary school from 1886 to 1932.[473] His classical books on veterinary pathology, translated into English, Russian, and Italian, marked him as the world leader of this discipline for many decades. (Gryuner, Krakht-Paleev)

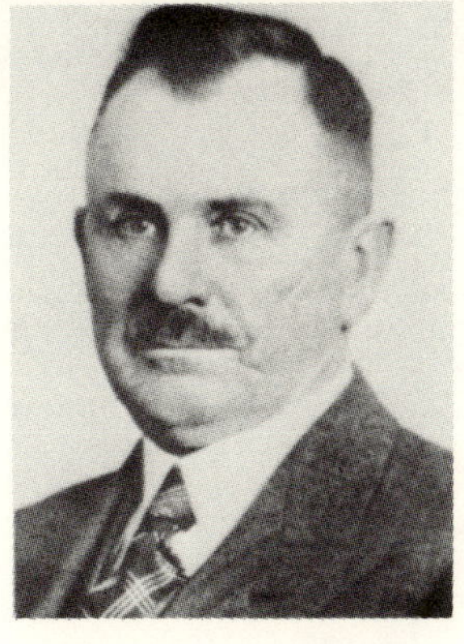

Karl Nieberle (1877–1946) taught pathology in the veterinary faculty of Leipzig University, as Joest's successor, from 1926 to 1944. His research on granulomatous diseases and his textbook of veterinary pathology (with Cohrs) brought him worldwide fame, and attracted postgraduate students from the United States as well as Russia. (Ivanov, Balzamentov)

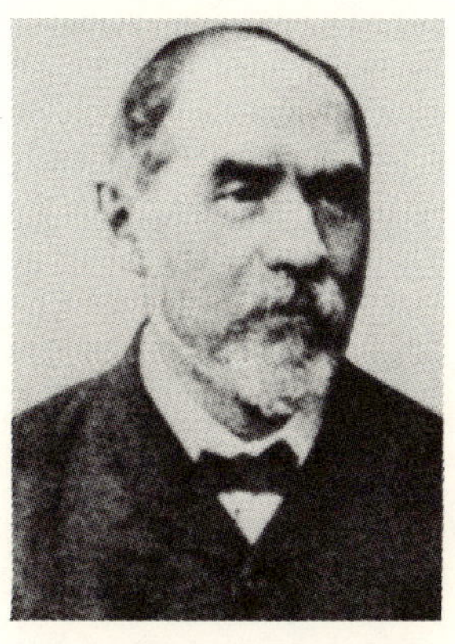

Feodor Zavarykin (1835–1899), a physician, taught histology and embryology at the Medico-Chirurgical Academy in St. Petersburg from 1867 to 1897. (Ravich, Raevskii)

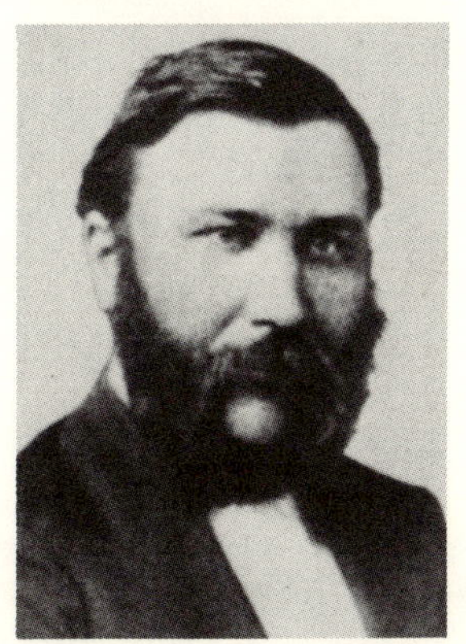

Mikhail Rudnev (1837–1878), Russian comparative pathologist. See biography in Chapter 4. (Lange, Novinskii, Raevskii, Vorontsov)

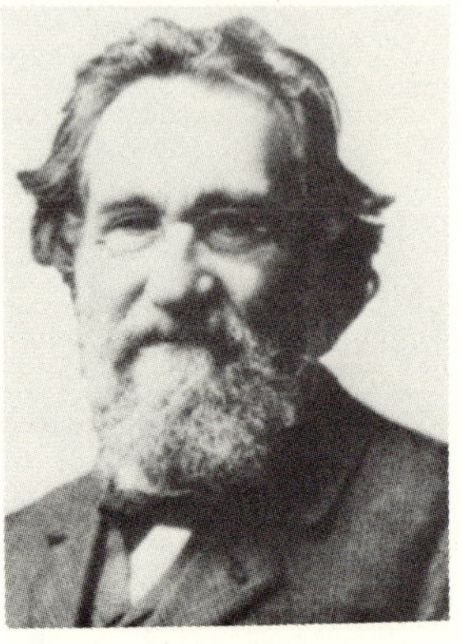

ILYA MECHNIKOV (1845–1916), Russian comparative pathologist. (Shukevich)

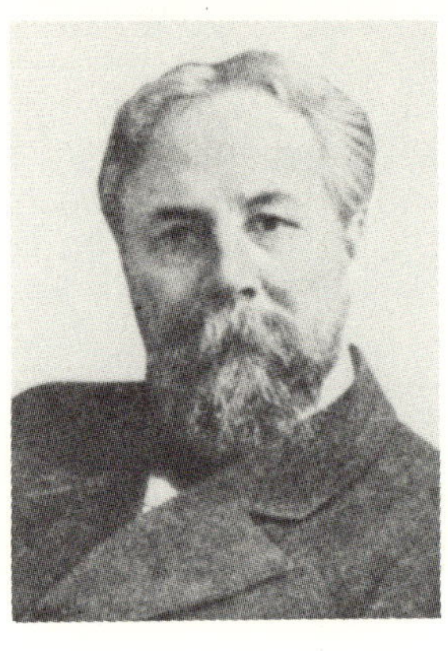

NIKOLAI LYUBIMOV (1852–1907) trained in Germany under von Recklinghausen and then taught pathology and bacteriology in the Medical Faculty of Kazan University from 1880 until his death.[345] His major interests were conducting research work on infectious diseases of man and animals. (Bohl, Karaulov, Polovinkin)

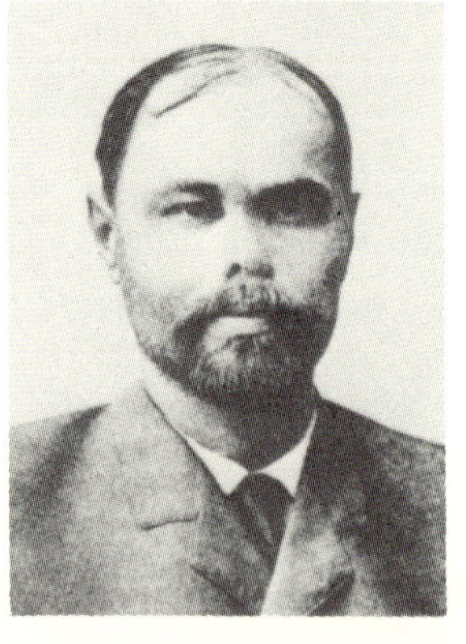

NIKOLAI MELNIKOV-RAZVEDENKOV (1866–1937) taught pathology in the medical faculties first of Moscow University and later of Kharkov (see biography in Chapter 5). (Krakht-Paleev, Petrov, Shukevich)

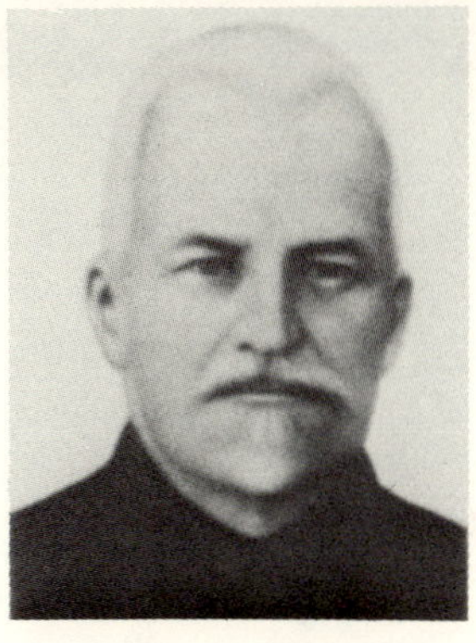

PAVLO KUCHERENKO (1882–1936) taught pathology in Kiev University from 1920 until his death; see biography in Chapter 5. (Pinus)

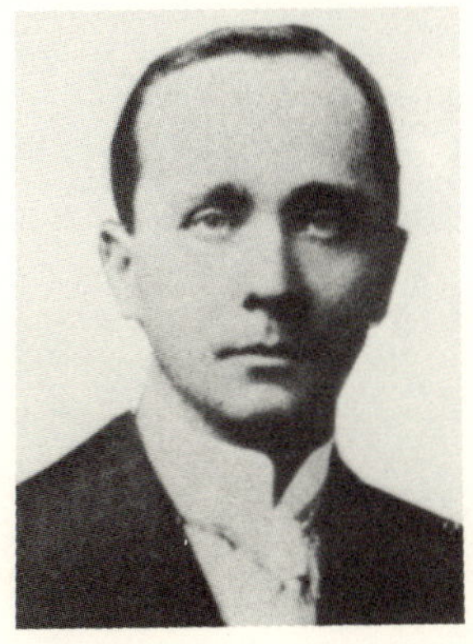

BENJAMIN KAUPP (1874–1954), American veterinarian, professor of pathology, Veterinary Division, Colorado Agricultural College, 1908–1912. Pioneer studies of equine encephalitis, but best known as first American poultry pathologist; professor of poultry science, North Carolina State College, 1914–1930. (Gryuner)

Sources of Illustrations

Grateful acknowledgment is made to those who provided illustrative material.

Journals

Arkhiv Veterinarnykh Nauk, Figs. 19 and 62
Century Magazine, Figs. 59, 63, and 64
Österreichische Monatsschrift Tierheilkunde, Fig. 60
Sbornik Rabot Kharkov., Vet. Inst., Figs. 56 and 70
Sovetskaya Veterinariya, Fig. 67
Ucheniye Zapiski Kazan. Vet. Inst., Fig. 39
Veterinariya, Frontispiece, Figs. 22, 37, 40, 51, and 52
Veterinary Journal, Fig. 24

Anonymous,[15] Fig. 34
Dr. K. Baresel, Hanover, Figs. 1, 43, and 44, and Verlag M. & H. Schaper, Hanover (for permission to reprint Figs. 43 and 44)
Bolshaya Meditsinskaya Entsiklopediya, Fig. 45
Chebotarev,[132] Fig. 38
Colange,[153] Fig. 11
Prof. Dr. E. Dahme, Munich, portrait of Theodor Kitt, P. 272
Dzanelidze,[164] Figs. 23 and 54
Prof. Dr. R. Fankhauser, University of Bern, portrait of Karl Guillebeau, p. 271
Free Library of Philadelphia, Fig. 26
Dr. W. Girolla, Vienna, Figs. 6, 7, 57, and 58
Prof. Dr. B. Hörning, University of Bern, Figs. 9, 14, 28, 31, 32, 41, 46, and 56
Ivanovskii,[217] Figs. 12, 13, and 16
Dr. I. Katić, Copenhagen, Figs. 4, 5, 8, and 10
Koropov,[265] Figs. 15 and 35
Kucherenko,[284] Fig. 55

Library of Congress, Figs. 50 and 65
Dr. G. Lucyszyn, Figs. 36 and 66
Mr. R. Mack, F.R.C.V.S., Figs. 68 and 69
Dr. H. Madissoo, Fig. 2
Millak,[354] Fig. 48
National Library of Medicine, Figs. 17 and 30
Shabad,[529] Figs. 18 and 20
Dr. M. Shimkin, Fig. 61
Tereshkov,[591] Fig. 25
Tolstova-Pariiskaya,[594] Fig. 33
Valdmann and Negotin,[609] Fig. 3
Veterinarnaya Entsiklopediya, Figs. 49 and 53
Dr. A. M. Watrach, Fig. 21
Dr. S. Young, portrait of Benjamin Kaupp, p. 275

References

While I have transliterated the names of most Russian authors and places into English, I have left those of Russian authors who published in French or German as they appeared in those languages. Because of the differences in the transliteration of Cyrillic names into English, German, and French, the same people may not always be recognizable as such at first glance. If the reader uses a little imagination and studies the following examples, however, he should have no problems.

Almeev, Almejew	= Алмеев
Chernyak, Tscherniak	= Черняк
Ravich, Rawitsch	= Равич

In his preface to the book *Russia under the Last Tsar,*[625] T. G. Stavrou wrote: "In a volume of this kind, transliteration presents great problems, especially when the names of many literary and revolutionary figures have been spelled in a variety of ways* and in some cases have been standardized despite violations of transliteration rules. Although no particular transliteration system has been followed faithfully, the effort was made to be as consistent as possible while simul-

*To illustrate this variety, I have found that И. И. Шукевич, when publishing in French, rendered his name (which in English we would transliterate as Shukevich) in the following ways: Schoulkevich, Choukevitch, Shoukevitch, and Choukewitch!

taneously trying to satisfy the transliteration idiosyncrasies of some of the contributors."

The difficulty of maintaining consistency in Russian transliteration against certain accepted practices which, although wrong, have become well entrenched, has also been described by Edmund Wilson.[635] In commenting on some work of Vladimir Nabokov's, Wilson took him to task for resorting to transliteration at all, saying: "He has elsewhere invariably transliterated the Russian—a procedure which is confusing and useless. Transliterated Russian means as little to anyone who does not read Russian as if it were printed in Russian characters, and for anyone who does read Russian it is an unnecessary nuisance to have to transpose it back into the Cyrillic alphabet before one can recognize it."

Wilson, of course, is not correct in saying that transliteration is useless; in medical writing, many Russian words become recognizable in transliteration because of their Greek and Latin roots. Furthermore, whatever may be true in other fields, in medical literature it is precisely the student who *does* read Russian who will need to resort to the transliterated references which follow. Such a student is unlikely to work in any Western library which has more than a fifth of these works, and will have to borrow the bulk of them elsewhere. Since our typewriters and teletype machines do not have Cyrillic keyboards, we must resort to the expedient of transliteration in order to obtain books and articles on loan from other libraries.

I offer this explanation for my seeming defiance of Wilson, whose erudition I respect. I have usually followed transliteration System I of those proposed by Shaw,[530] in which the hard and soft signs are omitted.

1. Abrikosov, A. I. Akademik Nikolai Fedotovich Melnikov-Razvedenkov. Sovet. Med. 2(2): 63–64, 1938.
2. Akulov, A. V. Osnovnye napravleniya i dostizheniya v rabote laboratorii

patologicheskoi anatomii VIEV za 1922–1972 g. [The principal trends and achievements in the work of the laboratory of pathologic anatomy of VIEV during the years 1922–1972.] Trudy VIEV *41:* 197–205, 1973.

3. Alekseev, A. [Biography of] E. M. Semmer. Vet. Delo (St. Petersburg) *9*(2): 1–5, 1891.
4. Almeev, Kh. Sh., and L. M. Krapivner. Nekotorye dannye po istorii patologicheskoi anatomii. [Some data on the history of pathologic anatomy.] Veterinariya *42* (5): 112–113, 1966.
5. Almejew, K. S. K. H. Bohl. Mhefte. Vet. Med. *14:* 391–392, 1959.
6. Andersohn, R. Beitrag zur Geschichte des Milzbrandes als Hausthierseuche. Oesterr. Vierteljschr. wiss. Veterinärk. *31:* 167–197, 1869.
7. Anonymous. First Report of the Commissioners Appointed to Inquire into the Origin and Nature &c. of the Cattle Plague. London, Her Majesty's Stationery Office, 1865, p. 128.
8. Anonymous. Third Report of the Commissioners Appointed to Inquire into the Origin and Nature &c. of the Cattle Plague. London, Her Majesty's Stationery Office, 1866.
9. Anonymous. Necrology of J. Ravich. Arch. Tierheilk. 2: 255–256, 1876.
10. Anonymous: Konstantin Gustavovich Blumberg†. Ustav Obshchestva Vet. Vrachei Kazan. Vet. Inst. 1897, p. 11. (Bound with Uchen. Zap. Kazan. Vet. Inst. *14,* 1897.)
11. Anonymous. Ravich, Iosif Ippolitovich, 1822–75. Entsiklopedicheskii Slovar, vol. 26, p. 59. St. Petersburg, Izdatel. Byvshee Brokhaus-Efron, 1899.
12. Anonymous. Doklad kommissii naznachennoi i konferentsiya Imperat. Voenno-Med. Akad. Po voprosu o sisteme prepodovaniya epizootiologii i veterinarnoi politsii. [Report of the commission appointed by the council of the Imperial Military-Medical Academy on the question of teaching epidemiology and veterinary sanitation.] Izvest. Imperat. Voenno-Med. Akad. 2(5): 576–579, 1901.
13. Anonymous. Rudolf Virchow. Vet. Obozrenie *4:* 719–728, 1902.
14. Anonymous. Meditsinski Fakultet Kharkovskago Universiteta za perviya 100 Let ego Sushchestvovaniya 1805–1905. [The Medical Faculty of Kharkov University during the first 100 years of its existence, 1805–1905.] Kharkov, Izdanie Universiteta, Tipografiya K. N. Gagarin, 1906. [Portrait of N. F. Melnikov-Razvedenkov on Plate 5.)
15. Anonymous. E. Semmer†. Przeglad Weterynarski *22:* 83, 1907.
16. Anonymous. Otchet o zagranichnoi komandirovke Prosektora P. N. Krakht-Paleeva. [Report on the official trip abroad of Prosector P. N. Krakht-Paleev.] Sborn. Trud. Kharkov. Vet. Inst. *11*: 64–71, 1914.

17. Anonymous. Ot redaktsii. [From the editorial office.] Kubanskiy Nauch. Med. Vestnik *4*: 5–10, 1924.
18. Anonymous. Prazdnovanie 50-letnego yubileya Kazanskogo Veterinarnogo Instituta. [The 50th jubilee of the Kazan Veterinary Institute.] Uchen. Zap. Kazan. Vet. Inst. *37*: 29–37, 1926.
19. Anonymous. Gryuner, Sergei Aleksandrovich. Sibirskaya Sovetskaya Entsiklopediya, vol. 1, p. 754. Novosibirsk, Sibirskoe Kraevoe Izdatelstvo, 1929.
20. Anonymous. Sorok let nauchno-pedagogicheskoi i obshchestvennoi deyatelnosti zasluzhennogo deyatelya doktora veterinarnykh nauk Professora K. H. Bol. [Forty years of scientific-pedagogical and public activity of meritorious scientific worker Professor K. H. Bohl, D.V.Sc.] Uchen. Zap. Kazan. Gosud. Zoovet. Inst. *47*: 8–12, 1937.
21. Anonymous. Podgotovka nauchnykh kadrov. [Training of scientific staff.] Uchen. Zap. Kazan. Gosud. Vet. Inst. *63*: 23–25, 1956.
22. Anonymous. Yubilei Prof. K. H. Bol. [Jubilee of Prof. K. H. Bohl.] Veterinariya *33*(10): 95–96, 1956.
23. Anonymous. Melnikov-Razvedenkov, N. F. Bolshaya Med. Entsiklop. *17*: 972, 1960.
24. Anonymous. Kucherenko, P. O. Ukrainska Radyanska Entsiklopediya 7: 530–531, 1962.
25. Anonymous. Pamyati Professora V. Z. Chernyak. [In memory of Professor V. Z. Chernyak.] Veterinariya *40*(9): 93, 1963.
26. Anonymous. Bauman, Nikolai Ernestovich. Great Soviet Encyclopedia, 3d ed., vol. 3, p. 81. New York, Macmillan, 1973.
27. Anonymous. Her Majesty's unnecessary guest. New Statesman *90*: 213, 1975.
28. Anonymous. Acta persecutionis. Frankf. allg. Zeitung, pp. 15–16, August 21, 1975.
29. Arndt, H. J. Bemerkungen zur Leberamyloidose bei russischen Pferden. Münch. tierärztl. Wschr. *79*: 321–323, 1928.
30. Arndt, H. J. Veterinärmedizinisches aus Sowjetrussland. Berl. tierärztl. Wschr. *45*: 222–224; 241–243; 257–258; 276–278; 292–293, 1929.
31. Aschoff, L. [Letter to the editor.] Kubanskiy Nauch. Med. Vestnik *4*: 11–12, 1924.
32. B., Yu. [Initials only.] Kursy usovershenstvovaniya vrachei. [Postgraduate course for doctors.] Vestnik Sovrem. Vet. *5*: 492, 1929.
33. Babel, I. You Must Know Everything, p. 62. New York, Farrar, Straus & Giroux, 1966.
34. Babel, I. Über Pferde, pp. 107–109 in his Werke, Bd. 2. Berlin, Verlag Volk und Welt, 1973.
35. Babris, P. J. Baltic Youth Under Communism, pp. 14–15. Arlington Heights, Ill., Research Publishers, 1967.

36. Ball, N. D. Patologo-anatomicheskoe izsledovanie protsessa zazhivleniya perelomov kostei u domashnikh ptits. [Pathologic-anatomic study of the healing process of fractured bone in the domestic chicken.] M.V.Sc. dissertation, Yuryev, 1899.
37. Ball, N. D. Mari, N. N., Prof. Osnovy Patologicheskoi Anatomii Domashnikh Zhivotnykh. Patologo-anatomicheskaya Diagnostika. [Review of book Fundamentals of the Pathologic Anatomy of Domestic Animals. Pathologic-anatomical Diagnosis.] Zhurnal Nauch. Prakt. Vet. Med. Izd. Yurev. Vet. Inst. *1*: 157–159, 1906.
38. Ball, N. D. Patologicheskii institut Berlinskoi vysshei veterinarnoi shkoly. [The pathological institute of the Berlin Veterinary College.] Zhurnal Nauch. Prakt. Vet. Med. Izd. Yurev. Vet. Inst. *1*: 205–222, 1907.
39. Ball, N. D. Obzor literatury po patologicheskoi anatomii za 1906 god. [Survey of literature on pathologic anatomy for the year 1906.] Zhurnal Nauch. Prakt. Vet. Med. Izd. Yurev. Vet. Inst. *2*: 163–192, 1909.
40. Ball, N. D. Sluchai rudimentarnago legkago v bryushnoi polosti telenka. [A case of rudimentary lungs in the abdominal cavity of a calf.] Trudy 2. Vserossiiskago Sezda Vet. Vrachei, Moskva, *2*: 548–559, 1910.
41. Ball, N. D. K patologicheskoi anatomii podagry. [On the pathologic anatomy of gout.] Izvest. Don. Vet. Inst. *1*(1): 1–12, 1919.
42. Ball, N. D. Sluchai amiloidnoi infiltratsii pecheni u koshki. [A case of amyloid infiltration in the liver of a cat.] Izvest. Don. Vet. Inst. *1*(2): 1–3, 1919.
43. Ball, N. D. Deyatelnost Gosudar. Instituta Eksperimentalnoi Veterinarii v 1922 godu. [Activity of the National Institute of Experimental Veterinary Medicine for the year 1922.] Trudy Gosud. Inst. Eksp. Vet. *1*: 304–323, 1923.
44. Ball, N. D., G. Ya. Belkin, and V. Z. Chernyak. Etiudy po sapu. 2. Gruppirovka form sapnogo porazheniya legikh u loshadei. [Study of glanders. Purulent form of glanders lesions in the lungs of horses.] Prakt. Vet. Konevodst. *1*(3): 10–14; (4): 22–28, 1924.
45. Ball, N. D. Deyatelnost studencheskikh nauchno-issledovatelskikh kruzhkov v 1927–28 akad. godu. [Activities of the students' scientific society for the academic year 1927–28.] Trudy Leningr. Gosud. Vet. Inst. *2*: 173–174, 1928.
46. Bater, J. H. St. Petersburg, Industrialization and Change, pp. 270–271; 392–393. London, Edward Arnold, 1976.
47. Balzamentov, A. D. Izmeneniya vymeni korov pri infektsii Bac. pyogenes. [Alterations in the bovine udder infected with B. pyogenes.] Uchen. Zap. Kazan. Gosud. Zoovet. Inst. *47*: 316–323, 1937.
48. Bazhenov, S. V. Pervy veterinarny zhurnal sovetskoi Ukrainy. [The

first veterinary journal in Soviet Ukraine.] Veterinariya *49*(5): 121–122, 1972.

49. Bederke, O. Tierärztliche Hochschulreform in Sowjetrussland. Berl. tierärztl. Wschr. *48*: 321–323, 1932.
50. Belkin, G. Y., & N. V. Pastukhov. Sluchai raka zheludka u loshadi. [A case of carcinoma of the stomach in a horse.] Trudy Gosud. Inst. Exp. Vet. *1*: 72–76, 1923.
51. Belkin, G. Leiomyoma der Leber nebst Bemerkungen über Leiomyoma im Magen, Darm und Vagina bei Hunden. Berl. tierärztl. Wschr. *41*: 829–830, 1925.
52. Belkin, G. Obzor dannykh vskrytii 85 trupov loshadei, unichtozhennykh kak sapnye. [Postmortem findings on 85 horse cadavers killed because of glanders.] Prakt. Vet. Konevodstvo 2: 26–36, 1925.
53. Berg, A. Geschichte der Mikroskopie, vol. 2, p. 230, Frankfurt, Umschau Verlag, 1964.
54. Beskhlebnov, Yu. A. Veterinarnye entsiklopedii, vol. 1, pp. 1023–1024, in Skryabin, K. I., ed., Veterinarnaya Entsiklopediya. Moscow, Izdatel. Sovet. Entsiklop., 1968.
55. Blumberg, C. Ueber das estnische Pferd und das Gestüt zu Torgel. Oesterr. Vierteljschr. wiss. Veterinärk. *47*: 99–148, 1877.
56. Blumberg, C. Ein Beitrag zur Tuberkulosefrage. Deut. Z. Thiermed. *5*: 319–325, 1879.
57. Blumberg, C. Ueber einen neuen Parasiten beim Hunde und der Katze (Cysticercus elongatus.). Deut. Z. Thiermed. *8*: 140–147, 1882.
58. Blumberg, K. O znachenii patologicheskoi zootomi v veterinarii. [On the significance of pathologic zootomy in veterinary medicine.] Arkh. Vet. Nauk *12*(Sect. 3): 167–191, 1882.
59. Blumberg, K. Materialy dlya patologicheskoi zootomii. [Data on pathological zootomy.] Arkh. Vet. Nauk *13*(Sect. 3): 73–94, 1883.
60. Blumberg, C. Der Sectionssaal des Kasan'schen Veterinärinstitutes. Deut. Z. Thiermed. *8*: 225–229, 1883.
61. Blumberg, K. K voprosu o gnilostnom otravlenii. [The question of putrid intoxication.] Uchen. Zap. Kazan. Vet. Inst. *1*: 21–39, 57–73; 176–188; 268–296; 334–353, 1883–1884. (Extensive abstract in Jahresb. Vet. Med. *4*: 53–54, 1884).
62. Blumberg, C. Experimenteller Beitrag zur Kenntniss der putriden Intoxicationen. Virchows Arch. *100*: 377–415, 1885.
63. Blumberg, K. K zarazitelnosti sushenoi mokroty chakhotochnykh. [The infectiousness of dried phthisic sputum.] Uchen. Zap. Kazan. Vet. Inst. 2: 267–273, 1885.
64. Blumberg, C. Fractur eines Hauers bei einem wilden Eber. Deut. Zschr. Thiermed. *12*: 42–45, 1886.
65. Blumberg, K. Otchet o vskrytiyakh za 1883–1885 goda. [Report of au-

topsies for the years 1883–1885.] Uchen. Zap. Kazan. Vet. Inst. *3*: 98–119, 1886.

66. Blumberg, C. Eine Krebsbildung in der vorderen Hohlvene und rechten Vorkammer einer Kuh. Deut. Zschr. Thiermed. *12*: 415–419, 1886.
67. Blumberg, K. O bakteriologicheskikh kursakh v gigienicheskom institute Berlinskago Universiteta. [On the bacteriological course in the Hygienic Institute of the University of Berlin.] Uchen Zap. Kazan. Vet. Inst. *4*: 266–270, 1887.
68. Blumberg, K. Eesti hobune. The Estonian Horse. Rakvere, Estonia, G. Kuhs, 1887.
69. Blumberg, C. Zur Wuthfrage. Cbl. Bakt. *6*: 766–767, 1890.
70. Blumberg, C. Zur Aufklärung eines durch die russische Bezeichnung des Anthrax ("sibirisches Pest") hervorgerufenen Missverständnisses. Deut. Zschr. Thiermed. *16*: 437–439, 1890.
71. Blumberg, K. Gnoiniki v pravom yaichnike i tazovoi polosti u kobyly. [Abscess in the right ovary and pelvic cavity of a mare.] Uchen. Zap. Kazan. Vet. Inst. *10*: 192–194, 1893.
72. Blumberg, K. K patologicheskoi anatomii pishchevoda. [On the pathological anatomy of the esophagus.] Uchen. Zap. Kazan. Vet. Inst. *11*: 215–219, 1894.
73. Blumberg, K. Sektsionnaya Tekhnika. Rukovodstvo k Patologo-Anatomicheskomu Vskrytiyu Domashnikh Zhivotnykh. [Autopsy Technique. Manual of Pathologic-Anatomic Dissection of Domestic Animals.] Kazan, Tipografiya B. L. Dombrovsky, 1895.
74. Blumberg, K. Materialy dlya patologicheskoi zootomii. [Data on pathological zootomy.] Uchen. Zap. Kazan. Vet. Inst. *13*: 276–298, 1896.
75. Bogdanov, M. M., and M. M. Pavlov. Nemetsko-Russkii Slovar dlya Meditsinkikh i Veterinarnykh Vrachei. [German-Russian Dictionary for Medical and Veterinary Physicians.] Kharkov, 1929. Cited in: Zbirnik Prats Kharkiv. Vet. Inst. *15*: 59, 1929.
76. Bogdanovich, V. V. Nauchnaya Makulatura. [Scientific "junk literature."] Vet. Obozrenie *4*: 767–774, 1902.
77. Bohl, K. K voprosu o patologo-anatomicheskikh izmeneniyakh spinnogo mozga pri chume sobak. [On the pathologic-anatomical changes in the spinal cord in canine distemper.] Uchen. Zap. Kazan. Vet. Inst. *16*: 1–21; 53–91; 115–228, 1899.
78. Bohl, K. K voprosu konservirovanii patologo-anatomicheskikh preparatov. [The conservation of pathologic-anatomical preparations.] Arkhiv Vet. Nauk *31*: 1004–1010, 1901.
79. Bohl, K. K voprosu o konservirovanii zhivotnikh parazitov. [The conservation of animal parasites.] Uchen. Zap. Kazan. Vet. Inst. *19*: 36–38, 1902.
80. Bohl, K. O sagovoi selezenkie u zhivotnykh. [On sago spleen in ani-

mals.] Uchen. Zap. Kazan. Vet. Inst. *19*: 489–491, 1902.

81. Bohl, K. Zur Frage der Wuthdiagnose. Arch. Tierheilk. *28*: 523–525, 1902.

82. Bohl, K. K kazuistiki zhivotnykh parazitov. [Case reports of animal parasitism.] Arch. Tierheilk. *21*: 378–381, 1904.

83. Bohl, K. K voprosii ob amiloidie pecheni u loshadu. [On amyloid in the liver of horses.] Arkh. Vet. Nauk *35*: 236–240, 1905.

84. Bohl, K. H. Otchet o vskrytiyakh, proizvedennykh v Kazanskom Veterinarnom Institute v 1904 godu. [Report of the autopsies conducted at the KVI in 1904.] Uchen. Zap. Kazan. Vet. Inst. *22*: 378–383, 1905.

85. Bohl, K. H. K patologo-anatomicheskoi kazuistike. [Pathologic-anatomic case reports.] Uchen. Zap. Kazan. Vet. Inst. *22*: 453–462, 1905.

86. Bohl, K. K patologii diabetes mellitus. [The pathology of diabetes mellitus [in dogs].] Arkh. Vet. Nauk *36*: 569–598, 1906.

87. Bohl, K. H. Razryvy selezenki na pochve amiloidnoi infiltratsii. [On rupture of the spleen following amyloid infiltration.] Arkh. Vet. Nauk *38*: 619–624, 1908.

88. Bohl, K. K ucheniya o biliarnom zirroze. [On biliary hepatic cirrhosis.] Arkh. Vet. Nauk *39*: 145–171, 1909.

89. Bohl, K. K kazuistikie amiloida koshek. [On amyloid in cats.] Uchen. Zap. Kazan. Vet. Inst. *26*: 14–25, 1909.

90. Bohl, K. H. K kazuistik novobrazovadim u zhivotnikh: carcinomatosis. [Case reports of new growths in animals.] Uchen. Zap. Kazan. Vet. Inst. *26*: 138–142, 1909.

91. Bohl, K. H. K patologo-anatomicheskoi kazuistiki. 1. Arteriitis et aneurysma aorti i eya razetlenii vizvannie Sclerostoma armatum. [Arteritis and aneurysm of a branch of the aorta caused by S. armatum.] Arkh. Vet. Nauk *40*: 138–147, 1910. 2. K ucheniyu o mistnoi eozinofilli fragmentatsiya serdtsa. [Eosinophilic fragmentation of the heart.] Ibid. *40*: 148–152, 1910.

92. Bohl, K. H. Polyposis tonkago kishechnika i adeno-carcino-chondro-osteoma obodochnoi kishki loshadi. [Polyposis of the small intestine and adeno-carcino-chondro-osteoma of the colon in the horse.] Arkh. Vet. Nauk *40*(8): 869–877, 1910.

93. Bohl, K. H. K patologo-anatomicheskoi kazuistike. [Pathologic-anatomic case reports.] I. Volvulus nodosus et strongulatio lipomatosa-ligamentosa tonkago kishechnika. Ruptura ventriculi. [Volvulus nodusus and strangulatio lipomatosa-ligamentosa of the small intestine.] Uchen. Zap. Kazan. Vet. Inst. 27: 77–78, 1910. II. Vypadenie i ushchemlenie tonkago otdyela kishechnika v grudnuyu polost cherez razryv diafragmy. [Prolapse and strangulation of the small intestine into the thorax through a diaphragmatic rupture.] Ibid. 79–80, 1910. III. Subperitonealnoe krovoizliyanie tochei

kishki u loshadi. [Subperitoneal hemorrhage of the jejunum in a horse.] Ibid. 80–82, 1910. IV. Hydrops vesicae felleae s. dilatatio vesicae congenitalis u telenka. [Congential hydrops vesicae felleae and dilatatio vesicae felleae in a calf.] Ibid. 82–83, 1910. VI. Pervichnyi razryvy selezenki loshadi. [Primary splenic rupture in horses.] Ibid. 85–87, 1910. VII. Urocystitia fibrino-purulenta et ruptura vesicae urinariae u loshadi na pochve cancroida penisa. [Urocystitis fibrino-purulenta and rupture of the urinary bladder in a horse following penile cancroid.] Ibid. 87–89, 1910. VIII. Hydronephrosis u sobaku. [Hydronephrosis in dogs.] Ibid. 89–94, 1910.

94. Bohl, K. H. Adenoma pochechnoi lokhanki, amiloidnaya infiltratsiya i atrofiya pochki loshadi. [Adenoma of the renal pelvis, amyloid infiltration, and atrophy of the kidney in horses.] Uchen. Zap. Kazan. Vet. Inst. 27: 169–174, 1910.

95. Bohl, K. H. K patologii roga. [On the pathology of the horns.] Vet. Vrach *5*(22): 342–345, 1910.

96. Bohl, K. H. K Patologo-anatomicheskoi Kazuistike. [Pathologic-Anatomic Case Reports.] St. Petersburg, Tipografiya M.V.D., 1910.

97. Bohl, K. H. K patologii nervnoi sistemi. [On the pathology of the nervous system.] Arkh. Vet. Nauk *41*: 29–43, 1911.

98. Bohl, K. H. Topografiya nervnykh kletok n. vagi i formirovanie ganglion jugulare i ganglion nodosum u domashnykh zhivotnykh. [Topography of the nerve cells in the vagus nerve and the form of the jugular ganglion and nodosal ganglion in domestic animals.] Arkh. Vet. Nauk *42*: 605–637, 1912.

99. Bohl, K. H. Osnovy Patologicheskoi Anatomii Domashnykh Zhivotnykh. [Principles of Pathologic Anatomy of Domestic Animals.] Kazan, Tipografiya D. M. Gran, 1913.

100. Bohl, K. H. Kak ne sleduet kormit loshad. [How not to feed the horse.] Uchen. Zap. Kazan. Vet. Inst. *46*: 127–131, 1919.

101. Bohl, K. K voprosu struktura soedinitelnaya tkan. [The structure of connective tissue.] Prakt. Vet. Kon. 5(7/8): 558–560, 1926.

102. Bohl, K. Krovoizliyaniya, ikh genesis i klassifikatsiya. [Hemorrhage, its genesis and classification.] Uchen. Zap. Kazan. Gosud. Vet. Inst. *37*: 38–48, 1926.

103. Bohl, K. Zur Frage über die Struktur des Bindegewebes. Anat. Anz. *61*: 404–406, 1926.

104. Bohl, C. [K.] Die Blutungen, ihre Entstehung und Klassifizierung. Deut. tierärztl. Wschr. *35*: 661–664, 1927. (Professor Bohl used the initial C interchangeably with K when he published in German.)

105. Bohl, K. H. Paratuberkulöse Darmentzündung der Rinder. Deut. tierärztl. Wschr. *35*: 725–727, 1927.

106. Bohl, K. H. Der Rotz beim Pferde. Deut. tierärztl. Wschr. *35*: 727–729, 1927.
107. Bohl, K. H. Amiloidoz slizistoi obolotchki nosovoi polosti u loshadi. [Amyloidosis of the nasal mucosa in a horse.] Uchen. Zap. Kazan. Vet. Inst. *38*: 92–95, 1929.
108. Bohl, K. Vospalennie. [Inflammation.] Uchen. Zap. Kazan. Gosud. Vet. Inst. *41*: 3–46, 1933.
109. Bohl, K. Prof. K. R. Viktorov, kak pedagog i obshchestvennyi rabotnik. [Prof. K. R. Viktorov, as teacher and public worker.] Uchen. Zap. Kazan. Gosud. Vet. Inst. *44*: 12–14, 1934.
110. Bohl, K. H. 60 let kafedry patologicheskoi anatomii pri Kazanskom Zooveterinarnom Institute. [Sixty years of the chair of pathological anatomy in the Kazan Zooveterinary Institute.] Uchen. Zap. Kazan. Gosud. Zoovetinst. *47*: 28–42, 1937.
111. Bohl, K. H. and B. K. Bohl. Osnovy Patologicheskoi Anatomii Selskokhozyaistvennykh Zhivotnykh. (The Basis of Pathologic Anatomy of Farm Animals.] 3d ed., Moscow, Gos. Izd. Selsk. Lit. 1961.
112. Bohlen, C. E. Witness to History, pp. 19, 27–28. New York, Norton, 1973.
113. Bollinger, O. Cited by Röll, M. F. Die Thierseuchen, p. 282. Wien, Braumüller, 1881.
114. Borisovich, F. K., and Yu. F. Borisovich. Nekotorye materialy k istorii V.I.E.V. (Nachalnyi period, 1917–1928 gg.). [Some data on the history of the All-Union Veterinary Research Institute (initial period, 1917–1928).] Trudy Vsesoyuz. Inst. Eksp. Vet. 22: 355–370, 1959.
115. Boczkowski, P. S. P. Alfred Krajewski. Wiadomosci Wet. *3*(1–5): 1–2, 1921.
116. Brauell, F. Dem Andenken Dr. Theobald Renner's, vormaligem Professor der Veterinair-Medicin in Moskau und Jena. Mag. ges. Thierheilk. *18*: 119–126, 1852.
117. Brauell, F. Das Wachstum der Hufwand. Zum funfzigjährigen Jubelfeste der Kaiserlichen Dorpater Universität. Dorpat, Druck von Heinrich Laakmann, 1852.
118. Brauell, F. Eine Beobachtung, betreffend eine eigenthümliche hypertrophische Entartung des Dreistigkeits-Organs. Deutsche Klinik *8*: 474, 1856.
119. Brauell, F. Versuche und Untersuchungen betreffend den Milzbrand des menschen und der Thiere. Virchows Arch. *11*: 132–144, 1857.
120. Brauell, F. Bemerkungen über Druck und andere Fehler. Mag. ges. Thierheilk. *23*: 374–379, 1857.
121. Brauell, F. Weitere Mittheilungen über Milzbrand und Milzbrandblut. Virchows Arch. *14*: 432–465, 1858.

122. Brauell, F. Neue Untersuchungen betreffend die pathologische Anatomie der Rinderpest. Dorpat, Verlag E. J. Karow, Universitäts-Buchhändler, 1862.
123. Brauell, F. Pathologisch-anatomische Notizen. Oesterr. Vierteljschr. wiss. Vetkde. *35*: 5–33, 1871.
124. Bray, R. G. A. de. Guide to the Slavonic Languages, pp. 69–73. 2d ed. London, Dent, 1969.
125. Brockhaus, F. A., and I. A. Efron. Ravich, I. I. Entsiklopedicheskii Slovar, *26*: 59. St. Petersburg, Tipografiya Akts. "Izdat. Dielo," 1899.
126. Brown, A. H. A voice from the Kremlin. Times Literary Supplement (London), p. 115, Jan. 31, 1975.
127. Budenny, S. M. Kovochnaya Bezgramotnost. [Incompetent farriery.] Prakt. Vet. Kon. *1*(3), 1924. [Original not seen, cited in Budenny, S. M. Krasnaya Konnitsa. Sbornik Statei. (Red Cavalry. Collected Papers), pp. 141–143. Moscow/Leningrad, Gos. Izd. Odtel. Voennoi Lit., 1930].
128. Budenny, S. M. Glavnomu redaktoru, redaktsionnoi kollegii, chitatelyam i korrespondentam zhurnala "Veterinariya." [To the chief editor, editorial board, readers, and authors of the journal "Veterinariya."] Veterinariya *41*(5): 2, 1964.
129. Bulgakov, M. The White Guard, p. 59. New York, McGraw-Hill, 1971.
130. Bulloch, W. The History of Bacteriology. Oxford, Oxford University Press, 1938.
131. Carmichael, J. A Cultural History of Russia, pp. 131, 232. London, Weidenfield and Nicolson, 1968.
132. Chebotarev, R. S. Ocherki po Istorii Meditsinskoi i Veterinarnoi Parazitologii. [Outline of History of Medical and Veterinary Parasitology.] Pp. 157–158. Minsk, Nauka i Tekhnika, 1965.
133. Chebotarev, R. S., and Yu. B. Ratner. Kratkii Parazitologicheskii Slovar. [Short Parasitological Dictionary.] P. 39. Minsk, Gos. Izd. Selskokhoz. Lit. Belorussk. S.S.R., 1962.
134. Cheredkov, V. Leningradskii Institut Usovershenstvovaniya Veterinarnykh Vrachei. [The Leningrad Institute for Postgraduate Training of Veterinarians.] Sovet. Vet. *16*(7): 91–92, 1939.
135. Chernogorov, A. Dvatsdatipyatiletie sluzhebnoi deyatelnosti ordinarnago professora Kazanskago Veterinarnago Instituta K. G. Blumberga. [Twenty-five years of service of ordinary professor of the KVI K. G. Blumberg.] Uchen. Zap. Kazan. Vet. Inst. *14*: 58–62, 1897.
136. Chernyak, V. Z. Beitrag zur Histologie der Lungenknötchen bei Pferden. Zeitchr. Infektkr. Haustiere 25: 140–143, 1923.
137. Chernyak, V. Z. Zur Histologie der durch den Parasiten Strongylus

edentatus hervorgerufenen Veränderungen. Zeitschr. Infektkr. Haustiere *28*: 295–299, 1925.

138. Chernyak, V. Z. Obzor dannykh vskrytiya 235 trupov loshadei, unichtozhennykh, kak bolnye sapom, i sopostavlenie etikh dannykh s dannymi klinicheskikh metodov issledovaniya. [A postmortem study of 235 horse cadavers affected by glanders, and correlation of the findings with clinical methods of examination.] Prakt. Vet. Kon. *2*(11/12): 26–39, 1925.

139. Chernyak, V. Z. Histologische Untersuchungen. Beilage II zu: Yakimoff, W. L. und I. G. Galouzo. Die Darmkokzidiose der Rinder in Russland. Cbl. Bakt. (Abt. 1, Orig.) *103*: 110–112, 1927.

140. Chernyak, V. Z. Sluchai mestnogo opukholepodobnogo amiloidoza slizistoi obolochki nosovoi polosti u loshadi. [A case of localized tumorlike amyloidosis of the nasal mucosa in a horse.] Prakt. Vet. Kon. *4*(12): 20–24, 1927.

141. Chernyak, V. Z. Curschmansche Spiralen in den Lungen von Pferden. Berl. tierärztl. Wschr. *44*: 399–403, 1928.

142. Chernyak, V. Z. Zur Histologie der parasitären Veränderungen bei Pferden. (4 Fälle von Wurmknötchen der Nieren.) Zeitschr. Infektkr. Haustiere *34*: 62–73, 1928.

143. Chernyak, V. Z. Zur Lehre von den Broncho-und Pneumonomykosen der Pferde. Arch. Tierheilk. *57*: 417–444, 1928.

144. Chernyak, V. Z. Ein Fall von sekundären Rhinomykose bei einem an Petechialfieber erkrankten Pferd. Deut. tierärztl. Wschr. *37*: 99–101, 1929.

145. Chernyak, V. Z. Zur Kasuistik der durch Rotz hervorgerufenen Veränderungen des Myokards und der Nebennieren bei Pferden. Berl. tierärztl. Wschr. *45*: 488–490, 1929.

146. Chernyak, V. Z., and S. Voronzov. Zur Frage der Herzmuskelverkalkungen bei Haustieren. Virchows Arch. *274*: 154–169, 1929.

147. Chernyak, V. Z. Ein Fall von Ruptur und Verkalkung der Harnblase beim Hunde. Tierärztl. Rdsch. *11*: 781–782, 1930.

148. Chernyak, V. Z., and N. A. Romanov. Zur Frage von der Verkalkung des Endokards bei Haustieren. Virchows Arch. *276*: 170–186, 1930.

149. Chernyak, V. Z. Veterinarnaya patologiya kak glava sravnitelnoi patologii. [Veterinary pathology as a part of comparative pathology.] Arkh. Patologii *21*(11): 82–89, 1959.

150. Chernyak, V. Z. Leningrad (Petersburg, Petrograd)—Rodina otechestvennoi nauchnoi veterinarii. [Leningrad, St. Petersburg, Petrograd—the birthplace of Russian veterinary science.] Sbor. Rabot Leningr. Vet. Inst. *19*: 13–31, 1959.

151. Chernyak, V. Uchenyi-organizator Nikolai Davidovich Ball (1872–

1930). [The scientist-organizer N. D. Ball.] Trudy 2d Konf. Pat. Anat. Selskokhoz. Zhivot. 465-468, 1961.

152. Chinchenko, I. M. Visoka veterinarna osvita v Ukraini. [Higher veterinary education in the Ukraine.] Zhur. Obednannya Amerikansko-Ukrainskikh Vet. Likariv *10*(2-3): 6-12, 1959.

153. Colange, L. D. Picturesque Russia and Greece. Troy, N.Y., H. B. Nims, 1886.

154. Conquest, R. The Great Terror, p. 551. New York, Macmillan, 1973.

155. Csokor, J. Vet. Wjestnik. Oesterr. Vierteljschr. wiss. Vetkde. *59*: 49-50, 1883.

156. Davydovsky, I. V. Problemy sovremennoi patologii. [Problems of contemporary pathology.] Trudy 2d Konf. Pat. Anat. Selskokhoz. Zhivot., 3-10, 1961.

157. Dementev, I. L. Saratovskii Zooveterinarnyi Institut. Veterinariya *53*(11): 111-112, 1977.

158. Dexler, H. Die pathologische Anatomie des Nervensystems und der Sinnesorgane der Haustiere. Ergebn. allg. Path. 7: 400-505, 1900.

159. Dobin, M. A., A. A. Avrorov, and A. M. Rakhmanov. Pamyati Professora Valentina Zakharovicha Chernyaka. [In memory of Professor V. Z. Chernyak.] Trudy 2. Vsesoyuz. Konf. Patol. Anat. Zhivot., pp. 490-493, 1964.

160. Dobin, M. A., P. I. Kokurichev, and A. A. Avrorov. Ball, Nikolai Davidovich, k 100-letiyu so dyna rozhdeniya. [N. D. Ball. On the 100th anniversary of his birth.] Veterinariya *49*(12): 109, 1972.

161. Drew, W. R. M. The challenge of the Rickettsial diseases. J. Roy. Army Med. Corps *111*: 95-105, 1965.

162. Dukat, A. Rudolf Virchow und die russischen Aerzte. Russ. Med. Rundschau *1*: 90-92, 1902.

163. Dvizhkov, P. P. Trudy Vsesoyuznoi Konferentsii Patologanatomov, 4-9 Iyulya 1954. [Proceedings of the All-Union Conference of Pathologic Anatomists.] Moscow, Medgiz, 1956.

164. Dzanelidze, Yu. Biograficheskii Slovar Professorov 1. Leningradskogo Meditsinskogo Instituta. [Biographical Dictionary of Professors of the 1st Leningrad Medical Institute.] Pp. 14; 140. Leningrad, Medgiz, 1947.

165. Eberbeck, E. Zur Pathologie der Rotzkrankheit. Zeitschr. Veterinärk. *28*: 353-364, 1916.

166. Eberbeck, E. Zur anatomischen Differentialdiagnose der Rotzkrankheit des Pferdes. Zeitschr. Veterinärk. *30*: 193-215, 1918.

167. Eberbeck, E., and R. Bierbaum. Infektionsversuche mit Rotzknoten vom Pferde. Zeitschr. Veterinärk. *30*: 385-404, 1918.

168. Eberbeck, E. Die Lokalisation der rotzigen und zooparasitären Veränderungen beim Pferde und ihre Bedeutung für die anatomische

Differentialdiagnose der Rotzkrankheit. Zeitschr. Veterinärk. *32*: 153–172, 1920.

169. Eberbeck, E. Bohl, K. H.: Der Rotz beim Pferde. [Abstract of article by this author.] Jahresb. Vet. Med. *47*: 820, 1927.
170. Eberbeck, E. Bohl, B. K.: Der Lungenrotz der Pferde. [Abstract of article by this author.] Jahresb. Vet. Med. *49*: 847, 1929.
171. Eichbaum, F. Grundriss der Geschichte der Thierheilkunde. pp. 167–172. Berlin, Paul Parey, 1885.
172. Elenevskii, Z. F. Patologicheskaya gistologiya i bakteriologiya gubnogo aktinomikoza krupnago rogatago skota. [Pathologic histology and bacteriology of labial actinomycosis in cattle.] Arkh. Vet. Nauk *31*: 793–812; 873–896, 1901. (With two color plates.)
173. Fateev, A. Gimnazicheskie i studentcheskie gody I. I. Mechnikova. [High school and student years of I. I. Mechnikov.] Vestnik Evropy *50*: 145–151, 1916.
174. Footman, W. C. Civil War in Russia, p. 77. New York, Praeger, 1962.
175. Friis, H. Biography of A. F. Følger. Dansk Biografisk Leksikon, *7*: 524–525, 1935.
176. Froboese, C. Rudolf Virchow†. 5.9. 1902. Ein Gedenk- und Mahnwort an die heutige Ärztegeneration 50 Jahre nach seinem Tode, pp. 39–40. Stuttgart, Gustav Fischer, 1953.
177. Gautier, R. Russia. Translated by F. Tyson. Philadelphia, J. C. Winston, 1905.
178. Genes, S. G. Otchet o deyatelnosti sektsii patologov Kharkov. Med. Obshchest. za 1936 g. [Report of the activities of the Section on Pathology of the Kharkov Medical Society for the year 1936.] Vrachebnoe Delo *19*: 165, 1937.
179. Gerlach, A. C. Die Rinderpest, pp. 39, 46, 56, 69–70. Hannover, Schmorl und von Seefeld, 1867.
180. Ginzburg, A. G., and A. D. Ivanov. Organizatsiya Veterinarnogo Dela. [Organization of Veterinary Medicine in the U.S.S.R.] Moscow, Gos. Izd. Selsk. Lit., 1962. (English translation, Office Tech. Serv. U.S. Dept. Commerce, Washington, 1963.)
181. Gizatullin, Kh. G., V. P. Shishkov, K. I. Vertinskii, N. G. Tolstova-Pariiskaya, and I. T. Trofimov. Karla Genrikovich Bol (K 100 letiyu so dnya rozhdeniya). [K. H. Bohl, on the one hundredth anniversary of his birth.] Veterinariya *48*(9): 123–125, 1971.
182. Gizatullin, Kh. G. Kazanskomu Veterinarnomu Institut—100 Let. [Kazan Veterinary Institute—100 years.] Veterinariya *50*(5): 3–9, 1973.
183. Gizatullin, Kh. G., and O. V. Nesmelova. Istoriya Kazanskogo Gosudarstvennogo Veterinarnogo Instituta imenii N. E. Baumana. [History of the Bauman Kazan State Veterinary Institute.] Kazan, Tatarskoe Knizhnoe Izdatelstvo, 1973.

184. Gordzialkowski, I. Znachenie dlya posmertnago diagnoza trupnykh izmenenii naruzhnykh pokrovov. [On the significance in postmortem diagnosis of alterations in the skin.] Sbornik Trudov Kharkov. Vet. Inst. *1*: 305–346, 1887.

185. Goreglyad, Kh. S. Razvitie veterinarnoi nauki i sovetskoi Belorussii. [Development of veterinary science in Soviet Belorussia.] Trudy Vsesoyuz. Ord. Lenina Inst. Eksp. Vet. *41*: 28–39, 1973.

186. Gradyushko, G. M. K 50-letiyu voennoi epizootologii. [On 50 years of military epizootiology.] Veterinariya *45*(2): 48–49, 1969.

187. Graham, L. R. The Soviet Academy of Sciences and the Communist Party, 1927–1932. Princeton, Princeton University Press, 1967.

188. Graham, S. Changing Russia. London, John Lane, 1915.

189. Greuning, E. The State of Alaska, pp. 94–97. New York, Random House, 1968.

190. Gryuner, S. A. Otchet po komandirovke zagranitsu, 1902. [Report of an official trip abroad.] Vet. Khronika Voronezh. Guberniya *1*, 1902. (Original not seen, cited by Gryuner.[200])

191. Gryuner, S. A. Finnoz severnago olenya. (K materialam patologii severnago olenya). [Cysticercosis of northern reindeer. Data on the pathology of northern reindeer.] Arkh. Vet. Nauk *40*: 952–957, 1910.

192. Gryuner, S. A. Russian review. Amer. Vet. Rev. *39*: 453–455; 686–693, 1911.

193. Gryuner, S. A. *Cysticercus rangiferi* in Alaska. Amer. Vet. Rev. *40*: 362–364, 1911.

194. Gryuner, S. A. Veterinary work in Russia. Amer. Vet. Rev. *39:* 537–546, 1911.

195. Gryuner, S. A. K tekhnike diagnosticheskoi proby na otklonenie komplementa pri sape. [On the technique of the complement fixation diagnostic test in glanders.] Arkh. Vet. Nauk *43*: 404–427, 1913.

196. Gryuner, S. A. Boini v Severo-Amerikanskikh Soedinennykh Shtatakh. [Abattoirs in the United States of America.] Arkh. Vet. Nauk *44*: 158–187, 1914.

197. Gryuner, S. A. Olenevodstvo v Alyaske. [Deer husbandry in Alaska.] Arkh. Vet. Nauk *44*(11): 1423–1460; (12): 1544–1588, 1914.

198. Gryuner, S. A. Trikhinoz dikikh zverei soderzhimykh v nevole. [Trichinosis in wild animals in captivity.] Arkh. Vet. Nauk *45*: 745–754, 1915.

199. Gryuner, S. A. Pamyati Nikolai Ernestovich Bauman. [In memory of N. E. Bauman.] Vet. Truzhenik *1*(12): 1–3, 1925.

200. Gryuner, S. A. Furunkulez ryb na Kamchatke. [Furunculosis of fish in Kamchatka.] Vet. Truzhenik *3*(4): 4–7, 1927.

200a. Gryuner, S. A. Vysshaya veterinarnaya i s.-x. shkola v Kopengagene.

[The Veterinary and Agricultural College of Copenhagen.] Vet. Truzhenik *3*(11): 4–10, 1927.

201. Gurin, G. I. Kratkoe rukovodstvo obshchei patologii zhivotnykh. St. Petersburg, Tipograf. A. I. Snegirovoi, 1912.

202. Gurlt, E., and A. Wernieh. Biographisches Lexikon der hervorragende Ärzte. 2d ed., vol. 3, p. 606, Berlin, Urban & Schwarzenberg, 1931.

203. Guschin, N. I. Etapy bolshogo puti. K 40-letiyu zhurnala "Veterinariya". [Stages of a big journey. Forty years of the journal Veterinariya.] Veterinariya *41*(5): 6–9, 1964.

204. Gutmann, W. Die Entwicklung des tierärztlichen Unterrichts am Dorpater Veterinär-Institut. Eesti Loomarstlik Ringvaade *1*: 10–16, 1925.

205. Hamperl, H. Werdegang und Lebensweg eines Pathologen. Stuttgart, F. K. Schatter, 1972.

206. Helmann, Kh. Diagnoz sapa posredstvom podkozhnavo vpriskivaniya vityazkhi sapnikh batsill. (Diagnosis of glanders by means of subcutaneous injections of extract of glanders bacilli.] Vestnik Obshchoi Vet. *3*: 67–70, 1891.

207. Hickman, R. W. Epizootic cerebro-spinal meningitis of horses, pp. 165–172 in Twenty-third Annual Report, Bureau of Animal Industry for the Year 1906. Washington, Government Printing Office, 1908.

208. Hingle, R. The Russian Mind, p. 254. New York, Scribner, 1977.

209. Hobday, F. T. G. Discussion of animal and vegetable pathology in relation to human disease. Vet. J. *78*: 393–403, 1922.

210. Hobday, F. T. G. A visit to some of the veterinary colleges and veterinary research institutes of the United Socialist Soviet Republic. Vet. Rec. *10*: 1189–1194, 1930.

211. Hoover, H. The Memoirs of Herbert Hoover, vol. 2, pp. 22–26. New York, Macmillan, 1952.

212. Hueck, W. Felix Marchand†. Verh. Deutsche Path. Gesellsch. *23*: 533–545, 1928.

213. Hutyra, F., and J. Marek. Die Orientalische Rinderpest. Jena, Gustav Fischer, 1916.

214. Ivanov, B. G. Osnovnye itogi nauchno-issledovatelskikh rabot v oblasti patologicheskoi anatomii selskokhozyaistvennykh zhivotnykh za 1918–1957 gg. [The main results of research in the field of pathological anatomy of livestock in the period 1918–1957.] Trudy Vsesoyuz. Inst. Eksp. Vet. *23*: 59–72, 1959.

215. Ivanov, S. A. O patologo-anatomicheskikh izmeneniyakh tsentralnoi nervnoi sistemy pri beshenstve. [The pathologic-anatomic changes in the central nervous system in rabies.] M.V.Sc. Dissertation, St. Petersburg, 1883; also in Arkhiv Vet. Nauk *13*(Sect. IV): 129–191, 1883.

216. Ivanovskii, N. P. Rechi, proiznesenniya torzhestvenkom otkrytii byusta pokoinago Professora M. M. Rudneva. [Occurrences and speeches during the unveiling of the bust of the deceased Professor M. M. Rudnev.] Vrach *2*: 805–808, 1881.
217. Ivanovskii, N. P. Istoriya Imperatorskoi Voenno-Meditsinskoi (byvshei mediko-khirurgicheskoi) Akademii za sto let 1798–1898. [History of the Imperial Military-Medical (formerly medico-chirurgical) Academy during the years 1798–1898.] St. Petersburg, Tipografiya Ministerstva Vnutrennikh Del, 1898.
218. Izmailov, A. S. Iosif Ippolitovich Ravich. Vestnik Obshchest. Vet. *6*(6): 174–178, 1894.
219. Jennings, W. E. Glanders. Pp. 264–292 in Diseases Transmitted from Animals to Man. T. G. Hull, ed. 5th ed. Springfield, Ill., Charles C Thomas, 1963.
220. Jessen, P. Sendschreiben an die österreichischen Veterinairkundigen. Mag. ges. Thierheilk. *31*: 116–128, 1865.
221. Joest E., and P. Kracht-Palejeff. Untersuchungen über die Frühstadien der Milchdrüsentuberkulose des Rindes. Zeitschr. Infektkr. Haustiere *12*: 299–320, 1912.
222. Kalning, O. K diagnozu sapa. [On the diagnosis of glanders.] Arkh. Vet. Nauk 21(Sect. V): 113–116, 1891.
223. Kalugin, V. I. Professor A. A. Raevskii. Veterinariya *28*(10): 60–62, 1951.
224. Kalugin, V. I. Zasluzhennyi Professor N. N. Mari (1858–1921). [Honored Professor N. N. Mari.] Veterinariya *36*(3): 89, 1959.
225. Kalugin, V. I. N. P. Savvaitov—vydayushchiisya uchenii-pedagog i organizator otechestvennoi veterinarii. [N. P. Savvaitov—eminent educator, teacher, and organizer of Russian veterinary medicine.] Veterinariya *38*(8): 85–87, 1961.
226. Kalugin, V. I. G. I. Gurin—Vydayushchiisya uchenyi-pedagog i propagandist zootekhnicheskikh i veterinarnykh znanii v S.S.S.R. [G. I. Gurin—teacher, propagandist, expert on livestock and veterinary science in the U.S.S.R.] Veterinariya *40*(3): 80–81, 1963.
227. Kalugin, V. I. 75 Let so dnya vykhoda pervogo nomera zhurnala Vestnik Obshchestvennoi Veterinarii. [Seventy-five years from the appearance of the first issue of the journal Vestnik Obshchestvennoi Veterinarii.] Veterinariya *41*(5): 116–117, 1964.
228. Kalugin, V. I., and V. V. Kalugin. I. I. Ravich—vydayushchiisya patolog-eksperimentator otechestvennoi veterinarii. [I. I. Ravich—eminent pathologist-experimenter of Russian veterinary medicine.] Veterinariya *39*(6): 85–88, 1962.
229. Kalugin, V. I., and V. V. Kalugin. E. M. Zemmer—Vydayushchiisya uchenyi otechestvennoi veterinarii. K 120-letiyu so dnya rozhdeniya. [E. M. Semmer, outstanding Russian veterinary scien-

tist. On the 120th anniversary of his birth.] Veterinariya *40*(12): 69, 1963.

230. Kanevskii, L. O. Osnovnye cherty razvitiya meditsiny v Rossii v period kapitalizma, 1861–1917. [Fundamental lines of development of medicine in Russia in the period of capitalism.] P. 37. Moscow, Medgiz, 1956.

231. Karaulov, F. V. O patologo-anatomicheskikh izmeneniyakh organov zhivotnykh pri zarazhenii batsilloi chumy cheloveka. [The pathologic-anatomical study of the organs of animals infected with human plague.] Uchen. Zap. Kazan. Vet. Inst. *16*: 92–108; 569–589; 1899; *17*: 1–89, 1900.

232. Karokhin, V. N. Sorok devyataya soyuznaya gelmintologicheskaya ekspeditsiya v Tenkovskii raion Tatrespubliki 17-VII—14-IX 1927 god. [Forty-ninth all Union helminthological expedition to Tenkovsky district of the Tartar Republic.] Uchen. Zap. Kazan. Gosud. Vet. Inst. *37*: 178–189, 1927.

233. Kashina, L. V chest vydayushchegosya uchenogo. [In honor of a distinguished scholar.] Veterinariya *54*(7): 125, 1977.

234. Katić, I. Breve fra Carl Mæhl til Harald Krabbe. [Letters from Carl Mæhl to Harald Krabbe.] Copenhagen, the author, 1975.

235. Katić, I. Breve fra Chr. Engelsen til H. Krabbe og B. Bang, 1884–1906. Nord. Vet. Med. *26,* Suppl. II, 1974.

236. Keller, W. East Minus West = Zero. Russia's Debt to the Western World. New York, Putnam, 1962.

237. Kennan, G. Adventures in Eastern Siberia. Century Magazine *39*: 88–116, 1890.

238. Kennan, G. A winter journey through Siberia. Century Magazine *42*: 643–658, 1891.

239. Kennan, G. My last days in Siberia. Century Magazine*42*: 803–820, 1891. (Appendix V is from pp. 651–653; plague picture p. 816.)

240. Kennan, G. Siberia and the Exile System. New York, Century Company, 1891.

241. Khomitskii, F. V. Pervyi rektor Donskogo Veterinarnogo Instituta. [The first rector of the Don Veterinary Institute.] Veterinariya *48*(2): 117–118, 1972.

242. Khrushchev, N. Khrushchev Remembers, pp. 110–114. Translated by S. Talbott, Boston, Little, Brown, 1970.

243. Khrushchov, G. K. Ilya Ilich Mechnikov, vol. 3, pp. 192–200. *In* Kuznetsov, I. V., ed., Lyudi Russkoi Nauki. Moscow, Gosud. Izdatel. Fiziko-Matemat. Lit., 1963.

244. Kiesseweter. Das russische Militär-Veterinärwesen unter Friedens- und Feldverhältnissen. Ergänzungsbände zur Zschr. Veterinärkd. Heft 6, 1932.

245. Kikiloff. Ueber Bau und Entwicklung der Neubildungen bei der Perlsucht der Rinder. Deut. Z. Thiermed. *7*: 28–32, 1882.
246. King, L. S. The Growth of Medical Thought, p. 220. Chicago, University of Chicago Press, 1963.
247. Klementeva, A. M. 8 Let. [8 years.] Sbornik Nauch. Statei Kazan. Zootech.-Vet. Inst., pp. 30–31. Kazan, Tatizdat, 1932.
248. Koch, A. Review of Sektsionnaya Tekhnika, by K. Blumberg. Oesterr. Mschr. Tierheilk. *21*: 31, 1896.
249. Koch, A. Prof. Eugen Semmer†. Österr. Mschr. Tierheilk. *31*: 322, 1907.
250. Kokurichev, P. I. Shpat loshadei. [Spavin of horses.] Uchen. Zap. Kazan. Gosud. Vet. Inst. *43*: 352–369, 1933.
251. Kokurichev, P. I. Razvitie veterinarnoi patologicheskoi anatomii v SSSR. [The development of veterinary pathologic anatomy in the U.S.S.R.] Veterinariya *44*(1): 17–18, 1968.
252. Kokurichev, P. Atlas patologicheskoi anatomii selskokhozyaistvennykh zhivotnykh. [Atlas of Pathologic Anatomy of Farm Animals.] Leningrad, Izdatelstvo "Kolos," 1973.
253. Kokurichev, P., and A. Yatsyshin. Pamyati professora Fedora Mikhailovicha Ponomarenko. [In memory of Professor F. M. Ponomarenko.] Materialy VI Vsesoyuz. Konf. Pat. Anat. Zhivotnykh 2: 282–283, 1974. Tartu, 1975.
254. Kolesnikoff, N. Pathologische Veränderungen im Nervensystem bei der Wuthkranheit. Centralbl. med. Wissensch. *13*: 853–854, 1875.
255. Kolessnikow, N. Pigmentiertes Rhabdomyom [Rhabdomyoma melanoides.] Virchows Arch. *68*: 554–575, 1876.
256. Kolessnikow, N. Die Histologie der Milchdrüse der Kuh und die pathologisch-anatomischen Veränderungen derselben bei der Perlsucht. Virchows Arch. *70*: 531–546, 1877.
257. Kolesnikov, N. O patologicheskikh izmeneniyakh golovnago i spinnago mozga sobaki pri lyssa. [On pathologic changes in the spinal cord and brain of dogs with rabies.] Arkh. Vet. Nauk *11* (Sect. III): 274–296; 345–395, 1881.
258. Kolessnikow, N. Ueber pathologische Veränderungen des Gehirns und Rückenmarks der Hunde bei der Lyssa. Virchows Arch. *85*: 445–503, 1882.
259. Kolesnikov, N. Ob Izmeneniyakh Golovnago i Spinnago Mozga Sobak pri Beshenstve. [On the changes in the spinal cord and brain of the dog with rabies.] M.D. dissertation, St. Petersburg, 1885.
260. Kolesnikov, N. F. Materialy k ucheniyu o sibirskoi yazve. [Contribution to the knowledge of anthrax.] Arkh. Vet. Nauk *19*(Sect. V): 65–70, 1889.
261. Kolesnikov, N. F. K kazuistike kishechnoi formy sibirskoi yazvy u

cheloveka. [Cases of intestinal anthrax in man.] Russkaya Med. *16*: 587–590; 600–604; 616–620; 634–637; 648–652; 666–668; 680–683, 1891.

262. Kolyakov, Ya. E. Rol Kharkovskogo Veterinarnogo Instituta v razvitii otechestvennoi mikrobiologii. [The role of the KVI in the development of domestic microbiology.] Sbor. Trud. Kharkov. Vet. Inst. 22: 30–38, 1954.

263. Konervesky, A. Letter to the editor. Vet J. (London) *78*: 265–266, 1922.

264. Koropov, V. M. Veterinarnoe Obrazovanie v S.S.S.R. [Veterinary Education in the U.S.S.R.] Moscow, Gosud. Izd. Selsk. Lit., 1949.

265. Koropov, V. M. Istoriya Veterinarii v S.S.S.R. [History of Veterinary Medicine in the U.S.S.R.] Moscow, Gosud. Izd. Selsk. Lit., 1954.

266. Koropov, V. M. Razvitie vysshego veterinarnogo obrazovaniya v Rossii i rol v etom Kharkovskogo Veterinarnogo Instituta. [Development of higher veterinary education in Russia and the role therein of the Kharkov Veterinary Institute.] Sbornik Rabot Kharkov. Vet. Inst. 22: 12–28, 1954.

267. Kostiuk, H. Stalinist Rule in the Ukraine. New York, Praeger, 1960.

268. Kowalenko, J.R. Die ersten Dekrete der Sowjetmacht zur Entwicklung des Veterinärwesens. Mhfte. Vet.-Med. *32*: 802–805, 1977.

269. Kracht-Paléjeff, P. N. Zur Anatomie und pathologischen Anatomie der Prostata des Hundes. Arch. Tierheilk. *37*: 299–308, 1911.

270. Kraevskii, A. Chuma sobak, eya zarazitelnost i perenosimost putem privivaniya. [Canine distemper, its transmission through inoculation.] Arkh. Vet. Nauk *11* (Sect. V): 268–288, 1881.

271. Kraevskii, A. K ucheniyu o perenosimosti kontagiya loshadinago sapa na plotoyadnykh zhivotnykh. [A study of the transmissibility of contagious equine glanders to carnivorous animals.] Arkh. Vet. Nauk *12* (Sect. V): 122–131, 1882.

272. Krajewski, A. A. Die irritativ-nervöse Form der Hundestaupe. Deut. Z. Thiermed. *13*: 324–340, 1887.

273. Krakht-Paleev, P. N. Otchet o zagranichnoi komandirovke. [Report of an official trip abroad.] Sbor. Trud. Kharkov. Vet. Inst. *11*: 39–54, 1912.

274. Krakht-Paleev, P. N. Patoloho-anatomichnyi kabinet. [Department of pathologic anatomy.] Zbirnik. Prats. Kharkiv. Vet. Inst. *15*(1): 41–46, 1929.

275. Krakht-Paleev, P. N. Osnovy Patolohichnoi Anatomii Sviiskikh Tvaryin i Ptakhiv. [Fundamentals of Pathologic Anatomy of Farm Animals and Birds.] Vol. 1, Kharkov, Derzhsilgospvidav, 1932; vol. 2, 1933.

276. Krakht-Paleev, P. N. Aktinomikoz u Cheloveka i Zhivotnykh. [Actinomycosis in Man and Animals.] Moscow, Medgiz, 1937.

277. Krapivner, L. M. Vydayuschiisya uchebnyi N. N. Mari. [Honored teacher N. N. Mari.] Veterinariya *39*(3): 84–86, 1962.

278. Krapivner, L. M. Professor N. N. Mari—Dostopamyatnyi Pitomets Kazanskogo Veterinarnogo Instituta. [Professor N. N. Mari—A memorable alumnus of the KVI] Uchen. Zap. Kazan. Vet. Inst. *90*: 189–197, 1964.

279. Krasnoperov, N. P. Patologo-anatomicheskaya kartina i gistologicheskie izmeneniya v tkanyakh, parazhennyikh Onchocerca cervicalis. [Pathologic-anatomic picture and histologic changes in tissues affected by *Onchocerca cervicalis*.] Trudy Kirov. Zoovet. Inst. *3*(2-3): 3–17, 1938.

280. Krause, A. Die Uebertragung des Milzbrandes von Thieren auf Menschen. Deutsche Klinik *8*: 253–254, 1856.

281. Kravchenko, G. O. Periodychni Vydannya URSR 1918–1950. [Periodicals Published in the Ukrainian Soviet Socialist Republic, 1918–1950.] Kharkov, Knyzhkovoye Palaty URSR, 1956.

282. Krylow, W., and W. Favr: Ueber die Trichinose in Russland. Deutsch Z. Thiermed. *2*: 320–331, 1876.

283. Kucherenko, P. Novy shlyakhi v patolohiye. [New pathways in pathology.] Zapiski Kiiv. Vet.-Zootekh. Inst. *3*: 136–139, 1925.

284. Kucherenko, P. O. Patolohichna Anatomiya. [Pathological anatomy.] Kiev, Derzhmedvidav, 1936.

285. Küchenmeistei, F., and F. A. Zürn. Die Parasiten des Menschen, pp. 24–30. 2d ed. Leipzig, Ambrosius Abel, 1878.

286. Kulbin, N. Ravich, Iosif Ippolitovich. Russkii Biograficheskii Slovar *15*: 365–369, St. Petersburg, Tipografiya Imperatorskoi Akademii Nauk, 1910.

287. Kulbin, N. Rudnev, Mikhail Matvievich. Russki Biograficheskii Slovar *17*: 418–423, Petrograd, Tipografiya Akts. O-va. "Kadima" Vas. Ostr., 1918.

288. Kuznetsov, G. S. Leningradskomu Veterinarnomu Institutu 50 let. [Fifty years of Leningrad Veterinary Institute.] Veterinariya *46*(8): 5–8, 1969.

289. Laas, A. Prof. Nikolai Ball†. Eesti Loomaarstlik Ringvaade *7*: 95–96, 1931.

290. Landa, N. V. K voprosu ob okostenemim serdtsa u loshadi. [The problem of ossification of the heart in horses.] Arkh. Vet. Nauk. *44*: 1333–1362, 1914.

291. Landa, N. V. Smeshchenie zheludka, selezenki, salnika, chasti 12-tiperstnoi kishki i podzheludochnoi zhelezy v grudnuyu polost u koshki. [Displacement of the stomach, spleen, omentum, part of the

duodenum, and subgastric glands into the thoracic cavity of the cat.] Trudy Gosud. Inst. Eksp. Vet. *2*: 59–63, 1924.

292. Landa, N. Zur Histologie parasitärer Bauchfellveränderungen bei Pferden. Zeitschr. Infektkr. Haustiere *29*: 49–58, 1926.

293. Laya, F., and Vau. Naibolee vydayushchiesya issledovaniya v Tartuskom (byvshei Yurevskom) Veterinarnom Institute. [The most prominent scientific research work at the Tartu (formerly Yuryev) Veterinary Institute.] Sborn. Nauch. Trudov Estonskoi Selskokhoz. Akad. *4*: 86–91, 1958.

294. Lepeshinskaya, O. Die neue Theorie von der Abstammung und der Entwicklung der Zellen aus der lebendigen Materie. Zschr. ärztl. Fortbldg. *45*: 339–342, 1951.

295. Lerner, I. M. Dialectical materialism and Soviet science. Quart. Rev. Biol. *47*: 313–316, 1972.

296. Levitsky, G. V. Biograficheskii Slovar Professorov i Prepodavatelei Imperatorskago, Byvshago Derptskago Universiteta 1802–1902. [Biographical Dictionary of the Professors and Instructors of the Imperial former Dorpat University 1802–1902.] Yurev, Tipografiya K. Mattisen, vol. 2, 1903. (Professor Deutsch, pp. 55–56 and p. 315, Professor Krause, pp. 126–127 and p. 318.)

297. Lindtrop, G. F. Razdelenniya selezenki plotoyadnykh. [Divided spleens in carnivores.] Zhur. Nauch. Prakt. Vet. Med. *7*: 32–73, 1913.

298. Lipnik, I. A. K voprosu o fragmentatsii miokarda u loshadei. [On fragmentation of the myocardium in horses.] Izvest. Don. Vet. Inst. *1*(1): 1–16, 1919.

299. Lisovetskii, V. S. et al. Pavlo Oleksandrovich Kucherenko. Radyanska Med. *1*: 21–22, 1936.

300. Lisovskii, N. M. Russkaya Periodicheskaya Pechat, 1703–1900 gg., p. 112. [Russian Periodical Publications, 1703–1900.] Petrograd, Tipografiya G. A. Shumakher and B. D. Bruker, 1915.

301. Liubarskii, A. Pamyati bolshogo uchenogo. [In memory of a great scientist.] Okhotnik i Rybak Sibiri 7(4): 50, 1931. (Obituary of Professor S. A. Gruyner.)

302. Lockhart, R. H. B. British Agent, p. 98. New York, Putnam, 1933.

303. Lockhart, R. B.: My Europe, p. 45. London, Putnam, 1952.

304. London, I. D. De-Stalinization in Soviet physiology. Science *138*: 16–17, 1962.

305. Long, E. R. A History of Pathology, pp. 101, 125, and 128. New York, Dover, 1964.

306. Longworth, P. The Cossacks, pp. 298–303. New York, Holt, Rinehart and Winston, 1969.

307. Lubarsch, O. Ein bewegtes Gelehrtenleben, pp. 491, 497. Berlin, Springer, 1931.

308. Lukashov, I. I. Kharkovskii Veterinarnyi Institut k XXXII godovshche Oktyabrskoi revolyutsii. [The KVI 32 years after the October Revolution.] Trudy Kharkov. Vet. Inst. *20*: 3–7, 1950.

309. Lvov, V. M. Leningradskomu Institutu Usovershenstvovaniya Veterinarnykh Vrachei 25 let. [Twenty five years of the Leningrad Postgraduate Veterinary Institute.] Veterinariya *33*(5): 91–93, 1956.

310. McFadyean, J. The lesions of contagious pleuro-pneumonia. The Veterinarian *65*: 80–95, 1892. (See p. 94.)

311. McGilvray, C. D. Glanders. Encyclopaedia Brittanica *10*: 391–392, 1960.

312. Mæhl, C. Brudstykker af Forhandlingerne ved den 2. russiske Veterinærkongres i Moskov d. 3.–12. Jan. 1910. [Report on deliberations at the second Russian Veterinary Congress in Moscow, 3–12 Jan. 1910). Maanedskr. Dyrlæg. *22*: 118–134; 147–155, 180–187, 1910.

313. Mæhl, K. Indtryk fra den russiske Dyrlægekongres i Charkow. [Impressions of the Russian Veterinary Congress in Kharkov.] Maanedskr. Dyrlæg. *26*: 179–190, 1914.

314. Magda, I. I. Rol Kharkovskogo Veterinarnogo Institua v razvitii klinicheskoi veterinarii. [The role of the Kharkov Veterinary Institute in the development of clinical veterinary medicine.] Sborn. Rabot Kharkov. Vet. Inst. 22: 39–49, 1954.

314a. Magda, I., and V. Ustimenko. Znachenie oftalmoskopii v diagnostike boleznei zhivotnykh. [The significance of ophthalmoscopy in diagnosis of animal diseases.] Vet. Dilo *8*(4): 36–46, 1930.

315. Magoun, H. W., L. Darling, and M. A. B. Brazier. Russian contributions to an understanding of the central nervous system and behavior—A pictorial survey, pp. 23–100, in Brazier, M. A. B., ed. The Central Nervous System and Behavior. New York, Josiah Macy Foundation, 1959. (See page 62.)

316. Makhulko-Gorbatsevich, G. Ukrainskoe Obshchestvo Patologov. [Ukrainian Society of Pathologists.] Vrachebnoe Delo *11*: 993, 1928.

317, Malitskii, S. A. Redkii yubilei. 10-letie prebyvaniya K. H. Bolya na postu rektora. [An unusual jubilee. Ten years of K. H. Bohl in the post of rector.] Uchen. Zap. Kazan. Vet. Inst. *38*(2): 314, 1929.

318. Mari, N. N. K voprosu o borbe s chumnoi epizootiei. [The question of the struggle against epizootic rinderpest.] Uchen. Zap. Kazan. Vet. Inst. 2: 319–336, 1885.

319. Mari, N. N. Rol sistemy ubivaniya i estestvennago immuniteta v borbe s chumnymi epizootiyami. [The role of the reticuloendothelial system in natural immunity in the fight against epizootic rinderpest.] Uchen. Zap. Kazan. Vet. Inst. *3*: 164–187, 1886.

320. Mari, N. N. Kazuistika skotoboini. [Abattoir case reports.] Vet. Vestnik *5*(Sect. 3): 55–61, 1886.

321. Mari, N. N. Povtornaya epizootiya anthraxa. [A recurrent outbreak of anthrax.] Vet. Vestnik *5*(Sect. 5): 232-240, 1886.

322. Mari, N. N. O znachenii trupnykh yavlenii pri sudebno-veterinarnom vskrytii. [The significance of putrefactive phenomena in the veterinary-forensic autopsy.] Uchen. Zap. Kazan. Vet. Inst. *5*: 142-162; 199-227, 1888.

323. Mari, N. N. Oftalmoskopiya i ee primenenie v veterinarnoi meditsine. [Ophthalmoscopy and its application in veterinary medicine.] Uchen. Zap. Kazan. Vet. Inst. *5*: 257-305; 345-391 + color plate, 1888.

324. Mari, N. N. Keratitis traumatica u loshadi. [Traumatic keratitis in the horse.] Arkh. Vet. Nauk *19*(Sect. III): 90-95, 1889.

325. Mari, N. N. K kazuistike blennorroinago konyunktivita u zhivotnykh. [Case reports of blennorhea and conjunctivitis in animals.] Uchen. Zap. Kazan. Vet. Inst. *6*: 205-214, 1889.

326. Mari, N. N. Materialy k ucheniyu ob aktinomikoze. [Contribution to the study of actinomycosis.] Uchen. Zap. Kazan. Vet. Inst. *7*: 157-179; 255-284; 294-369; 371-398, 1890.

327. Mari, N. N. Ueber die Lippenaktinomykose. Cbl. Bakt. *12*: 854-855, 1892.

328. Mari, N. N. Etyudy po obshchei etiologii. [The study of general etiology.] Arkh. Vet. Nauk *25*(Sect. II): 35-43; 79-89; 109-115; 161-175, 1895.

329. Mari, N. N. Louis Pasteur. (A biographical article, bound with) Arkh. Vet. Nauk *25*: separate pages 1-10, 1895.

330. Mari, N. N. Osnovy Patologo-anatomicheskoi Diagnostike. [Fundamentals of Pathologic-Anatomic Diagnosis for Veterinarians.] Vol. I. [The Outer Inspection of the Cadaver.] 46 drawings. Warsaw, the author, 1896. Vol. II, Warsaw, 1898. 2d ed., Warsaw, the author, 1900. 3d ed., St. Petersburg, Izd. Prakt. Vet., 1906; 4th ed., 1913.

331. Mari, N. N. K voprosu bakteriologie v chumy sobak. [On the bacteriology of canine distemper.] Vet. Obozrenie *1*: 663-666, 1899.

332. Mari, N. N. K voprosu ob izsledovanii spermy po sposobu Florence'a. [On the question of investigation of sperm by the Florence reaction.] Russkii Arkhiv Patol., Klin. Med. i Bakt. *10*: 63-79 + 1 plate, 1900.

333. Mari, N. N. Chetyre sluchaya postoronnikh vklyuchenii vnutr kurinykh yaits. [Four cases of foreign body in hen eggs.] Russkii Arkhiv Patol., Klin. Med. i Bakt. *9*: 283-288, 1900.

334. Mari, N. N. Varshavskii Veterinarnyi Institut. Arkh. Vet. Nauk *31*: 171-190, 1901.

335. Mari, N. N. Sovremennoe sostoyanie voprosa o sootnoshenii bugorchatki cheloveka i zhivotnykh. [Contemporary status of the question

of correlation of tuberculosis in man and animals.] Russkii Vrach *1*: 994–997, 1057–1060, 1902.

336. Mari, N. N. O zadachakh sravitelnoi patologii. [On the tasks of comparative pathology.] Russkii Vrach *1*: 1517–1521, 1902.

337. Mari, N. N. O edinstve bugorchatki cheloveka i zhivotnykh. [On the unity of tuberculosis in man and animals.] Izvest. Imperat. Voenno-Med. Akad. *8*: 1–25, 1903.

338. Mari, N. N. Osnovy Patologicheskoi Anatomii Domashnikh Zhivotnykh. 3d ed. St. Petersburg, Izd. Prakt. Vet., 1906. (This is the 3d edition of item #330, with a change of title.)

339. Mari, N. N. Myasovedenie. Rukovodstvo po Osmotru Myasa dlya Vrachei i Studentov. [Meat Hygiene. Guidelines for Meat Inspection for Physicians and Students.] St. Petersburg, 1913; 2d (posthumous) ed., edited by P. N. Andreev. Moscow, Novaya Derevnya, 1929.

340. Mari, N. N. Gorodskaya tsentralnaya skotoboinya v g. Lvov (Galitsiya). [The central city stockyards in Lvov (Galicia).] Arkh. Vet. Nauk. *45*: 908–924, 1915.

341. Mari, N. N. Etyudi po obshchei patologii. [The study of general pathology.] Izvest. Don. Vet. Inst. *1*(1): 1–4, 1919; 2(1): 21–24, 1920.

342. Matsulevich, N. Izmeneniya spinnago mozga pri chume sobak. [Changes in the spinal cord in canine distemper.] Arkh. Vet. Nauk *14*(Sect. III): 1–27, 1884.

343. Maurer, F. D., T. C. Jones, B. Easterday, and D. DeTray. The pathology of rinderpest. Proc. 92d Ann. Meeting Amer. Vet. Med. Assn., 201–211, 1955.

343a. Melegari, V. The World's Great Regiments, p. 134. London, Spring Books, 1972.

344. Melnikow-Raswedenkow, N. Studien über den Echinococcus alveolaris. Beitr. path. Anat. *22*: Suppl. 4, 1–295, 1901.

345. Melnikov-Razvedenkov, N. Pamyati Nikolaya Matveevicha Lyubimova. [Obituary of N. M. Lyubimov.] Kharkov. Med. Zhur. *1*: 349–352, 1906.

346. Melnikov-Razvedenkov, N. O. znachenii Kievskogo sezda patologov. [On the significance of the Kiev conference of pathologists.] Vrachebnoe Delo *10*: 1582, 1927.

347. Melnikov-Razvedenkov, N. F. Ukrainskoe Obshchestvo Patologov. 19-oe zasedanie 12 Maya 1927 i. bylo posvyashcheno Prof. A. P. Ostapenko po sluchaya 50-letiya ego nauchnoi i obshchestvennoi deyatelnosti. [Ukrainian Society of Pathologists. 19th meeting, May 12, 1927, dedicated to Professor A. P. Ostapenko on the occasion of 50 years of scientific and public activity.] Vrachebnoe Delo *11*: 163, 1928.

348. Melnikov-Razvedenkov, N. F. trudy pervogo vsesoyuznogo sezda patologov (Pamyati R. Virkhova) v Kieve 15-20 Sentyabrya 1927 g. [Proceedings of the First All-Union Congress of Pathologists (in Memory of R. Virchow) in Kiev, September 15-20, 1927.] Kharkov, Nauchnaya Mysl, 1929. 338 pp. (Pages 271-316 contain abstracts of the Second Russian Congress of Pathologists in Moscow, September 13-18, 1925, edited by A. I. Abrikosov.)
349. Melnikov-Razvedenkov, M. F. Spohadi pro Pavla Oleksandrovich Kucherenka. [In memory of P. O. Kucherenko.] Radyanska Med. *1*: 23-24, 1936.
350. Melvin, A. D. Twenty-Third Annual Report of the Bureau of Animal Industry for the Year 1906, pp. 97-98. Washington, Government Printing Office, 1908.
351. Metchnikoff, Olga. Life of Elie Metchnikoff, 1845-1916, p. 99. London, Constable, 1921.
352. Metelkin, A. I. Iz istorii tuberkulina i malleina. [The history of tuberculin and mallein.] Zhur. Mikrob. Epidem. Immun. (11): 69-76, 1951.
353. Miessner, H. Wissenschaft und Wirtschaft in der Sowjet-Union. Deut. tierärztl. Wschr. *41*: 225-234; 242-251, 1933. (See p. 233.)
354. Millak, K. Historia prasy weterynaryjnej w Polsce. [History of the veterinary press in Poland.] Medycyna Wet. *15*: 394-412, 1959.
355. Millak, K. Słownik Polskich Lekarzy Weterynaryjnych 1394-1918. [Dictionary of Polish Veterinarians 1394-1918.] Pp. 63-64. Lublin, 1963.
356. Millak, K. Uczelnia Weterynaryjna w Warszawie 1840-1965. [The Veterinary Institute in Warsaw.] Warsaw, Państwowe Wydawnictwo Relnicze i Leśne, 1965.
357. Miller, J. Ernst Ziegler. Jour. Path. Bact. 77: 378-382, 1906.
358. Minett, F. C. Glanders. Chapter 8, pp. 296-309 in Infectious Diseases of Animals, A. W. Stableforth and I. A. Galloway, eds. New York, Academic Press, 1959.
359. Ministry of Agriculture, Fisheries and Food. Animal Health, a Centenary, 1865-1965. London, Her Majesty's Stationery Office, 1965.
360. Moldawsky, A. Ein Brief aus Südrussland. Berl. tierärztl. Wschr. *40*: 543, 1924.
361. Monas, S. The political police. Pp. 189-190 in C. E. Black, ed., The Transformation of Russian Society. Cambridge, Harvard University Press, 1967.
362. Moore, V. A. Annual Report of the State Veterinary College for 1916-1917, p. 24. Albany, N.Y., 1918.
363. Müller. R. 80 Jahre Seuchenbakteriologie. Zbl. Bakt. (Abt. 1, Orig.) *115*: 1-17, 1929.
364. Nepryakhin, G. G. 100 Let kafedry patologicheskoi anatomii

Kazanskogo Gosudarstvennogo Ordena Trudovogo Krasnogo Znameni meditsinskogo Instituta im. S. V. Kurashova (1865–1965). [One hundred years of the chair of pathologic anatomy at the Kazan State S. V. Kurashov Medical Institute, 1865–1965.] Arkh. Patol. *28*(12): 56–60, 1966.

365. Nepryakhin, G. G. Kratkaya istoriya Kafedry patologicheskoi anatomii Kazanskogo Gosudarstvennogo Ordena Trudovogo Krasnogo Znameni meditsinskogo Instituta im. S. V. Kurashova. [History of the chair of pathologic anatomy of the Kazan S. V. Kurashov Medical Institute.] Trudy Kazan. Gos. Med. Inst. *23*: 3–13, 1967.
366. Neumann, L.-G. Biographies Vétérinaires, pp. 296–298. Paris, Asselin et Houzeau, 1896.
367. Nevodoff, A.-P. Des vaccinations anticharbonneuses en masse, d'après le procédé de Besredka. Compt. Rend. Soc. Biol. *94*: 170–171, 1926.
368. Nieberle, K. Vergleichende pathologische Anatomie und Pathogenese des Milzbrandes bei Tieren und beim Menschen. Ergebn. allg. Path. *21*: 611–685, 1926.
369. Nieberle, K. Ernst Joest†. Verh. Deutsche Gesellsch. Path. *22*: 316–317, 1927.
370. Nocard, E. Compte Rendu des Séances du Ve Congrès International de Médecine Vétérinaire Tenu à Paris du 2 au 8 Septembre 1889, pp. 436–437. Paris, Asselin et Houzeau, 1890.
371. Nöller, W. Bericht über die Reise des Professors Dr. Nöller durch die Sowjetunion. Berlin, 1929. (Unpublished manuscript in possession of Professor Dr. B. Hörning, Berne.)
372. Nosik, A. F. Stoletie Kharkovskogo Veterinarnogo Instituta. [One hundred years of the Kharkov Veterinary Institute.] Sborn. Trud. Kharkov. Vet. Inst. *21*: 3–24, 1952.
373. Osipov, I. P., and D. I. Bagaleya. Fiziko-Matematicheskii Fakultet Kharkovskago Universiteta za perviya sto let ego sushchestvovaniya, 1805–1905. [The Physico-Mathematical Faculty of Kharkov University in the first one hundred years of its existence.] Kharkov, Tipografiya Adolf Darre, 1908.
374. Ostapenko, A. P. K voprosu o proiskhozhdenii gomogennykh mochevykh tsilindrov. [The question of the origin of homogeneous urinary casts.] Arkh. Vet. Nauk *11* (Sect. II): 121–138, 1881.
375. Ostapenko, A. P. Dva sluchaya sarkom u domashnikh zhivotnykh. [Two cases of sarcoma in domestic animals.] Arkh. Vet. Nauk *12* (Sect. III): 291–298, 1882.
376. Ostapenko, A. P. Teratologicheskie materialy. [Teratological materials.] Arkh Vet. Nauk *12* (Sect. II): 1–14, 1882.
377. Ostapenko, A. P. Kratkoe Rukovodstvo k Patologo-Anatomicheskomu Vskrytiyu Trupov Domashnikh Zhivotnykh. [Short Manual on Pathologic-Anatomic Examination of the Cadaver of Domestic

Animals.] Kharkov, Tipo-Litografiya Okruzhnago Shtaba, 1882.

378. Ostapenko, A. P. Sluchai sarkomatoznoi kakheksii sobaki. [A case of sarcomatous cachexia in a dog.] Arkh. Vet. Nauk *13*(Sect. III): 54–60, 1883.

379. Ostapenko, A. P. Patologo-anatomicheskie materialy. [Pathologic-anatomical materials.] Arkh. Vet. Nauk *17*(Sect. III): 1–5; 68–78, 1887.

380. Ostapenko, A. P. Perocephalus aprosopus. [Malformation in a calf.] Arkh. Vet. Nauk *18*(Sect. III): 69–71, 1888.

381. Ostapenko, A. P. Neskolko sluchaev novoobrazovanii i kamen v mochevom puzyre loshadi. [Some cases of neoplasms and stones in the urinary bladder of horses.] 1890. (Original not seen, cited by Pinus,[417] p. 460.)

382. Ostapenko, A. P. Rukovodstvo k Veterinarnomu Akusherstvu. 576 pp. Kharkov, Tipografiya V. S. Biryukov, 1891. (Russian translation from French of St. Cyr and Violet's Veterinary Obstetrics.)

383. Ostapenko, A. P. Rukovodstvo k Klinicheskim Metodam Izsledovaniya dlya Veterinarnykh Vrachei i Studentov. 300 pp. Kharkov, Tipografiya A. N. Gusev, 1892. (Russian translation from German of Friedberger and Froehner's Methods of Clinical Diagnosis for Veterinarians and Students.)

384. Ostapenko, A. P. Rukovodstvo k Patologicheskoi Anatomii i Gistologii Domashnikh Zhivotnykh. [Manual of Pathologic Anatomy and Histology of Domestic Animals.] Kharkov, N. B. Petrov, 1901.

385. Ostapenko, A. P. Kratkii istoricheskii ocherk razvitiya veterinarnoi meditsiny. [Brief historical sketch of the evolution of veterinary medicine.] Paper given at Vserossiiskago Sezda Vet. Vrachei [First All-Russian Convention of Veterinarians], St. Petersburg, 1903. (Not published in the proceedings, reference no. 465.)

386. Ostapenko, A. P. Kratkii obzor deyatelnosti Kharkovskikh gorodskikh boen s 1908 po 1912 god vklyuchitelno. [A brief sketch of the activities at the Kharkov City abattoir between the years 1908 to 1912 inclusive.] Arkh. Vet. Nauk *42*: 1588–1612, 1912.

387. Ostapenko, A. P. Patologo-anatomicheskie materialy muzeya Kharkovskikh gorodskikh boen. [Pathologic-anatomic material from the museum of the Kharkov city abattoir.] Arkh. Vet. Nauk *45*: 601–621, 1915.

388. Ostapenko, A. P. Materialy k veterinarnoi ekspertize. [Veterinary-sanitary case reports.] Arka. Vet. Nauk *45*: 988–1007, 1915.

389. Ostapenko, A. P. Patologoanatomicheskie materialy muzeya Kharkovskikh gorodskikh boen. [Pathologic case reports from the museum of the Kharkov city abbatoir.] Arkh. Vet. Nauk *46*: 915–928, 1916.

390. Parry, A. The Russian Scientist, pp. 12–13. New York, Macmillan, 1973.

391. Pashin, Helene. Hoover Institution Library, Stanford University, personal communication, December 1975.
392. Patzevich, B. L., and K. I. Tsvetkov. Sravnitelnye opyty vaktsinatsii morskikh svinok protiv sibirskoi yazvy. [Comparative studies of vaccination of guinea pigs against anthrax.] Prakt. Vet. Kon. *2*(11/12): 16–22, 1925. (Abstract in Jahresb. Vet. Med. *46*: 966, 1926.)
393. Pavlovski, P. Iz istorii periodicheskoi pechati po veterinarii [From the history of the periodical press in veterinary medicine.] Veterinariya *41*(5): 116–118, 1964.
394. Pavlovskii, E. N. et al. Nekrolog Karl Genrikovich Bohl. Uchen. Zap. Kazan. Vet. Inst. *76*: 199–201, 1959.
395. Pearlstien, E. W. Revolution in Russia, pp. 272, 278. New York, Viking Press, 1967.
396. Peebsen, E. Istoricheskie dannye po issledovaniyu vozbuditelya sibirskoi yazvy Professorom byvshei Tartuskoi Veterinarnoi Shkoly F. Brauelem. [Historical data on research into the cause of anthrax by the professor of the Tartu Veterinary School, F. Brauell.] Sborn. Nauch. Trudov Estonskoi Selskokhoz. Akad. *4*: 10–17, 1958.
397. Penskii, E. "Audiatur et altera pars." [Let's also listen to the other party.] Arkh. Vet. Nauk *18*(Sect. VI): 130–132, 1888.
398. Perroncito, E. Ueber das epizootische Typhoid der Hühner. Arch. Tierheilk. *5*: 22–51, 1879.
399. Petropavlovskii, N. I. Patologicheskii materialy patologo-anatomicheskago kabineta Kharkovskago Veterinarnago Instituta. [Pathological material in the pathology department of the KVI] Arkh. Vet. Nauk *28*(Sect. II): 312–325, 1898.
400. Petropavlovskii, N. I. Endocarditis ulcerosa u sobaki. [Ulcerative endocarditis in a dog.] Arkh. Vet. Nauk 28 (Sect. II): 393, 1898.
401. Petropavlovskii, N. I. Patologo-anatomicheskie materialy. Arkh. Vet. Nauk *28*(Sect. II): 107–122, 1898.
402. Petropavlovskii, N. I. K voprosu ob anomaliyakh nekotorykh organov u domashnikh zhivotnykh. [The problem of anomalies in some of the organs of domestic animals.] Arkh. Vet. Nauk *35*(Sect. II): 119–136, 1905.
403. Petropavlovskii, N. I. K voprosu o bronkhoektaziyakh u rog. skota. [The problem of bronchiectasis in cattle.] Arkh. Vet. Nauk *36*(Sect. I): 14–19, 1906.
404. Petrov, A. M. Zur pathologischen Histologie der distomatösen Lebercirrhose des Rindes. Centralbl. allg. Path. *21*: 667, 1910.
405. Petrov, A. M. Ob otnoshenii distomatoznogo tsiroza pecheni rogatogo skota k pechenochnym tsirozam cheloveka. [On the relationship between distomal cirrhosis of the liver in cattle and hepatic cirrhosis in man.] Kharkov. Med. Zhur. *11*: 263–276, 1911.
406. Petrov, A. M. Ob izmeneniyakh 12-perstnoi kishki u loshadei

(duodenitis larvaris) pri vnedrenii lichinok osobago vida ovoda. [On the alterations in the duodenum of the horse in the presence of bot-fly larvae.] Kharkov. Med. Zhur. *11*: 277-285, 1911.

407. Petrov, A. M. K patologicheskoi anatomii distomatoza cheloveka i domashnikh zhivotnykh. [On the pathologic anatomy of distomiasis in man and in domestic animals.] Sborn. Trud. Kharkov. Vet. Inst. *11*: 27-95, 1912.

408. Petrov, A. M. Tkaneviya izmeneniya pecheni rogatogo skota pri *Bilharzia haematobia* Cobb. [Tissue alterations in the liver of cattle from *Bilharzia haematobia*.] Vet. Obozrenie *14*: 413-416, 1912.

409. Petrov, A. M. Morfologicheskoe ponimanie diagnosticheskikh reaktsii na sap po patologo-anatomicheskim dannym. [Morphologic aspects of the glanders diagnostic reaction from pathologic anatomic information.] Vet. Delo *3*(14/15): 89-92, 1925.

410. Petrov, A. M. Novye eksperimentalnye dannye po regeneratsii tkanei v prakticheskom primenenii pri zazhivlenii pan. [New experimental data on regeneration of tissue and its practical application to healing.] Vet. Delo *4*(2-3): 28-31, 1926.

410a. Petrov A. M. Tanatologiya i patolgicheskaya anatomii. [Thanatology and pathologic anatomy] Vet. Delo 5(1): 44-47, 1927.

411. Petrov, A. M. 50-Letie nauchnoi i obshchestvennoi deyatelnosti Prof. Patolog. Anatomii Khark. Vet. I-ta A. P. Ostapenko. [50 years of scientific and public activity of professor of pathologic anatomy in the Kharkov Veterinary Institute A. P. Ostapenko.] Vrachebnoe Delo *11*: 163, 1928.

412. Petrov, A. M., and B. M. Gurvich. O lipoidakh v sapnykh uzelkakh. [On lipoid in glanders nodules.] Prakt. Vet. Kon. *3*(10); 1-12; (11):33-36, 1926.

413. Petrow, A. M. and B. M. Gurwitsch. Die Oxydasereaktion in den Rotzknötchen bei Pferden. Zeitschr. Infektkr. Haustiere *31*: 290-294, 1927.

414. Petrov, N. P. Bibliograficheskii Ukazatel Russkikh Dissertatsii po Meditsine i Veterinarii, 1860-1892. [Bibliographic Index of Russian Dissertations in Medicine and Veterinary Medicine, 1860-1892.] St. Petersburg, Tipografiya Departmenta Udelov, 1892.

415. Pinus, A. Zur Frage des Vorkommens von Lipoiden in Rotzknötchen der Pferdelunge. Zeitschr. Infektkr. Haustiere *30*: 1-7, 1927.

416. Pinus, A. Dostizheniya sovetskikh uchenykh v oblasti patologicheskoi anatomii zhivotnykh. [Achievements of Soviet scholars in the realm of pathologic anatomy of animals.] Veterinariya *24*(11): 34-38, 1947.

417. Pinus, A. A. K istorii veterinarnoy patologicheskoy anatomii. Iz istorii razvitiya veterinarnoy patologicheskoy anatomii v dorevolutsionnoy

Rossii. [The history of veterinary pathological anatomy. History of development of veterinary pathological anatomy in prerevolutionary Russia.] Trudy 2d Konf. Pat. Selskokhoz. Zhivot. pp. 455–463, 1961.

418. Pinus, A. and N. Romanov. Prof. N. D. Ball (1872–1930). Nekrolog. Praktichesk. Vet. 7(11–12): 1003–1004, 1930.
419. Plushch, V. Materialy do Istoriy Ukrainskoi Meditsiny. [Contributions to the History of Ukrainian Medicine.] Vol. 1, pp. 109 and 158. New York-Munich, Ukrainian Medical Association, 1975.
420. Podgaez, H. The past, present and future of veterinary education and of the profession in Russia. Vet. J. *29*: 309–314, 1922.
421. Podgaez, H. Glanders in man from eating infected horseflesh. Vet. J. *29*: 430–431, 1922.
422. Podolskii, N. S., and N. F. Poryvaev. Nikolai Matveevich Lyubimov kak uchenyi i obshchestvennyi deyatel. K 50-letiyu so dnya smerti. [N. M. Lyubimov, studies of his educational and public activities. On the 50th anniversary of his death.] Arkh. Patol. *18*(5): 99–100, 1956.
423. Polovinkin, F. P. K patologii epithelioma contagiosum golubei. [On the pathology of epithelioma contagiosum of pigeons.] Uchen. Zap. Kazan. Vet. Inst. *17*: 247–292, 1900.
424. Polowinkin, P. Beitrag zur pathologischen Anatomie der Taubenpocken. Arch. Tierheilk. 27: 86–109, 1901.
425. Ponirovskii, N. G. Voprosy i perspektivy veterinarnogo obrazovaniya. [Problems and perspectives in veterinary education.] Vet. Dilo (2–3): 64–74, 1926.
426. Ponirovskii, N. G. Novy etap v oblasti veterinarnogo obrazovaniya na Ukraine. [A new stage in the field of veterinary education in Ukraine.] Vet. Dilo (11–12): 1–18, 1926.
427. Ponirovskii, M. G. [N. G.] Pratsya fakulteskikh orhaniv Kharkovskoho Veterinarnoho Instituta za chas isnuvannya U.S.S.R. [Work of the faculties of the Kharkov Veterinary Institute at the time of founding of the Ukrainian Soviet Socialist Republic.] Zbirnik Prats Kharkiv. Vet. Inst. *15*: 5–25, 1929. (Ponirovskii's given name begins with an N when written in Russian but with an M in Ukrainian.)
428. Pustovar, Ya. P. Korotkyi Kurs Zahalnoyi Patolohichnoyi Anatomiyi Silskohospodarskikh Tvaryn i Ptytsi. [Short Course of Pathologic Anatomy of Farm Animals and Birds.] Kharkiv, Derzhsilhospvidav, 1935.
429. Raevskii, A. O. stroenii i roste kopyt domashnikh zhivotnykh. [On the Structure and Growth of the Hoof in Domestic Animals.] M.V.Sc. dissertation, Military-Medical Academy, St. Petersburg, 1872.
430. Raevskii, A. A. Patologicheskaya anatomiya domashnikh zhivotnykh. [Pathologic anatomy of domestic animals.] Arkh. Vet. Nauk 7(Sect.

III): 73–125; 209–257; 413–460, 1877; *8*(Sect. III): 78–134; 191–238; 370–418, 1878.

431. Raevskii, A. A.: Rukovodstvo k Izucheniyu Patologicheskoi Anatomii i Gistologii Domashnikh Zhivotnykh dlya Veterinarnykh Vrachei i Studentov. [Manual for the Study of Pathologic Anatomy and Histology of Domestic Animals for Veterinary Doctors and Students.] St. Petersburg, Tipografiya Yakov Trei, 1879.

432. Raevskii, A. A. Kratkii istoricheskii ocherk 50-letiya Kharkovskago Veterinarnago Instituta. (A brief historical sketch of 50 years of the Kharkov Veterinary Institute). Sborn. Trud. Kharkov. Vet. Inst. *10*(5/6): 54–86, 1912.

433. Raikov, B. E. Karl Ernest von Baer, 1792–1876. Sein Leben und sein Werk. Acta Historica Leopoldina, No. 5, p. 356, 1968.

434. Rammul, A. Geschichte der Universität Dorpat-Jurjeff. Russ. med. Rundschau *1*: 378–382; 540–549, 1902.

435. Rawitsch, J. Etwas über die Scrophel- und Tuberkelkrankheiten der Hausthiere. Mag. ges. Thierheilk. *27*: 337–363, 1861.

436. Ravich, J. Einige Worte über die Pathogenese der Rotz- und Wurmkrankheit des Pferdes. Virchows Arch. *23*: 33–48, 1862.

437. Ravitsch, J. Ueber den feinern Bau und das Wachsthum des Hufhorns. Mag. ges. Thierheilk. *28*: 444–479, 1862.

438. Ravitsch, J. Ueber das Vorkommen von quergestreifter Muskelfasern in Oesophagus der Hausthiere. Virchows Arch. *27*: 413, 1863.

439. Ravitsch, J. Neue Untersuchungen über die pathologische Anatomie der Rinderpest. Mag. ges. Thierheilk. *29*: 313–356, 1863. (Also published as a book with this title, Berlin, August Hirschwald, 1864.)

440. Ravitsch, J. Zur Lehre von der putriden Infection und deren Beziehung zum sogennanten Milzbrande. 118 pp. Berlin, August Hirschwald, 1872.

441. Renault, Mary. History in fiction. Times Lit. Suppl., pp. 315–316, March 23, 1973.

442. Revo, M. I. I. Mechnikov. Zapiski Kiiv. Vet.-Zootekh. Inst. *4*: 279–285, 1926.

443. Robinson, V. Pathfinders in Medicine, p. 764. New York, Medical Life Press, 1929.

444. Röll, M. F. Amtlicher Bericht über den zweiten internationalen Congress von Thierärzten zu Wien am 21.–27. August 1865, pp. 150–157. Wien, W. Braumüller, 1865.

445. Röll, M. F. Die Tierseuchen, p. 124. Vienna, W. Braumüller, 1881.

446. Romanovich, M. I. I. Shukevich. Vet. Vestnik *1*(2): 100–102, 1922.

447. Rubeli, T. O. Die Tierärztliche Lehranstalt zu Bern, p. 178. Bern, Druck der Haller'schen Buchdruckerei, 1906.

448. Rudnev, M. M. O trikinakh v Rossii. [On trichinosis in Russia.] Med.

Vestnik (St. Petersburg) *6*: 193–196; 204–206; 213–215; 225–227; 237–240, 1866.
449. Rudnev, M. K ucheniyu o sobachem beshenstve. Rabies canina. Tollwuth. Wasserscheu. [On canine rabies.] Zhur. Norm. Patol. Gistol. Farmakol. i Klin. Med. (St. Petersburg) *3*: 201–204, 1871.
450. Rudnev, M. M. Trikhiny v S.-Peterburge, 1875. (Cited by Shumakovich[548].)
451. Rudnew. Zur pathologischen Anatomie der Wuthkrankheit der Hunde. Centralb. med. Wissensch. *9*: 321–322, 1871.
452. Rukhlyadev, N. Dostizheniya Professora Karla Henrikovicha Bola, zasluzhennogo deyatelya nauki, d-ra veterinarii. [The achievements of Professor K. H. Bohl, meritorious scientific worker and doctor of veterinary science.] Uchen. Zap. Kazan. Gosud. Zoovet. Inst. *47*: 13–14, 1937.
453. Sacharoff, G. P. Rudolf Virchow und die russische Medizin. Virchows Arch. *235*: 329–378, 1921.
454. Samodelkin, N. I. Otchet o zagranichnoi komandirovke v 1910–1911 godu. [Report on an official trip abroad during the years 1910–1911.] Sborn. Trud. Kharkov. Vet. Inst. *10*(5/6): 1–38, 1912.
455. Samodelkin, N. I. Khronicheskii deformiruyushchii artrit chelyustnogo sochleneniya loshadi. [Chronic deforming arthritis of the mandibular joint in the horse.] Sborn. Trud. Kharkov. Vet. Inst. *11*(4): 1–27, 1912. (Also published as separate monograph, Kharkov, Tipograf. A. Darre, 1912.)
456. Samodjelkin, N. I. Arthritis chronica deformans des Kiefergelenks des Pferdes. Mhefte. prakt. Tierheilk. *23*: 367–389, 1912.
457. Samodelkin, N. I. Tridermoma testis loshadi. [Teratoma of the testis in a horse.] Sborn. Trud. Kharkov. Vet. Inst. *13*(5): 1–8 + 6 plates on unnumbered pages, 1916.
458. Sarkisov, A. Kh. Stakhibotriotoksikoz. [Stachbothriotoxicosis.] Pp. 63–109 in Mikotoksikozy [Mycotoxicoses.] Moscow, Gosud. Izd. Selsk. Lit., 1954.
459. Saunders, L. Z. Book review of Handbuch der Virusinfektionen bei Tieren, Jena, Fischer, 1968. Path. Vet. 7: 84–85, 1970.
460. Saunders, L. Z. Some historical aspects of the neuropathology of canine distemper. Schweiz. Arch. Neurol. *112*: 341–352, 1973.
461. Savvaitov, N. P. Materialy dlya Izsliedovaniya S.-Peterburga v Sanitarnom, Zoogigienicheskom i Veterinarno-Statisticheskom Otnosheniyakh. [Research data on St. Petersburg from the sanitary, zoohygienic, and veterinary-statistical aspects.] St. Petersburg, 1897.
462. Savvaitov, N. P. Sluchai srostaniya pereloma predplechya u loshadi. [A case of fracture of the forearm in a horse.] Arkh. Vet. Nauk *31*: 919–922, 1901.
463. Savvaitov, N. P. Karies poyasnichnago pozvonka u loshadi, vyzvavshii paralich. zadnikh nog (patologo-anatomicheskaya zametka). [Caries

of the lumbar vertebrae in a horse, with paralysis of the hind leg–pathologic-anatomic note.] Arkh. Vet. Nauk *31*: 923–926, 1901.

464. Savvaitov, N. P. K kazuistike novoobrazovanii na naruzhnykh pokrovakh konechnostei u loshadi. [Cases of cutaneous neoplasms on the extremities of horses.] Arkh. Vet. Nauk *31*: 1113–1116, 1901.
465. Savvaitov, N. P. Trudy Pervago Vserossiiskago Veterinarnago Sezda v S.-Peterburge. [Proceedings, First All-Russian Veterinary Convention in St. Petersburg.] St. Petersburg, Tipografiya Trenke i Fyusno, 1903.
466. Scheffer, P. Augenzeuge im Staate Lenins, pp. 70, 83, 86, 88. München, R. Piper, 1972.
467. Schmaltz, R. Jubiläum des Veterinär-Instituts zu Dorpat. Berl. tierärztl. Wschr. *14*: 79–81, 1898.
468. Schmaltz, R. Die Wiedereröffnung der tierärztlichen Hochschule in Dorpat. Berl. tierärztl. Wschr. *34*: 387, 1918.
469. Schmaltz, R. Tagesgeschichte. Der Letzte der Pioniere. Berl. tierärztl. Wschr. *36*: 624–628, 1920.
470. Schmaltz, R. Gefährdung des alten Dorpater Veterinär-Institutes. Berl. tierärztl. Wschr. *40*: 229–230, 1924.
471. Schmaltz, R. Fünfzigjähriges Dozentenjubiläum. Berl. tierärztl. Wschr. *48*: 815, 1932.
472. Schütz, W. Die Thierärztliche Hochschule zu Berlin, 1790–1890, pp. 255–256. Berlin, August Hirschwald, 1890.
473. Seifried, O. Theodor Kitt zum 75. Geburtstag. Münch. tierärztl. Wschr. *84*: 495–497, 1933.
474. Semmer, E. Die Schlundmuskeln der Hausthiere. M.V.Sc. dissertation, Dorpat Veterinary Institute, 1865. (Semmer's name appeared as Zemmer in articles published in Russian; however, since he was not a Russian, I have ignored this transliteration and amalgamated all of the references to his published work under the letter S.)
475. Semmer, E. Resultate der Injectionen von Pilzsporen und Pilzhefen in's Blut der Thiere. Virchows Arch. *50*: 158–160, 1870.
476. Semmer, E. Iz Derptskago Veterinarnago Instituta. [From the Dorpat Veterinary Institute.] Arkh. Vet. Nauk *1* (Sect. III): 65–72, 1871.
477. Semmer, E. Vozrazheniya protiv zamiechanii redaktsii na stati... [Objection against the reproof by the editor on the article... (see reference[476])]. Arkh. Vet. Nauk *1* (Sect. V): 173–177, 1871.
478. Semmer, E. Uebertragungsversuche der Perlsucht der Rinder auf Fleischfresser und Pferde. Oesterr. Vierteljschr. wiss. Veterinärk. *36*: 174–180, 1872.
479. Semmer, E. Zur Pathologie des Milzbrandes. Oesterr. Vierteljschr. wiss. Veterinärk. *38*: 21–23, 1872.
480. Semmer, E. Pathologisch-anatomische Mitteilungen mit besonderer

Berücksichtigung der bösartigen Neubildungen der Haustiere. Oesterr. Vierteljschr. wiss. Veterinärk. *40*: 10–23, 1873.

481. Semmer, E. Über die Beziehungen der pathologisch-anatomischen Erscheinungen bei den contagiösen Krankheiten zu den Contagien. Oesterr. Vierteljschr. wiss. Veterinärk. *41*: 134–136, 1874.
482. Semmer, E. Ueber die pathologische Anatomie der Rinderpest. 78 pp. Dorpat, Druck von C. Mattiesen, 1875.
483. Semmer, E. Ueber die Staupe der Hunde. Deutsche Z. Thiermed. *1*: 204–207, 1875.
484. Semmer, E. Ein Beitrag zur Tuberkelfrage. Deutsche Z. Thiermed. *1*: 207–209, 1875.
485. Semmer, E. Ueber die Ursache der Furunkel. Deutsche Z. Thiermed. *1*: 214–215, 1875.
486. Semmer, E. Versuche über die Uebertragbarkeit der Tuberkulose (Perlsucht) der Rinder auf andere Thiere. Deutsche Z. Thiermed. *2*: 209–220, 1876.
487. Semmer, E. Zur pathologischen Anatomie der Wuth. Deutsche Z. Thiermed. *2*: 221–223, 1876.
488. Semmer, E. Über Tuberkulose des Gehirns. Deutsche Z. Thiermed. *2*: 223–224, 1876. (4 cases among 40 autopsies of tuberculous cattle.)
489. Semmer, E. Versuche über die Uebertragbarkeit des Rotzes von Thier auf Thier. Deutsche Z. Thiermed. *2*: 351–354, 1876.
490. Semmer, E. Zur Genesis der septischen Blutzersetzungen. Virchows Arch. *70*: 371–378, 1877.
491. Semmer, E. Zur Frage über die Geniessbarkeit des Fleisches und der Milch perlsüchtiger Rinder. Revue Thierheilk. Thierzucht 1: 17–24, 1878.
492. Semmer, E. Über die Hühnerpest. Deutsche Z. Thiermed. *4*: 244–250, 1878.
493. Semmer, E. Zhiroviya embolii v legkikh. [Fat emboli in the lungs.] Arkh. Vet. Nauk *9*(Sect. III): 1–3, 1879.
494. Semmer, E. Fettembolien in der Lunge in Folge ausgedehnter eitriger Infiltration des Oberschenkels beim Pferde. Deutsche Z. Thiermed. *5*: 213–214, 1879.
495. Semmer, E. Über die Bedeutung der Haustiere für den Nationalreichtum. Baltische Wochenschrift, 1879.
496. Semmer, E. Zur Diagnose des Lungenrotzes. Revue Thierheilk. Thierzucht. *3*: 113–117, 1880.
497. Semmer, E. Tuberculose und Perlsucht. Virchows Arch. *82*: 546–551, 1880.
498. Semmer, E. Sarcomatose bei einem Vorsteherhunde, der an Diabetes insipidus gelitten hatte. Deutsche Z. Thiermed. *6*: 224–225, 1880.
499. Semmer, E. Eine verschluckte Nähnadel als Todesursache bei einem jungen Hunde. Deutsche Z. Thiermed. *6*: 226–228, 1880.

500. Semmer, E. Die Priorität der Entdeckung der Bakterien in der Hühnercholera, dem Milzbrand und der Rinderpest. Virchows Arch. *82*: 549-551, 1880.

501. Semmer, E. Skotovodstvo Rossii sravnitelno s skotovodstvom, Evropy, Ameriki i Avstralii [Cattle husbandry in Russia compared with it in Europe, America, and Australia.] Trudy Imper. Voln. Ekonon. Obshchestva 2: 448-451, 1880.

502. Semmer, E. Tuberculose und Perlsucht. Virchows Arch. *82*: 546-547, 1880; *83*: 555-556, 1881.

503. Semmer, E. Die Rinderpest und das Rinderpest-Contagium. Revue Thierheilk. Thierzucht *4*: 65-71; 83-88; 97-105; 113-122; 129-134; 145-150; 161-168, 1881.

504. Semmer, E. Putride Intoxication und septische Infection, metastatische Abscesse und Pyämie. Virchows Arch. *83*: 99-116, 1881.

505. Semmer, E. Die contagiöse Pyämie der Kaninchen. Centralb. med. Wissensch. *19*: 737-738, 1881.

506. Semmer, E. Der gegenwärtige Standpunkt der Lehre über den Milzbrand mit Berücksichtigung der Schutzimpfungen gegen denselben. Revue Thierheilk. Thierzucht *5*: 145-150; 161-165; 177-180; 1882; *6*: 12-13; 47-48; 57-61; 68-73; 1883.

507. Semmer, E., and C. Raupach. Beitrag zur Lehre von der Immunität und Mitigation. Deutsche Z. Thiermed. 7: 347-363, 1882.

508. Semmer, E. Der Milzbrand und das Milzbrandcontagium. Jena, Dege & Haenel, 1882.

509. Semmer, E. Melanosarcomatose und Melanämie bei Schimmeln. Deutsche Z. Thiermed. *9*: 89-90, 1883.

510. Semmer, E., and A. Archangelski. Ueber das Rinderpestcontagium und dessen Mitigation. Centralb. med. Wissensch. *21*: 306-307, 1883.

511. Semmer, E. Chetvertyi internatsionalnyi veterinarnyi kongress v Bryussele. [The Fourth International Veterinary Congress in Brussels.] Vet. Delo 2: 11-13, 1884.

512. Semmer, E. Po povodu referata staty Prof. N. F. Kolesnikova o spirillakh v krovi chumnykh zhivotnykh. [Apropos of the abstract of the article of Prof. N. F. Kolesnikov on spirilla in the blood of animals with pest.] Novosti Vet. Lit. 2(11): 12-13, 1884.

513. Semmer, E. Geschichte der Veterinärmedizin, vol. 3, pp. 537-574 in Encyklopädie der gesammten Tierheilkunde und Tierzucht. Wien, Moritz Perles, 1886.

514. Semmer, E. Neskolko slov o 5-m Mezhdunarodnom Veterinarnom Kongresse v Paris v 1889 g. [Some words on the Fifth International Veterinary Congress in Paris, 1889.] Arkh. Vet. Nauk *20*(Sect. VI): 8-9, 1890.

515. Semmer, E. O progressakh veterinarii v poslednem stoletii [The prog-

ress of veterinary medicine in the last hundred years.] Arkh. Vet. Nauk *21* (Sect. VI): 25-30, 1891.

516. Semmer, E. Sur la valeur diagnostique des injections de malleine. Arkh. Biol. Nauk (St. Petersburg) *1*: 746-771, 1892.

517. Semmer, E. Ueber gutartige heilbare Formen des Rotzes. Deutsche Z. Thiermed. *20*: 59-66, 1894.

518. Semmer, E. Zur Frage über die Aetiologie und Bekämpfung der Rinderpest. Deutsche Z. Thiermed. *22*: 32-46, 1895.

519. Semmer, E. O sapnom gribke. [On the fungus of glanders.] Uchen. Zap. Kazan. Vet. Inst. *12*: 202-205, 1895,

520. Semmer, E. Über die Tuberkulose in Russland. Berichte und Verhandl. 6. Int. tierärztl. Kongr. 335-345, 1896.

521. Semmer, E. Zur Frage der thierärztlichen Bildung im Allgemeinen und insbesondere in Russland. Oesterr. Mschr. Thierheilk. *20*: 258-262, 1896.

522. Semmer, E. Ueber den Einfluss des Alters, der Quantität und Qualität des Malleins und Tuberkulins auf die Wirkung dieser Substanzen. Oesterr. Mschr. Tierheilk. *29*: 53-58, 1901.

523. Semmer, E. Ueber Hielbarkeit des Rotzes und der Tuberkulose und über Immunität gegen diese Krankheiten. Oesterr. Mschr. Tierheilk. *29*: 193-196, 1901.

524. Semmer, E. Aus den Sitzungs-Protokollen des kleinen tierärztlichen Vereines in St. Petersburg. Tierärztl. Zbl. *26*: 229-231, 1903.

525. Seton-Watson, H. From Lenin to Malenkov, pp. 85, 89. New York, Praeger, 1953.

526. Seton-Watson, H. The Russian Empire, 1801-1917, pp. ix; 386, 496-497, 640. Oxford, Clarendon Press, 1967.

527. Seton-Watson, H. Reaction, reform and revolution. Pp. 281-290 in A. Briggs, ed., The Nineteenth Century. New York, McGraw-Hill, 1971.

528. Seton-Watson, H. Intelligentsias in east-central Europe. Times Lit. Suppl., No. 3817, p. 483, May 2, 1975.

529. Shabad, L. M. M. A. Novinskii, pp. 145-151. Moscow, Izd. Akad. Med. Nauk SSSR, 1950.

529a. Shatsillo, B. A. Professor Aleksandr Vasilevich Reprev. Odesskii Med. Zhur. *3*: 333-334, 1928.

530. Shaw, J. T. The Transliteration of Modern Russian for English-Language Publications. Madison, University of Wisconsin Press, 1967.

531. Shchurevskii, V. E. Professor B. G. Ivanov (1898-1959). Trudy 2d Konf. Pat. Anat. Selsk. Zhivot., pp. 475-479, 1961.

532. Shchurevskii, V. E. K 100-letiyu so dnya rozhdeniya N. D. Balla. [100 years since the birth of N. D. Ball.] Trudy Vsesoyuz. Inst. Eksp. Vet. *40*: 395-397, 1972.

533. Shifanovich, G. L. Otkrytie Instituta Usovershenstvovaniya Vetvrachei. [Opening of the Postgraduate Veterinary Institute.] Vestnik Sovrem. Vet. *6*: 529–530, 1930.
534. Shimkin, M. G. M. A. Novinsky: A note on the history of transplantation of tumors. Cancer *8*: 652–655, 1955.
535. Shishkov, V. P., ed. Itogi Nauchno-Pedagogicheskoi Raboty. [Review of scientific-pedagogical work.] 210 pp. Moscow, "Kolos," 1969. (See pp. 83–87 for data on the pathology department of the Moscow Veterinary Institute.)
536. Shukevich, I. I. K ucheniyu ob aktinomikoze rogatogo skota. [The study of actinomycosis in cattle.] Uchen. Zap. Kazan. Vet. Inst. *19*: 193–230; 231–335, 1902.
537. Shukevich, I. I. K voprosu ob amiloidnom pererozhdenii i razryvakh pecheni u loshadei. [The question of amyloid degeneration in rupture of the liver in horses.] Vet. Obozrenie 7: 57–62; 97–106; 145–151, 1905.
538. Shukevich, I. I. De la dégénérescence amyloide chez le ehevaux. Arch. Sci. Biol. (St. Petersburg) *12*: 190–196, 1906.
539. Shukevich, I. I. Otchet ob ekspeditskii dlya obsledovaniya po chume zarazhennykh rainov Kirgizkoi stepi. [Report on an expedition for the study of rinderpest infection on the Khirgiz steppes.] Arkh. Vet. Nauk *43*: 47–77; 145–167, 1913.
540. Shukevich, I. I. O metastaticheskikh pnevmoniyakh loshadei. [Metastatic pneumonia in the horse.] Arkh. Vet. Nauk *43*: 1900–1102, 1913. (Abstract in Jahresb. Vet. Med. *33*: 156, 1913.)
541. Shukevich, I. I., M. I. Romanovich, A. P. Uranov, and A. N. Petrovsky. Otchet o deyatelnosti patologo-anatomicheskago odtela Veterinarnoi Laboratorii M.V.D. s l iyulya 1911 g po l yanvarya 1914 g. [Report on the activities of the pathologic-anatomic department of the Veterinary Laboratory of the Ministry of Internal Affairs from July 1, 1911, to January 1, 1914.] Arkh. Vet. Nauk *44*: 413–447; 543–563, 1914.
542. Shukevich, I. I. O tripanozomoze verblyudov v Uralskoi oblasti. [On trypanosomiasis of camels in the Ural region.] Arkh. Vet. Nauk *44*: 1320–1321, 1914.
543. Shukevich, I. and A. Petrovsky. Ob amiloidnom pererozhdenii u verblyudov. [On amyloid degeneration in camels.] Arkh. Vet. Nauk *45*: 773–780, 1915.
544. Shukevich, I. I. Izsledovanie po bakteriologii gangrenoznykh protsessov. [A study of the bacteriology of the gangrenous process.] Russkii Vrach *14*: 1071–1076, 1915.
545. Shukevich, I. I., M. Romanovich and A. Uranov. Patologoanatomicheskiya izmeneniya u loshadei, otravlennykh parami

khlora. [Pathologic-anatomic alterations in horses poisoned by chlorine fumes.] Arkh. Vet. Nauk *46*: 137–182, 1916.

546. Shukevich, I. I. Gemorragicheskie enterity gurtovogo skota. [Hemorrhagic enteritis in a cattle herd.] Arkh. Vet. Nauk vol. 47, 1917.(Cited by Romanovich[446]).

547. Shukevich, I. I., M. Romanovich and A. Uranov. Gastroenterit gurtovogo skota. [Gastroenteritis in a cattle herd.] Trudy Gosud. Inst. Eksp. Vet. 2: 109–119, 1926. (Posthumous publication.)

548. Shumakovich, E. E. Obshaya i Veterinarnaya Gelmintologiya [General and Veterinary Helminthology.] P. 235. Moscow, Izdatel. "Nauka," 1965. (This is a bibliographic listing of papers in helminthology by Russian authors from the eighteenth century until 1960.)

549. Sikorskii, A. N. Professor S. A. Gryuner. Veterinariya *41*(2): 118, 1964.

550. Skomorokhov, A. Iz inostrannoi zhizni. [From foreign life.] Vestnik Sovrem. Vet. *6*: 280–289, 1930.

551. Skryabin, K. I., B. L. Isachenko, and S. Vyshelesskii. Aleksandr Aleksandrovich Vladimirov. Mikrobiologiya *16*: 545–546, 1947.

552. Skryabin, K. I., ed. Bohl, K. H., biography. Vet. Entsikloped. *1*: 701–702, 1968. Moscow, Izd. Sovet. Entsikloped., 1968.

553. Skryabin, K. I. Moya Zhizn v Nauke. [My life in science.] Moscow, "Politisdat," 1969.

553a. Skryabin, K. I., ed. Gryuner, S. A. biography. Vet. Entsikloped. 2: 683, 1969.

554. Skryabin, K. I., ed. Mari, N. N., biography. Vet. Entsikloped. *3*: 1037, 1972.

555. Skryabin, K. I., ed. Ravich, I. I., biography. Vet. Entsikloped. *5*: 264–266, 1975.

556. Skryabin, K. I., ed. Tartakovskii, M. G., biography. Vet. Entsikloped. *5*: 1005–1006, 1975.

557. Skryabin, K. I., ed. Shukevich, I. I., biography. Vet. Entsikloped. *6*: 543–544, 1976.

558. Smirnov, I. K voprosu ob aktinomikoze u sviny. [The question of actinomycosis in swine.] Uchen. Zap. Kazan. Vet. Inst. *35*: 221–226, 1918.

559. Smirnov, I. Glanders of the nasal chambers. Vestnik Sovrem. Vet. 2(11): 10–11, 1926. (Original not seen, abstract in Jahresb. Vet. Med. *46*: 931–932, 1926.)

560. Smith, F. The early History of Veterinary Literature and its British Development. Vol. 3, p. 77 (Blaine); Vol. 4, pp. 65–68 (rinderpest); pp. 82–85 (Simonds). London, J. A. Allen, 1976.

561. Sobelevskii, V. S. Bibliografiya. Arkh. Vet. Nauk *25*(Sect. IV): 325–326, 1895.

562. Sobelsohn. Exzellenz Prof. Dr. E. M. Semmer†. Tierärztl. Zbl. *30*: 301–302, 1907.

563. Soloveev, B. M. I Vsesoyuzni Sezd Patologov. [The First All-Union Congress of Pathologists.] Vrachebnoe Delo *9*: 1582–1584, 1927.

564. Solzhenitsyn, A. I. The Gulag Archipelago, pp. xi, 27–37. New York, Harper & Row, 1974.

565. Soshestvenskii, N. A. Anatomiya i gistologiya pishchevoda, myagkago nëba glotki i cardia loshadi. [Anatomy and histology of the esophagus, soft palate, pharynx, and stomach of the horse.] Uchen. Zap. Kazan. Vet. Inst. 27: 123–191, 1910.

566. Soshestvenskii, N. A. K patologo-anatomicheskoi kazuistike. [Pathologic-anatomic case reports.] Arkh. Vet. Nauk *43*: 1102–1110, 1913.

567. Soshestvenskii, N. A. Kratkii Kurs Patologicheskoi Gistologii. [Short course in pathologic histology.] Uchen. Zap. Kazan. Vet. Inst. *30*: 1–85; 117–135; 249–322; 377–387, 1913; *31*: 1–75; 142–161; 191–269, 1914.

568. Strukov, A. I., P. P. Dvizhkov, R. D. Shtern and G. G. Avtandilov. Patologicheskaya anatomiya v SSSR za 50 let, 1917–1967. [Pathologic anatomy in the USSR for 50 years, 1917–1967.] Arkh. Patol. *29*(10): 1–98, (11): 99–197, 1967. (See p. 141 for reference to Belkin.)

569. Stubbs, E. L. Langdon Frothingham. Path. Vet. *3*: 565–567, 1966.

570. Studentsov, A. P., and I. M. Sabin. Vvedenie, istorii veterinarnogo obrazovaniya v SSSR. [Data on the history of veterinary medicine in the USSR.] Uchen. Zap. Kazan. Gosud. Vet. Inst. *63*: 3–8, 1956.

571. Suponitskaya, F. M. Ukrainskoe Obshchestvo Patologov. [Ukrainian Society of Pathologists.] Vrachebnoe Delo *11*: 77, 1928.

572. Tartakovskii, M. G. Izsledovanie ob etiologii chume rogatago skota. [Research on the etiology of rinderpest.] Arkh. Biol. Nauk *4*: 279–308, 1895.

573. Tartakovskii, M. G. K voprosu o vospriimchivosti verblyudov k chume rogatago skota. [On the question of susceptibility of camels to rinderpest.] Arkh. Vet. Nauk 27(Sect. II); 109–118, 1897.

574. Tartakovskii, M. G. Afrikanskii sap loshadei. [Epizootic lymphangitis of horses.] Arkh. Vet. Nauk 27(Sect. II): 171–218, 1897.

575. Tartakovskii, M. G. Povalnoe vospalenie legkikh u morskikh svinok. [Epidemic inflammation of the lungs in guinea pigs.] Arkh. Vet. Nauk 27(Sect. II): 235–245, 1897.

576. Tartakovskii, M. G. Kontagioznaya pnevmoniya morskikh svinok. Novaya infektsionnaya bolezn. [Contagious pneumonia in guinea pigs. A new infectious disease.] M.V.Sc. dissertation, Dorpat Veterinary Institute, 1898.

577. Tartakovskii, M. G. Eksperimentalniya danniya k voprosu o vospriimchivosti verblyudov k chume rogatago skota. [Experimental findings on the question of susceptibility of camels to rinderpest.] Arkh. Vet. Nauk *29*(Sect. II): 228–254, 1899.

578. Tartakovskii, M. G. K etiologii nekotorykh nagnoenii u rogatago skota. [The etiology of certain purulent infections in cattle.] Arkh. Vet. Nauk *30*(Sect. II): 89–108, 1900.

579. Tartakovskii, M. G. Ob odnoi infektsionnoi bolezni kanareek. [On an infectious disease of canaries.] Arkh. Vet. Nauk *31*: 989–1004, 1901.

580. Tartakovskii, M. G. Parazitologicheskie zametki. O legochno-glistnoi bolezni u zaitsev. [Parasitological note. On pulmonary worm disease in a hare.] Arkh. Vet. Nauk *31*: 1043, 1901.

581. Tartakovskii, M. G. Linguatulosis u morskikh svinok. [Linguatulosis in the guinea pig.] Arkh. Vet. Nauk *31*: 1049–1053, 1901.

582. Tartakovskii, M. G. Plevropneimoniya morskikh svinok. [Pleuropneumonia of guinea pigs.] Arkh. Vet. Nauk *31*: 1097–1107, 1901.

583. Tartakovskii, M. G. Eksudativnyi tif ili chuma kur. [Exudative typhoid or fowl cholera.] Arkh. Vet. Nauk *34*: 545–575; 617–666, 1904.

584. Tartakovskii, M. G. Materialy k voprosu ob etiologii kontagioznoi plevropneivmonii i skhodnykh zabolevanii loshadei. [Contribution to the problem of the etiology of contagious pleuropneumonia and similar disease in the horse.] Arkh. Vet. Nauk *34*: 765–787; 875–933, 1904.

585. Tartakovskii, M. G. Tsirkulyarnoe obrashchenie i nastavlenie selskokhozyastvenno-bakteriologicheskoi laboratorii. [Circular of instruction for the Agricultural-Bacteriologic Laboratory.] Trudy Selskokhoz. Bakt.-Lab. (Petrograd) *6*(6): 244–254, 1916. (Deals with collection and study of ectoparasites of farm animals.)

586. Tartakovskii, M. G. Predvaritelnye itogi raboty ekspeditsii po izucheniyu voprosov borby s peripnevmoniei. [Preliminary results of the work of the expedition to study the campaign against pleuropneumonia.] Sovet. Vet. *9*(13/14): 17–21, 1932.

587. Tartakovskii, M. G. Iz raboty ekspeditskii po peripnevmonii. [From the work of the expedition on pleuropneumonia.] Sovet. Vet. *9*(17/18): 15–20, 1932.

588. Taylor, A. J. P. Fiction in history. Times Lit. Suppl., pp. 327–328, March 23, 1973.

589. Tehver, J. Einiges aus der Geschichte der Dorpater Veterinärschule und des Veterinär-Instituts. Eesti Loomarstlik Ringvaade 7: 97–179, 1931.

590. Tehver, J. and J. Parre. Kõrgema Veterinaarhariduse ajaloost Tartus 1848–1973. [On the History of Higher Veterinary Education in Tartu, 1848–1973.] Tallinn, "Valgus," 1973.

591. Tereshkov, F. G. K 100-Letiyu so dnya rozhdeniya I. I. Shukevicha. [The 100th anniversary of the birth of I. I. Shukevich.] Trudy Vsesoyuz. Inst. Eksp. Vet. *39*: 412–413, 1971.

592. Timofeef, P. P. Das Weissrussische Staatliche Veterinärinstitut zu

Witebsk. Deut. tierärztl. Wschr. *38*: 400 (and photograph on cover), 1930.

593. Tolstova-Pariiskaya, N. G. and I. T. Trofimov. K. H. Bohl—Osnovatel Kazanskoi skoly veterinarnykh patologoanatomov. [K. H. Bohl—founder of the Kazan school of veterinary pathologic anatomists.] Trudy 2d Konf. Pat. Anat. Selskokhoz. Zhivot., 469-473, 1961.

594. Tolstova-Pariiskaya, N. G. K 100-letiyu kafedry patologicheskoi anatomii Kharkovskogo Zooveterinarnogo Instituta. [One hundred years of the chair of pathologic anatomy at the Kharkov Zooveterinary Institute.] Materialy VI Vsesoyuznoi Konferentsii po Patologicheskoi Anatomii Zhivotnykh *1*: 102-106, 1977.

595. Tolstova-Pariiskaya, N. G. and G. P. Demkin. Borodulina, Natalya Andreevna. Materialy VI Vses. Konf. Pat. Anat. Zhivot. 2: 284-286, 1977.

596. Topchiev, I.: 50-Letnii yubilei Kharkavskago Veterinarnago Instituta. [The 50th jubilee of the Kharkov Veterinary Institute.] Arkhiv Vet. Nauk *31*: 929-964, 1901.

597. Trofimov, I. T. Kafedra patanatomii Kazanskogo Veterinarnogo Instituta. za 50 let Sovetskoi vlasti. [The chair of pathologic anatomy at the K.V.I. during 50 years of Soviet power.] Uchen. Zap. Kazan Vet. Inst. *100*: 165-175, 1968.

598. Trofimov, I. T. Shkola veterinarnykh patologoanatomov. [Schools of veterinary pathology.] Veterinariya *49*(5): 13-15, 1973.

599. Trotsky, L. The Revolution Betrayed, pp. 17, 209. Garden City, N.Y., Doubleday Doran, 1937.

Tscherniak, W. S.: see Chernyak, V. Z.

600. Tsimofeew, P. P. Da yubileyu Praf. Evg. Frenera i Praf. Vilhelma Ellenbergera. [The birthdays of Prof. Eugene Froehner and Prof. Wilhelm Ellenberger.] Belarusk. Vet. *5*: 26-29, 1928.

601. Tsvetkov, N. E. and V. Z. Chernyak. Sap. [Glanders.] 2d edition. Moscow, Ogiz-Selkhoghiz, 1947.

602. Turkevich, J. Fifty years of Soviet science. Pp. 244-261 in Drachkovich, M.M., ed., Fifty Years of Soviet Science State College, Penna. State Coll. Press, 1968.

603. Ulam, A. B. Stalin, the Man and his Era, p. 439. New York, Viking, 1973.

604. Unterberger, F. Mittheilungen aus dem Innern von Russland, zunächst für Pferdeliebhaber. Dorpat, Schünmann's Witwe, 1853.

605. Unterberger, F., J. Rawitsch, and P. Jessen. Pp. 150-157 in Amtlicher Bericht 2. Int. Congress Thierärzten zu Wien, 1865. Vienna, W. Braumüller, 1865.

606. Unterberger, F. Das erste Jubiläum der Dorpater Veterinärschule. Repert. Tierheilk. *34*: 267-273, 1873.

607. Unterberger, F. Izvlechenie iz otcheta Derptskago Veterinarnago Uchilitshchaza 1872 god. [Extract from report of the Dorpat Veterinary College for the year 1872.] Voenno-Med. Zhur. *118*(v): 1-4, 1978.

608. Uspensky, D. Stroenie i Razvitie Sapnykh Uzlov Legkikh. [The Structure and Development of Glanders Nodules in the Lungs.] M.D. dissertation, St. Petersburg, Military-Medical Academy, 1880.

Valdman, I.: see also Waldmann, J.

609. Valdman, I. and Ya. Negotin. Albom Immatrikulirovannykh v Derptskom, nyne Yurevskom Veterinarnom Institute 1848-1898. [List of Matriculants in the Dorpat, now Yurev Veterinary Institute 1848-1898]. Yurev, 1898. (Pp. 42-48, Semmer; 61-62, Blumberg; 87-88, Waldmann; 179-180, Gryuner; 194, Tartakovskii; 282, Ball; 327, Ravich).

610. Valdman, I. Prof. E. M. Zemmer†. Zhurnal Nauch. Prakt. Vet. Med. Izd. Yurev. Vet. Inst. *1*: 147-156, 1906.

611. Vasilev, K. G. and A. E. Segal. Istoriya Epidemii v Rossii. Moscow. Medgiz, 1960.

612. Vau, E. Nauchnaya deyatelnost Professora F. Brauelya v Tartuskoi Veterinarnoi Shkole v 1848-1868 gg. [Scientific activities of Professor F. Brauell at the Tartu Veterinary School during the years 1848-1868]. Sborn. Nauch. Trudov Estonskoi Selskokhoz. Akad. *4*: 3-9, 1958.

613. Vereshchagin, M. N. Rol i deyatelnost Professora K. H. Bohl v organizatsii borby s infektsionnymi boleznyami s.-x. zhivotnykh v Tatarii. [Role and activity of Professor K. H. Bohl in the organization of the struggle against infectious diseases of agricultural animals in the Tatar ASSR.] Uchen. Zap. Kazan. Gosud. Zoovet. Inst. *47*(2): 15-21, 1937.

614. Vertinskii, K. I., N. A. Naletov and V. P. Shishkov. Patologicheskaya Anatomiya Selskokhozyaistvennykh Zhivotnykh. [Pathologic Anatomy of Farm Animals.] Moscow, Kolos, 1973.

615. Viktorov, K. R. K istorii Kazanskogo Veterinarnogo Instituta po pobodu 50-letiya ego sushchestvovaniya (1874-1924 gg.). [The history of the Kazan Veterinary Institute on the occasion of the 50th year of its existence.] Uchen. Zap. Kazan. Gosud. Vet. Inst. *37*: 5-30, 1926.

616. Viktorov, K. K. H. Bohl—k 35-Letiyu nauchno-uchebnoi deyatelnosti. (K. H. Bohl—35 years of scientific-educational activity.] Kazan. Med. Zhur. 27: 1061-1062, 1931.

617. Villents, G. G. Melkaya khronika. [Small chronicle.] Vet. Zhizn. *3*: 544, 1909.

618. Vinogradoff, I. The ancien régime. Times Lit. Suppl. No. 3951; p. 1468, Dec. 16, 1977.

619. Virchow, R. Ueber die Standpunkte in der wissenschaftlichen Medicin. Arch. path. Anat. *70*: 1–10, 1877.
620. Virchow, R. Zur Statistik von Rotz und Wurm in Preussen. Arch. path. Anat. *70*: 291–292, 1877.
621. Virchow, R. Die Uebertragbarkeit der Perlsucht durch die Nahrung. Virchows Arch. *82*: 550–551, 1880.
622. Virchow, R. Erwiderung auf die Bemerkungen des Herrn Professor Semmer. Virchows Arch. *83*: 557, 1881.
623. Völker-Carpin, R. Rudolf Virchow und die Veterinärmedizin. Verhandl. 20. Int. Congr. Hist. Med., Berlin, 588–595, 1966.
624. Vucinich, A. Science in Russian Culture: A History to 1860, pp. 333; 365. Stanford, Stanford University Press, 1963.
625. Vucinich, A. Politics, Universities and Science. Pp. 154–178 in Stavrou, T. G., ed., Russia under the Last Tsar. Minneapolis, University of Minnesota Press, 1969.
626. Vucinich, A. Science in Russian Culture, 1861–1917, pp. 5; 302–304. Stanford, Stanford University Press, 1970.
627. A. W. Biographie. Semmer (1843–1906). Rev. Gén. Méd. Vét. *10*: 431–433, 1907.
628. Waldmann, J. Abstract of paper by N. D. Ball: Pathologisch-anatomische Untersuchungen des Heilprocesses der Knochenbrüche beim Hausgeflügel. Jurjew, 1897. Zschr. Thiermed. *3*: 353–357, 1897. [See also Ball.[36]]
629. Wehenkel, J.-M. Compte Rendu du IVe Congrès International de Médecine Vétérinaire, pp. 31–32. Brussels, 1864.
630. Weissman, B. M. Herbert Hoover and Famine Relief to Soviet Russia, 1921–1923. Stanford, Hoover Institution Press, 1974.
631. Werth, A. Russia, the Post-War Years, pp. 349–379. New York, Taplinger, 1971.
632. Westwood, J. N. A History of Russian Railways, p. 123. London, George Allen & Unwin, 1964.
633. Westwood, J. N. Endurance and Endeavour, Russian History, 1812–1971. Oxford, Oxford University Press, 1973.
634. Wetzel, R. Bericht über die Fachtierärztetagung zur Bekämpfung der Aufzuchtkrankheiten in Jena vom 1. bis 4. Oktober 1927. Deut. tierärztl. Wschr. *36*: 51–55, 1928.
635. Wilson, E. A Window on Russia, p. 219. New York, Farrar, Straus & Giroux, 1972.
636. Wilson, E. Muscovy. Russia Through Foreign Eyes, 1553–1900, p. 305. New York, Praeger, 1970.
637. Wladimiroff, A. Malleus. Vol. 5, Chapter 17, pp. 1120–1183 in W. Kolle and A. von Wasserman, eds., Handbuch der pathogenen Mikroorganismen. 2d ed. Jena, Gustav Fischer, 1913.

638. Yanov, A. Behind the Soviet Union's grain purchases. New York Times, p. 36, Dec. 31, 1975.
639. Yanovskii, A. G. Uchastie veterinarnykh rabotnikov v revolyutsii 1905-1907. [Participation of veterinary workers in the revolutions of 1905-1907.] Veterinariya *49*(6): 107-108, 1973.
640. Yefremenko, A. A. From the history of Russian-German scientific relationships. Jour. Hyg. Epidem. Microb. Immunol. (Prague) *12*: 498-505, 1966.
641. Zabolotnov, P. Nikolai Matveevich Lyubimov, kak professor i uchenyi. [N. M. Lyubimov, as professor and scholar.] Kazan. Med. Zhur. 7: 1-17, 1907.
642. Zagrodzki, K. W. Organizacja służby weterynaryjnej i walka z chorobami zakaźnymi w Rosji sowieckiej. [Organization of the veterinary service and the campaign against contagious diseases in Soviet Russia.] Przegl. Wet. *34*(11-12): 315-328, 1921.
643. Zagrodski, K. W. La médecine vétérinaire sous la régime bolchevique. Rev. Gén. Méd. Vét. *31*: 609-619, 1922.
644. Zagrodski, K. W. Die Organisation des Veterinärdienstes und die Bekämpfung der Tierseuchen in Sowjetrussland. Berl. tierärztl. Wschr. *38*: 246-248; 258-260; 270-271, 1922.
645. Zakharevskaya, M. A. K 50-Letiyu 1 Vserossiiskogo Sezda Patologov. [Fifty years since the First All-Russian Congress of Pathologists.] Arkh. Patol. *35*(10): 84-87, 1973.
646. Zakharov, M. V. (chief editor). 50 Let Vooruzhennykh Sil SSSR. [Fifty Years of the Armed Forces of the USSR.] Moscow, Voennoe Izdatelstvo Ministerstva Oborony, SSSR, 1968.
647. Zalewsky. Das Schicksal der tierärztlichen Hochschule zu Dorpat. Berl. tierärztl. Wschr. *34*: 321-324, 1918.
648. Zangger, R. Amtlicher Bericht über den dritten internationalen Congress von Thierärzten zu Zürich am 2.-7. September 1867, pp. 23-41. Zurich, 1869.
649. Zavarykin, F. N. Rechi, proiznesennyiya pri torzhenstvennom otkrytii byusta pokoinago Professora M. M. Rudneva. [Occurrences and speeches during the unveiling of the bust of the deceased Professor M. M. Rudnev.] Vrach 2: 821-822, 1881.
Zemmer: see Semmer.
650. Ziman, J. The problem of Soviet scientists. Nature *246*: 322-323, 1973.
651. Zolotovskii, A. L., A. Unterberger, and F. I. Bostrom. Josif Ippolitovich Ravich. Arkh. Vet. Nauk *5*: 1-9, 1875.

Index

Veterinary Pathology
in Russia, 1860–1930

Designed by Richard E. Rosenbaum.
Composed by The Composing Room of Michigan, Inc.
in 11 point Baskerville V.I.P., 3 points leaded,
with display lines in Baskerville.
Printed offset by Thomson/Shore, Inc. on
Warren's Olde Style 60 pound basis.
Bound by John H. Dekker & Sons, Inc.
in Holliston book cloth.

Library of Congress Cataloging in Publication Data

Saunders, Leon Z 1919–
Veterinary pathology in Russia, 1860–1930.

Bibliography: p.
Includes index.
1. Veterinary pathology—Russia—History. I. Title.
[DNLM: 1. Pathology, Veterinary—History—Russia. SF769 S257v]
SF769.S28 636.089'607'0947 79-52502
ISBN 0-8014-1191-2

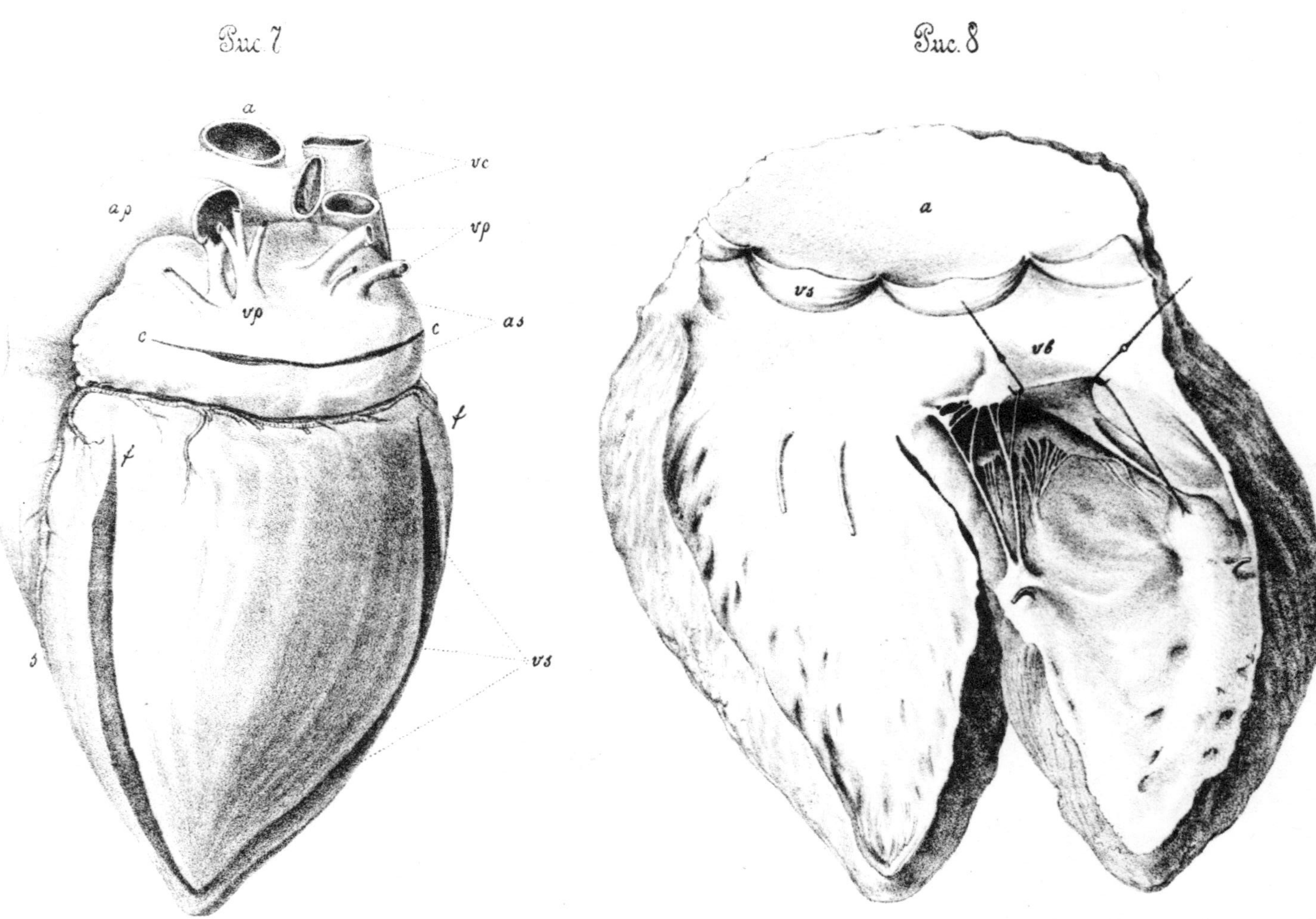
Рис. 7
a
vc
ap
vp
vp
c
c
as
f
f
vs
Рис. 8
a
vs
vb